D1327891

WITHDRAWN

GEORGE ELIOT CENTRE LIBRARY

T03841

T03841

6582
B

SPINAL MANIPULATION

Spinal Manipulation

J. F. Bourdillon FRCS, FRCS (C)
Past President, North American Academy of
Manipulative Medicine
Formerly Consultant Orthopaedic Surgeon to the
Gloucestershire Royal Hospital, UK
Clinical Professor, Department of Physical Medicine
and Rehabilitation, College of Osteopathic Medicine,
Michigan State University, USA

E. A. Day MD, FRCP (C)
Specialist in Physical Medicine and Rehabilitation, Ottawa, Canada

M. R. Bookhout MS, PT
Specialist in Orthopaedic Physical Therapy and
Lecturer in Manual Medicine, Michigan
State University, USA

Fifth Edition

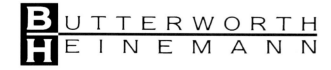

Butterworth-Heinemann Ltd
Linacre House, Jordan Hill, Oxford OX2 8DP

 A member of the Reed Elsevier plc group

OXFORD   LONDON   BOSTON
MUNICH   NEW DELHI   SINGAPORE   SYDNEY
TOKYO   TORONTO   WELLINGTON

First published 1970
Second edition 1973
Revised reprint 1975
Third edition 1982
Fourth edition 1987
Reprinted 1988
Fifth edition 1992
Reprinted 1994, 1995

© J.F. Bourdillon, E.A. Day and M.R. Bookhout 1992

All rights reserved. No part of this publication
may be reproduced in any material form (including
photocopying or storing in any medium by electronic
means and whether or not transiently or incidentally
to some other use of this publication) without the
written permission of the copyright holder except in
accordance with the provisions of the Copyright,
Designs and Patents Act 1988 or under the terms of a
licence issued by the Copyright Licensing Agency Ltd,
90 Tottenham Court Road, London, England W1P 9HE.
Applications for the copyright holder's written permission
to reproduce any part of this publication should be addressed
to the publishers

British Library Cataloguing in Publication Data
A catalogue record for this book is available from the British Library

ISBN 0 7506 0576 6

Composition by Scribe Design, Gillingham, Kent
Printed in Great Britain by The Bath Press, Avon

Contents

Preface to the Fifth Edition

The fifth edition has again been expanded. Two entirely new chapters have been added on exercise therapy with particular reference to adjunctive and self treatment for those for whom the manipulative approach by itself is inadequate to produce long lasting relief. These have been written by Mark R. Bookhout, MS, PT whose master's degree is in orthopaedic physical therapy and who has been teaching in the courses on manual medicine at Michigan State University for the last five years. He has made a special study of exercise therapy and this addition is believed to be the first that has been incorporated in any text of this kind. He comments that he has tried to provide the practitioner with the background information necessary to examine and treat patients for muscle imbalances in the trunk and pelvis as well as specific exercises for self help for those who have chronic problems. Chapter 14 concentrates on evaluation and treatment of faulty movement patterns and imbalances of muscle length and strength. Chapter 15 gives instructions for self mobilising exercises.

The chapter on anatomy has been changed and now brings together many of the additional pieces of anatomical detail which previously were spread in various chapters. The technique chapters have been very largely rewritten and have many new illustrations. In addition several new techniques are described, and illustrated, and problems not previously addressed have been included so that the book is now inclusive of the large majority of currently recognised spinal, pelvic and rib joint problems that may respond to manual treatment. There are, of course, a large number of other techniques used in treatment but those selected for this book have the benefit of having been taught to physicians and physical therapists over the last 13 years and in the process have been tested and refined.

Thrusting techniques for the cervical spine have been reintroduced because it is clear that there are patients who do not respond adequately to other types of manual approach. The techniques described are not the same as those described in and before the third edition but the senior author has reason to feel that those previously described were in fact safe if used as outlined.

Particular thanks are due to Dr Barbara Briner, DO for her help with the paragraphs on craniosacral treatment, to Dr Edward Stiles, DO for his help with the description of indirect treatment and to Dr Robert Ward, DO for his help over the myofascial treatment description.

A new index has been prepared which is much more complete and will render the text easier to use for reference. The new illustrations have almost all been prepared from black and white negatives and show significantly greater detail. My thanks are due for these to Mr Elwood Miles who prepared all the new prints for the publishers. Several of the new illustrations have been copied from other texts and the authors' thanks are due for permission to do this. In particular thanks are due to:

The Librairie Maloine and Dr I. A. Kapandji for permission to reproduce Figs 2.1, 2.8b, 2.9, 2.11, 2.13, 4.2 and 10.4, from *The Physiology of the Joints.*

Dr R. Frederick Becker, PhD for Figs 2.5a and b, 2.7, 2.8a and 2.16, from *The Anatomical Basis of Medical Practice.*

The Oxford University Press for Figs 2.6a and b, from *Cunningham's Textbook of Anatomy.*

Dr Philip E. Greenman, DO from whose personal collection of slides Figs 2.14 and 2.15 were prepared.

Dr Robert E. Irvin, DO for Figs 3.18a and b, from his article in the *Journal of the American Osteopathic Association*, January, 1991.

Dr Malcolm B. Carpenter, MD and Messrs Williams and Wilkins for Fig. 2.16, which was originally published in Dr Carpenter's *Human Neuroanatomy.*

Thanks are also due to the various people, some patients, some students, some friends who have allowed us to use them as models and to those who have helped by criticism, corrections and encouragement not least of whom is my wife.

It is perhaps unexpected to find a man trained as an orthodox orthopaedic surgeon (JFB) writing as a protagonist of manipulative therapy of the kind described in this book, and a brief explanation is appropriate. My early interest in the subject was stimulated by a series of coincidences which led to an appreciation of its importance in spite of the early 'brainwashing' to which I was subjected.

While still a preclinical student I sustained a severe strain of my lumbar spine as a result of a motorcycle accident, and I continued to suffer symptoms from this almost continuously for a number of years and at intervals ever since. I was treated initially first by one and then by a second very well-known orthopaedic surgeon, but the treatments which I received had no effect whatever on the condition other than to give me temporary relief at the time of administration of heat and massage. I well remember the black looks I used to get from the ward sister on teaching rounds in St Thomas's Hospital in the days when Dame Lloyd-Still was matron. When I stood for more than 10 minutes at a time my back began to ache so badly that I found it necessary to rest my buttocks on some sort of support and the neighbouring bed was by far the easiest. This disarranged the bed cover and was the cause of the sister's displeasure.

During my war service with the Royal Air Force, I was well grounded in the treatment of acute trauma but the chronic back condition was relatively rare and my introduction to these came after my return as senior registrar to St Thomas's Hospital, where I quickly learned the then new operation of removal of the protruded intervertebral disc. At first it seemed that this might be the answer to the problem, but disillusionment very quickly followed in the wake of negative exploration and unsatisfactory postoperative results. Like many others, I had originally been taught that manipulation under general anaesthetic of a patient with backache was dangerous and the more so if there was coexistent sciatica. In my case the teaching resulted from the unfortunate experience of two of my tutors, in which the manipulation under anaesthetic of the spine of a doctor's wife produced a permanent cauda equina paralysis.

I completed my training in Cambridge, where I learned from R. W. Butler his technique for manipulating spines under general anaesthetic with good results and without any accidents. Working for him I naturally observed and followed his techniques, often with a very satisfactory measure of success. One of the basic points that he taught was a strict avoidance of forced flexion of the spine. The manipulation consisted of traction, rotation and extension only.

I had the good fortune to be called to see a woman with a recurrence of old back trouble. She described how her general practitioner relieved her by a simple manipulation and explained to me how he did it. The movement was similar to one that I had been using under anaesthesia but was accomplished easily and almost without pain. She obtained immediate relief and only required one treatment. Later I discovered the need of repeated treatment in many cases in order to give lasting relief.

By this time I was using techniques similar to those used by Butler but without anaesthesia because I found it to be unnecessary and because of the need for repeated treatment. I have now come to believe that the use of anaesthesia is a great mistake except for very exceptional circumstances. The intense muscle spasm over destructive lesions is a very valuable ally because it prevents damage being done even if one should misdiagnose such a lesion in the early stages and manipulate it. Anaesthesia will, of course, diminish or even abolish the muscle spasm.

When I first started manipulating spines I was doing it solely for problems in the back itself. I quickly began to find that I was relieving pain in the arms or legs at the same time, even when the symptomatology had not been such as to make me feel that the pain was a referred one. At that time I still believed in the theory that pressure on nerves was the chief cause of referred pain. My continuing experience led me to have serious doubts and at least tended to make me think.

My interest in the other schools of manipulative therapy was stimulated by a number of patients whose backs I had manipulated without success, who were kind enough to let me know that subsequent visits to non-medically qualified manipulators had given satisfactory relief. This naturally made me wish to study the methods used by these practitioners. The rules of the profession made this somewhat difficult until by chance I met the late Dr Donald Turner, then a general practitioner in Folkestone, who himself had learnt the techniques after being relieved of a severe sciatica by an osteopath. He was kind enough to teach me what he knew and from this and other medical manipulators I developed the system which I described in earlier editions under the heading of semi-specific or 'simpler'. I have subsequently been exposed to much more specific techniques, chiefly by members of the osteopathic profession and have come to believe that these are so much more satisfactory that the 'simpler' techniques are no longer included as I have come to regard them as second best and not worth the time that it takes to learn them.

As mentioned later, my thanks for this instruction are due to many who have helped, in particular Dr Philip E. Greenman DO, FAAO, Dr Paul E. Kimberly, DO, FAAO, Dr Fred L. Mitchell, jnr., DO, FAAO and Dr Edward G. Stiles, DO, FAAO. My hope and that of my co-authors is that this book will help those who are looking for better ways of treating patients with pain of musculoskeletal origin at least when the cause is connected with the axial skeleton.

Preface to the First Edition

So many people have helped me in my efforts to produce this book that it would be impossible to mention them all.

I must gratefully acknowledge the permission given by the *British Medical Journal* for the extracts from a 1910 Editorial; from H. K. Lewis & Company Limited to quote from Timbrell Fisher's *Treatment by Manipulation*; from the J. B. Lippincott Company for permission to quote from an article by Dr Horace Gray in the *International Clinics*, and from the Editors of *Brain* and the *Anatomical Record* for permission to reproduce the dermatome charts in the papers by Sir Henry Head and by Drs Keegan and Garrett respectively.

It is invidious to thank individuals but I must express my gratitude for the cheerful and untiring help which I have received from the British Columbia Medical Library Service and from the Staff of the Records Department of the Gloucestershire Royal Hospital.

I cannot leave out my secretary who has typed, typed and retyped every word that is here written, nor indeed, my wife, who has in turn typed, criticised, encouraged and proof read. Finally, it would be very discourteous not to mention both my long suffering model and her husband who took the photographs.

I have endeavoured to shed light on the mystery that surrounds manipulation, to explain how to do it in terms that I hope will be easy enough to understand, to produce a working hypothesis as a basis for argument and a guide for research, and to show some of the reasons why I believe that it is essential that Medicine should incorporate this teaching into its structure.

Vancouver, B.C.   J.F.B.
1970

Chapter 1

Introduction

In this chapter, in order to save words and make meanings clear, the initials MD will be used when referring to the orthodox medical profession in general and its practitioners in spite of the fact that, in the United Kingdom, MD is a higher degree.

The art of manipulation of the spine is a very old one. It has been practised since prehistoric times and was known to Hippocrates and the physicians of ancient Rome.

Bone setters have existed for as long as there are records, and in many countries, including England, they still existed, at least in the 1960s. In the library of the Royal College of Surgeons in London is a book dated 1656 which is a revision by one Robert Turner of a work by an Augustinian monk, Friar Moulton, entitled *The Compleat Bone Setter*.

In 1745 the surgeons eventually separated from the old City of London Company of Barbers and Surgeons and formed a new company which, in the early nineteenth century became the Royal College of Surgeons of England. Prior to this time it is probable that the bone setters were regarded as the orthopaedic surgeons of their day, but for reasons that are unknown they became less and less respected as the art of medicine and surgery gradually became more scientific.

The art of bone setting appears often to have been passed from father to son, and there is some evidence to suggest that an hereditary trait is of some value. Certainly it is accepted that some learn the art of manipulation much more easily than others. The art was not at any time supported by adequate scientific investigation, but experience with patients previously handled by bone setters shows that these practitioners are sometimes surprisingly skilful. Unfortunately their explanation to their clients of what they do is often quite unacceptable to the medical profession and reflects their almost total lack of knowledge of anatomy, physiology or pathology.

The advent of routine radiography, the research into the anatomy of the intervertebral joint and of the disc, and operative findings have conclusively shown that there is not 'a little bone out of place'. The orthodox medical profession has, therefore, found itself unable to accept the manipulator's claims. Unfortunately, the rejection of these claims has provided the profession with a most convenient cloak behind which to hide its refusal to acknowledge the manipulators' success and its dislike of anything new or strange. This, however, is a poor excuse for failure to investigate, test and research into the treatment which these practitioners use, even if it were less successful than it is known to be.

It is easy in this modern day to forget that only a few generations ago medicine itself was an art and the large majority of medical and surgical treatments were based on the results of practical experience rather than on firm scientific foundation. There are still many procedures being carried out without ever being subjected to scientific scrutiny. Carotid endarterectomy was singled out in the fourth edition as such a procedure and, at the time of writing, investigation is under way. Medicine is in many ways still an art. There are many patients for whom the truly scientific approach has nothing constructive to offer but who do not have the signs of the neurotic. For such people it is kinder to be prepared to try to help, even if there is no proven benefit from the proposed treatment, than to send them away with no hope of relief or, worse, with the implied or explicit feeling that their complaints are unreal. It is interesting to look back to one's early days as a physician and to find how, with experience and increasing knowledge, many of those who in the early days were branded as neurotics or worse have genuine treatable organic conditions which one had failed to recognise.

There have been many reasons for the failure of the orthodox medical profession to accept that manipulators might be of value to their patients. The result of this has been serious, it has caused the emergence of several schools of therapy separate from the main stream. This is sad because there is only one possible ethical object for anyone in the healing profession, namely the welfare of the patient. Only one of these schools has embraced the main body of knowledge of the medical profession and its members are recognised, in the United States at least, as fully qualified physicians.

At a time when bone setters were well known in England there was evidence of rejection of their work. The celebrated John Hunter was quoted by Timbrell Fisher[1] as having said:

> Nothing can promote contracture of a joint so much as motion before the disease is removed. . . . When all inflammation has gone off and healing has begun, a little motion frequently repeated is necessary to prevent healing taking place with the parts fixed in one position.

This, unfortunately, was interpreted by Hunter's successors in such a way that they felt justified in allowing adhesions to form in a joint and relying on their ability afterwards to mobilise them. Immobilisation is still accepted as being of the greatest value in infective arthritis. Unfortunately, the concept was extended to joints stiffened by injury and it is now well known that in such patients early movement of the injured joint is a much more reliable method of restoring function.

It must be remembered that at that time there were no X-rays, tuberculosis was common in England, and diagnosis presented serious difficulties. The standard of orthodox treatment for joint disease was far from satisfactory, many ending up with a joint excision or amputation. At the same time the fear of litigation against bone setters was almost non-existent and there can be no doubt that patients were injured by forcible manipulation of infected joints.

The famous British surgeon Sir James Paget was one of the few of his day who appreciated the value of manipulative therapy and in his lecture published in the *British Medical Journal*[2] he gave the following advice:

> Learn then, to imitate what is good and avoid what is bad in the practice of bone setters . . . too long rest is, I believe, by far the most frequent cause of delayed recovery of injured joints, and not only to injured joints, but to those that are kept at rest because parts near them have been injured.

The medical profession of the time paid little heed to Paget's advice. Hugh Owen Thomas used to teach that an overdose of rest was impossible, an idea that appears to have taken root at a time when he had a bitter quarrel with his father who, like his grandfather, was a bone setter. He is quoted by Timbrell Fisher[1] as having written a letter in reply to Paget's lecture in which he said

> For many years after the commencement of my experience in surgery I had the opportunity of observing the practice of those who had acquired a good reputation for skill as successful manipulators. . . . I cannot find suitable cases on which I would perform the deception known as passive motion.

Later, however, his own sufferings led Thomas to visit one of the most celebrated bone setters of the nineteenth century and the following passage in another letter, quoted by Timbrell Fisher, reflects the change of heart produced by personal experience.

> In my own case, after submitting to Mr Hutton's manipulation, I was instantly relieved of that pain, tension and coldness in the joint that I had suffered for six years and was able to walk. . . . Professional men accounted for the manifest change in my condition on one hypothesis or another, whilst all affected to smile at my ignorance and delusion. . . . I had been lame and in pain and could now walk and was at ease . . . and had the whole College of Surgeons clearly demonstrated to their entire satisfaction that I could not possibly have been benefited by Mr Hutton's treatment, my opinion would not have been in the smallest degree shaken by it.

Since as long ago as 1871 there have been those within the medical profession who have tried to understand and make use of the skills of the bone setters. Dr Wharton Hood MD, MRCS[3] gave a description of the treatment and relief in his presence of two patients by Mr Hutton and described what he had learned from Hutton and had afterwards used in his own practice. He was given the opportunity to do this because his father, Dr Peter Hood, had attended Hutton in a long illness but did not charge him. He is said to have done this because Hutton himself was in the habit of treating the poor for nothing.

Dr Hood reported that Hutton himself said that he had a plain education and was 'entirely destitute of anatomical knowledge'. He was fully convinced that he was putting something back in place and the sound, followed by relief made his patients feel that he was correct. Dr Hood suggested that rupture of adhesions was more likely to be the true effect. He describes, in some detail and with illustrations, the type of manipulation which Hutton used on limb joints and on page 631 answers a letter from a Mr Prall describing fatal complications from treatment by a bone setter. He concludes reasonably 'that professional discrimination must be exercised in the selection of cases'.

One of the difficulties arises from the fact that the symptoms from a spinal joint derangement (dysfunction) can be surprisingly diverse and are often manifest at a distance from the spine rather than in the spine itself. Another arises from the anatomy, the spinal joint being situated deep beneath powerful muscles so that it is only indirectly available to the examining finger. A possible third is that the art of successful spinal manipulation comes much more easily to some people than to others. It is a skill that comes with training and perseverance but, as with any other skill demanding manual dexterity, some people find it more difficult than others.

Another factor in the neglect of this branch of work by the medical profession has been the claims of manipulators that they were able to cure all manner of diseases by manipulation of the spine. This claim was so obviously unacceptable that it tended to blind the medical profession to what the manipulators were really doing. The effect of these extravagant claims was so to alienate the medical profession that its members were unprepared to accept anything the manipulators said, nor were they even prepared to believe the patients who said that they had benefited. The reason that claims were made by manipulators in this way may not be entirely their own fault. Macdonald and Hargrave-Wilson[4] describe several cases of abdominal symptoms that had been thought to be either of gastric or cholecystic origin but which were relieved completely by manual treatment of the thoracic spine. If such a patient with one of those diagnoses had been relieved by a manipulator without medical training, would it be more the fault of the manipulator if he claimed to have cured a case of cholecystitis (or ulcer) or more the fault of the physician who failed to make the correct diagnosis?

The general public is notorious for pursuing the unorthodox, even when experience later shows the stupidity of this action. In the case of manipulators, however, experience has shown that the public could obtain genuine relief from the symptoms of spinal joint derangement by their treatments and this natural tendency to pursue the unorthodox was greatly reinforced. Because of this public demand, irregular practitioners have persisted and increased in numbers.

One of the authors (EAD) has had the experience of using manipulative methods on patients from as diverse places as Mexico and Iran only to have the patient say that there was someone in the village at home who did that too!

In the last 100 years two major schools of manipulative therapy have developed and their practitioners are widespread through many parts of the world. In spite of this, there are still large numbers of practising 'natural' manipulators, the successors to the old bone setters, and some of these may still be found without basic scientific training of any kind.

From time to time the voices of highly respected and competent doctors of medicine have been raised in favour of manipulative treatment, but until after the Second World War the number of such medical manipulators was small and they were generally despised by their colleagues.

One of the author's (JFB) own early experiences highlight the scepticism and open prejudice sometimes displayed by members of the medical profession towards manipulative treatment. As a medical student at Oxford University he was encouraged to attend a special meeting of the medical society (the Osler Society) which was addressed by a famous physician of the time, who, it seems apparent in retrospect, attempted to prejudice listeners against manipulators and their art. Later, when training at St Thomas's Hospital in London, where manipulative treatment was practised by Dr James Mennell in the physiotherapy department, and intending to enter the field of orthopaedic surgery, the author was strongly advised by the orthopaedic surgeons to avoid any contact with Dr Mennell's department. Even within his own hospital he (and later his successor, Dr James Cyriax) was considered almost an outcast. It is interesting for this author to look back over more than 40 years of manipulative practice since the Second World War to find that the attitudes of large sections of the medical profession still show the same kind of prejudice. This in spite of the fact that there has always been evidence that patients have felt themselves to have been materially helped by manipulators and this often after the failure of more orthodox treatment.

Osteopathy

The two modern manipulative schools are probably derived in part from the bone setters, in spite of some claims that they were started *ab initio* by their respective founders. The first of these was the Osteopathic school which was started by Dr Andrew Taylor Still (1828–1917). Although there has been some doubt about his training, Dr Still was registered as a medical practitioner in Missouri. Northup says that he entered the Kansas City College of Physicians and Surgeons but, with the advent of the civil war, dropped out to enlist. The rest of his training appears to have been at his physician father's side by preceptorship, a method common in the United States at that time. Hildreth[5] reproduces copies of two certificates, one of registration in Adair county in 1883 and the other dated 1893 stating that he was on the role of physicians and surgeons in Macon county as early as 1874.

Gevitz[6] agrees that Still's training was largely at his father's side and from books on anatomy, physiology and materia medica, and goes on to say that much of medical treatment at that time was brutal and often ineffective which made Still very dissatisfied. This dissatisfaction was increased when the best efforts of a fellow practitioner failed to save three of his family who were dying of cerebrospinal meningitis.

It is interesting to note that there was a well known family of bone setters in that part of the United States at the time and it is recorded that Still's ideas began to crystallise after he had had a woman patient with shoulder problems for which he had mobilised the spine and rib joints. She came back relieved but later returned to tell him that the asthma, from which she had suffered for a long time, had also gone. Downing[7] records that Still's interest in manual therapy started from a personal observation. He is said to have obtained relief from a severe headache, by lying on the ground with his head supported by a rope hung from a tree, the rope was under the upper neck, evidently close to the point where direct pressure on muscle is described as a partial treatment for headache in Chapter 6.

Unfortunately Dr Still appears to have antagonised the profession of his day which did little to further the acceptance of manipulative treatment. He founded the American School of Osteopathy in 1892, but Gevitz suggests that the training there in the early days was not what would now be recognised as adequate. The school is now the Kirksville College of Osteopathic Medicine and, in addition to training in the manual medicine field, its students, like those in all the other US colleges of osteopathy, receive a full medical education.

In the United States doctors of osteopathy (DOs) trained in US schools are equally licensed with MDs and often practise in the same hospitals and share medical practices with MDs. Indeed many DOs are to be found in all branches of medicine, not necessarily involved in the manipulative field. In other countries the term Osteopath is used by a variety of practitioners of whom many (e.g. graduates of the British School of Osteopathy) are not fully trained physicians. They are trained in anatomy etc. and learn manual techniques.

Chiropractic

The second manipulative school is that of chiropractic, which was started in 1895 in Davenport, Iowa, USA by D. D. Palmer who is described as a 'self-educated erstwhile grocer' in a book on chiropractic published in 1962[8].

The start of chiropractic is said to date from a specific incident when Palmer manipulated the thoracic vertebrae of a Negro porter and by this means cured him of deafness from which he had suffered for some years. On the face of it this is a fantastic and totally unacceptable claim. As a result of personal experience, however, there is no doubt in the mind of at least one of the authors that dysfunction in joints in the upper thoracic spine can affect the function of the inner ear, presumably by way of its sympathetic innervation.

For the present argument, the fact that Palmer claims at that time to have manipulated a specific vertebra indicates at least a modicum of knowledge and experience of manipulative treatment. That incident is considered to be the starting point of chiropractic, but it is clear that Palmer must have been working on his ideas for some years before. It seems likely that he actually learned techniques from some other person, either an osteopath or a bone setter. It is said that he was at one time in Kirksville but it does not seem to be known to what extent he might have been exposed to Dr Still or his ideas.

Unlike the osteopaths, chiropractors are not qualified physicians and even in some relatively modern books on chiropractic there are passages which are completely unacceptable to the medical profession, MDs or DOs. In spite of this the art of chiropractic has spread far and wide, not only in North America but in Europe and most other parts of the world. It is well known that it is impossible to 'fool all of the people all of the time' and the continued existence and spread of chiropractic is evidence that they are giving relief to at least a reasonable proportion of those who seek their help. It seems a pity that at the present time there are several different 'schools' (in the sense of methods and teachings) of chiropractic with widely varying treatments. This is sad, both for the profession itself (Matt. 12, 25: 'a house divided against itself cannot stand') and for patients, in particular for those who move to a different area and wish to continue to receive the same kind of therapy.

With chiropractic again the MDs appear largely to have hidden behind the unacceptability of some of their theories and failed to see that there is probably something of value that should be investigated and, if found to be of value, developed. There is no doubt that 'burying their heads in the sand' in that manner will not make the problem go away.

Progress

In 1910 in an issue in which a Dr Bryce had written about osteopathy the editorial in the *British Medical Journal*[9] was an example of broad-mindedness that is often lacking in the profession and indeed which has since then sometimes been lacking in the pages of the same professional journal. It read:

> In the sphere of medicine there is a vast area of 'undeveloped land' which Mr Lloyd George has somehow failed to include in his budget. It comprises many methods of treatment which are scarcely taught at all in the schools, which find no place in textbooks and which consequently the 'superior person' passes with gown uplifted to avoid a touch that is deemed pollution. The superior person is, as has more than once been pointed out, one of the greatest obstacles to progress.
>
> Rational medicine should take as its motto Molière's saying 'Je prends mon bien ou je le trouve'; whatever can be used in this warfare against disease belongs to it of right. . . . Now Dr Bryce has witnessed the mysteries of osteopathy and tells us what he saw in a paper published in this week's issue. . . . The results recorded by him are of themselves sufficient to justify us in calling attention to the method. Not to go so far back as Harvey, who was denounced by the leaders of the profession in his day as a circulator or quack, we need only recall how the open-air treatment of consumption was ridiculed when the idea was first put forward by Bebbington . . . famous physicians refused to listen to Pasteur because he was not a medical man; Lister was scoffed at; the laryngoscope was sneered at as a physiological toy; the early

ovariotomists were threatened by colleagues with the coroner's court; electricity was looked upon with suspicion; massage, within our own memory, was looked upon as an unclean thing. But even now the vast field of physiotherapy is largely left to laymen for exploitation.

In an address to the Pacific Interurban Clinical Club in 1938, Dr Horace Gray[10] quoted Sir Robert Jones, nephew of Hugh Owen Thomas:

> . . . forcible manipulation is a branch of surgery that from time immemorial has been neglected by our profession, and as a direct consequence, much of it has fallen into the hands of the unqualified practitioner. Let there be no mistake, this has seriously undermined the public confidence, which has on occasion amounted to open hostility. If we honestly face the facts this should cause us no surprise. No excuse will avail when a stiff joint, which has been treated for many months by various surgeons and practitioners without effect, rapidly regains its mobility and function at the hands of an irregular practitioner. We should be self-critical and ask why we missed such an opportunity ourselves. The problem is not solved by pointing out mistakes made by the unqualified, the question at issue is their success. Reputations are not made in any walk of life simply by failures. Failures are common to us all and it is a far wiser and more dignified attitude on our part to improve our armamentarium than dwell upon the mistakes made by others.

In Great Britain in the early 1930s there was a move on behalf of osteopaths to obtain licensing but the 1935 report of a House of Lords Select Committee, appointed for the purpose, showed such grave deficiencies in the practice of some of the so-called osteopaths that the move was dropped. Since that time the British School of Osteopathy has trained large numbers of students who practice in the field of manual medicine and are established all over the country. Their position in Britain is similar to that of the chiropractors both in the USA and elsewhere. There is still no full licensure as physicians in the United Kingdom even for US-trained DOs. The unethical practices which were a major part of the problem in 1935 have been dealt with by the profession.

Much research in the field has been done by the MD profession but, although the percentage of back pain patients with surgical lesions is well under 10%, there remains an enormous preponderance of papers concerned with the surgical approach in almost all conferences and journals concerned with the spine.

There has been much research also from both osteopaths and chiropractors and much more is now known about the biomechanics of the spine and the function of the various parts of the intervertebral and other joints.

Several attempts have been made by each group to produce a controlled study to compare treatment by manipulation with other methods. The difficulty has proved to be greater than expected, in particular:

1. The nature of the treatment is such that it is almost impossible to make the study double blind.

2. There is a wide variety of different dysfunctions, and all of them require their own specific treatment. Because of this several of the trials have been invalidated as the treatment given was a standardised one unrelated to the specific diagnosis for the individual.

3. There is a very wide range of ability between different operators making comparison difficult.

It is likely that in time these difficulties will be overcome but in the meantime those with personal experience either as a patient or as an operator in a dramatic case will have no doubt about the possibilities of good manual therapy.

The challenge

The challenge remains. There is not dichotomy but trichotomy in the healing profession even if we neglect traditional Chinese and other variations on the healing theme.

The sick person comes to one of the healers looking for help, not looking for the random application of a theory that may not be flawless. It is urgent that the differences between the branches of the profession should be healed. It will hurt. Practitioners of any of the three branches under consideration will lose part of their 'heritage'. One of the problems is the feeling among some groups that their territory is being invaded and that they stand to lose patients and, in consequence, some of their financial reward. This is certainly a possibility and perhaps could be advanced as an argument in favour of salaried rather than fee for service medicine. The only territory likely to be invaded is the edge where the specialty has thought that their treatment was best and have failed to recognise that something better was available.

The seniority of the MD section does not necessarily give them pride of place. The gaps in the training of the DCs does not commend them as the nucleus, however good some of their treatments may be. The DOs in the United States have the advantage that they have both exposure to manual methods in their training and a full medical curriculum. Unfortunately the same is not true of DOs trained elsewhere. The physiotherapists are also involved in treatment of the musculoskeletal system, as indeed are the massage therapists, and some of those interested in manual medicine have acquired a high degree of skill but they are not trained in the whole spectrum of medical care.

The DOs also have had the experience in California when, as a result of accepting MD degrees, they ceased to be 'visible' in the sense that patients wanting manual treatment (or to be treated by an osteopath for some other reason) were unable to find them. To do nothing more than to give all DOs MD degrees would not be a satisfactory answer. What appears to be required is that all medical students should be exposed to methods of manual treatment during their time as undergraduates and that there should be a specialty like orthopaedic surgery or neurology whose practitioners would be experts in manual medicine. In the meantime there is room for much closer cooperation between MDs and DOs as well as between both of them and the chiropractors. The latter would be easier if the chiropractors could find a way back to being one rather than several different groups.

What is the manipulator doing?

One of the patients relieved by the Dr Turner referred to in the preface was a woman still crippled by symptoms in spite of having disc protrusions removed by one of the authors (JFB) at both L5–S1 and, later, L4–5. Dr Turner succeeded in relieving her by mobilising one of her sacroiliac joints and subsequent recurrences responded to similar treatment given by the same author.

The suggestion that a sciatic radiation of pain could arise from the sacroiliac joint was difficult for the author to accept, believing as he then did that referred pain was due to direct interference with nerves or their roots. The results in this case and the author's subsequent experience have convinced him that a sacroiliac strain can indeed be a cause of sciatic radiation of pain. No satisfactory proof of the mechanism has been demonstrated experimentally.

There are, of course, two joints in the spine that have no intervertebral disc, namely the occipitoatlantal and that between the 1st and 2nd cervical vertebrae. As a result of practical experience, the authors are also satisfied that joint derangements of both the occipitoatlantal and atlantoaxial joints can cause pain both locally and referred. These findings in the occipitoatlantal, atlantoaxial and sacroiliac joints strongly suggest that the disc itself is not the only important source of symptoms, and possibly not even the most important.

Many authors have arrived by similar means at similar conclusions and have developed theories of their own. Our theories and the reasons for them will be discussed, but for the moment the manipulative techniques can be thought of as a means of getting muscle to let go and putting a stiffened joint through a range of movement rather than anything more complicated.

Stiffness of the involved joints can be demonstrated both clinically and radiologically. The radiological demonstration requires a comparison of films taken in sidebending right and left or flexion and extension, preferably with application of some stress to enhance the overall range. By this means those joints that are completely stiff and those with restricted motion can be seen. A knowledge of the normal range of motion is required and it is useful to remember that when one joint does not move fully, one or more of the neighbouring joints may well become overmobile in compensation.

The clinical demonstration depends on the appreciation of abnormalities in joint movement and of tension differences in the soft tissues around them. These are not easily felt by untrained fingers and this may make the demonstration unconvincing for the newcomer to the field. Some people have tissues through which it is easy to feel but there are those whose subcutaneous tissues are dense and apparently fibrous. Severe obesity also causes increased difficulty. For the sceptical beginner it may be important to find a model (or patient) with the thin type of soft tissue through which to feel until his (or her) palpatory skill is better developed.

The soft tissue changes are various but one of the most important is hypertonus in muscle. It was suggested, in earlier editions, that the muscle changes were the fundamental cause of the problems. The present feeling is that they are important manifestations of a more fundamental change, partly in the central nervous system (as if a rogue program had got into the computer) and partly in the other soft tissues including the fascial investment of the muscles. From the point of view of treatment it makes a reasonable start to work as if hypertonic muscle were the main source of symptoms.

The thrusting techniques are not new, they have been used in some form for at least 100 years, and techniques of a kind for very much longer. One of the earliest British books describing similar techniques of which the authors are aware was published in 1934 by Dr Thomas Marlin[11]. He was in charge of what later became the physiotherapy department at University College Hospital in London and had gone to learn osteopathic techniques in the United States. He records that, following one of his demonstrations, a colleague told him that similar techniques had been practised in England 40 years before.

How slowly we learn!

Before proceeding it must be emphasised that what is being described is not a new system of medicine. Manual treatment does not stand alone and it should only be done in the context of total patient care, even if much of the care is more directly the responsibility of another practitioner. One of the advantages of the system in which patients are only seen by specialists in consultation with or on referral by the referring physician is that the practitioner of manual medicine has the opportunity to obtain a past history from the other physician in addition to that given by the patient. That advantage is lost if the patient does not bring a letter giving details unless, of course, the referring physician has previously communicated the details.

1. Timbrell Fisher A.G. (1948). *Treatment by Manipulation*, 5th edn. London: Lewis.
2. Paget Sir James (1867). Cases that bone setters cure. *Brit. Med. J.;* **1**:1–4.
3. Hood Wharton (1871). On the so-called 'Bone-setting,' its nature and results. *Lancet*, **1**: 336–338, 372–374, 441–443 and 499–501.
4. MacDonald G., Hargrave-Wilson W. (1935). *The Osteopathic Lesion*. London: Heinemann.
5. Hildreth A.G. (1938). *The Lengthening Shadow of Dr. Andrew Taylor Still*. Macon, Missouri: Hildreth.
6. Gevitz N. (1982). *The D.O.s, Osteopathic Medicine in America*. Baltimore: Johns Hopkins University Press.
7. Downing C.H. (1935). *Osteopathic Principles in Disease*. San Francisco: Orozco.
8. Homewood A.E. (1962). *The Neurodynamics of Vertebral Subluxation*. Publisher not cited.

 9. Editorial (1910). *Brit. Med. J.;* **2**:638.
10. Gray H. (1938). Sacro–iliac joint pain. *Int. Clin.;* **2**:54–96.
11. Marlin T. (1934). *Manipulative Treatment.* London: Edward Arnold.

Chapter 2

Anatomy and biomechanics

Practitioners in their training acquire a basic working knowledge of the anatomy of the spinal column and pelvis. The objects of this chapter are to refresh the reader's memory on points that he or she may have forgotten, to go into detail about specific points that are often neglected and to present evidence that some standard anatomical beliefs should be changed in the light of recent research. In trying to understand the reasons for the success of manual therapy, it is of the utmost importance to have as clear as possible a picture of the structure and normal function of the joint concerned. If one wishes to try to use manual treatment, the need is even greater.

It is the clinical experience of countless manipulators that patients obtain relief from certain symptoms after manipulation, not only of spinal joints themselves, but of the joints of the pelvis, including the pubic symphysis, and also of the joints between the ribs and the vertebrae. The fact that symptoms can be caused by dysfunction of rib joints is not well recognised by MD physicians, but experience suggests that they can be important sources of chest wall and arm pain. Early recognition of these dysfunctions might both hasten relief for the sufferer and reduce the need for costly cardiac investigations.

The classical paper of Mixter and Barr[1] stimulated the interest of the medical profession in the structure of the intervertebral joint. Since that time many papers have been published and much research work carried out, but it is important to remember the work that had been done before and an excellent review of that work is given by Armstrong[2] in his introduction. There is a summary of more recent research on the low back with a comprehensive list of references in Bogduk and Twomey's *Clinical Anatomy of the Lumbar Spine*[3] and those who plan to work in the field would be well advised to read this work.

THE ANATOMY OF THE PELVIS

The pelvis is a three-part bony ring with two diarthrodial joints posteriorly – the sacroiliac joints – and a so-called symphysis anteriorly. The term 'so-called' is used because there is often a synovial cavity and there is an upward and downward gliding movement, albeit of small excursion. The upward glide of the pubis on the side on which weight is being borne is illustrated by Fig. 2.1, reproduced, with permission, from Kapandji[4].

Fig. 2.1 'Vertical' shear of pubic symphysis (after Kapandji).

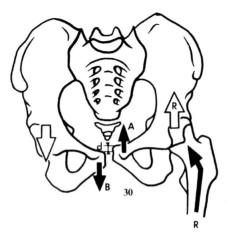

The paired innominate bones are regarded by many as being lower limb bones rather than belonging to the trunk. Their function is very much influenced by the muscles of the hip and thigh. Each innominate is formed by the fusion of three bones, the ilium anterior and superior, the ischium inferior and posterior and the pubis inferior and anterior. In diagnosis we shall need to find the anterior and posterior superior iliac spines (ASIS and PSIS), the ischial tuberosity and the superior ramus and tubercle of the pubis.

The midline sacrum is formed by the fusion of five (sometimes six) vertebral elements and may show incomplete fusion at one or more levels. The sacrum is broad at its base and narrows to its apex postero-inferiorly. On either side at the apex is the inferior lateral angle (ILA) which is, developmentally, the transverse process of S5. The shape of the ILA is quite variable, there may be an obvious angle or it may be rounded which can make it more difficult to identify (see Fig. 2.4).

THE SACROILIAC JOINT

The sacroiliac joints have an irregular articular surface, it is rare to find that the shape is the same on the two sides in the same patient, and there is marked variation in the details of shape between different subjects. This may be part of the reason for the variations in pelvic dysfunction seen in the patient population. Fryette[5] describes three main types of sacral shape. The first (type A) has the most typical shape of the first segment with the transverse measurement of the dorsum wider than that on the ventral surface. The second (type B) has a wider ventral than dorsal transverse measurement of the first segment and the third (type C) has the articular surface sloping down and in on one side and down and out on the other (Fig. 2.2). He found that the sacrum wider on the dorsum is usually associated with coronal facing facets (thoracic type) at the L5–S1 joint while the sacrum wider on the ventral aspect tends to have sagittal facing facets (lumbar type). In the type C sacrum the facet on the side

Posterior

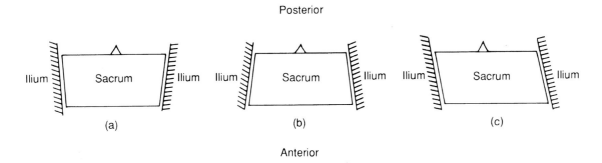

Anterior

Fig. 2.2 Diagram of types of sacral shape in transverse section. (a) Fryette type A; (b) Fryette type B; (c) Fryette type C.

with the 'down and in' slope (the type A slope) is likely to be coronal and that on the side with the type B slope sagittal. Below the second segment the ventral surface is typically wider than the dorsum. The typical shape of upper and lower segments is what would be expected on mechanical grounds as giving the best resistance to the tendency of the superincumbent weight to force the sacrum into the anteriorly nutated position (with the sacral base anterior and caudad and the apex superior and craniad).

In 10–15% of specimens the bevel change is absent. This absence of bevel change is necessary for the development of 'shear' dysfunctions of the innominates and in a series of chronic back pain patients the incidence of superior innominate shear is close to that figure[6]. There is another, less common variation. The usual sacral auricular surface is concave from antero-inferior to postero-superior while that of the ilium is convex. That shape prevents rotation of the ilia about an axis along the length of the sacrum. The less common shape is with the concavity on the ilial side (Fig. 2.3a and b). When this is the shape of the joint the flare dysfunctions become possible, the ilium on one side rotating forwards and that on the other side backwards about an abnormal longitudinal sacral axis. Treatment, of course, is only required when the joint becomes restricted in the rotated position.

In spite of the development of anatomical thought in the last half century, there remains in the mind of many physicians the idea that the sacroiliac joint is neither mobile nor likely to be a source of symptoms. In this connection it may be worth mentioning the blank disbelief in the mind of one of the authors (JFB) in 1953 at the first suggestion that symptoms could arise from the SI joint! The anatomical evidence is that

Fig. 2.3 Concave–convex relationship at the sacroiliac joint. (a) Typical; (b) unusual, thought to be required for flare dysfunctions.

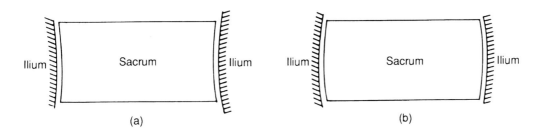

it is a mobile diarthrodial joint and according to Brooke[7] 'the old description of fibrous or bony ankylosis was a description of a pathological change'. Brooke, working on laboratory specimens, located the centre of motion in the short posterior sacroiliac ligament but emphasised that the movement had both rotatory and gliding components. Weisl[8], using live subjects with the pelvis restrained in a special apparatus, had X-ray pictures taken in various positions of the trunk and lower limbs. He reported:

> In a minority of subjects the sacral displacement was such that the sacral line remained parallel to its position at rest. Angular displacement occurred much more frequently and it was possible to locate an axis of rotation. It was situated approximately 10 cm below the promontory in the normal subjects, both recumbent and standing, and was placed a little higher in puerperal women. Contrary to the belief of previous authors, the site of this axis was variable in a majority of subjects, either the axis moved more than 5 cm following various changes of posture, or angular and parallel movement occurred in the same subject . . ..
>
> The position of this axis of rotation differed from that described by earlier authors who based their opinions only on the examination of the sacroiliac joint surfaces . . ..

In 1936 Pitkin and Pheasant[9] described referred pain to the gluteal and sacral regions and to the lower extremities originating in the sacroiliac and lumbosacral joints and their accessory ligaments and coined the name 'sacrarthrogenic telalgia'. They drew the following conclusions:

1. That sacroiliac mobility can be demonstrated *in vivo* by measuring the movements of the ilia.
2. That in the standing position all motions of the trunk, with the exception of flexion and extension, are normally associated with unpaired antagonistic movements of the ilia about a transverse axis that passes through the centre of the symphysis pubis.
3. That rotation and lateral bending of the sacrum do not normally occur alone, but as correlated motions that are coincidental to antagonistic movements of the ilia.
4. That the syndrome is not the result of irritation or compression of trunks of peripheral nerves but more from abnormal ligament tension associated with altered sacroiliac mobility.

The differences in the conclusions of Brooke and Weisl are striking and the probability is that both are at least partially correct. Consideration of the mechanics of the SI joint, and in particular the interosseous portion of the posterior ligament suggests that any rotatory motion *not* centred in that area must be very small. Also the irregularities in the auricular surface itself must restrict gliding motion or rotation about an antero-inferior axis. It seems certain that there are both rotatory and gliding movements and therefore there cannot be any fixed axis and it may be that, when certain restrictions are imposed, the axis appears to be where Weisl found it. There is no doubt that one innominate must be able to move on the other about an axis through or near the pubic symphysis. Is this perhaps the motion recorded by Weisl?

In a study of the anatomy of 40 sacroiliac joints from embryonic life to the eighth decade, Bowen and Cassidy[10] found that, at all ages studied, the sacral articular cartilage was hyaline, but that on the ilium was fibro-cartilage. The sacral cartilage was about three times as thick as that on the ilium and they noted relatively early degenerative changes more marked on the ilial side. There was a capsule with an inner synovial layer and an outer layer of dense fibrous tissue. They also give a short bibliography on the subject.

The body weight is transmitted from the sacrum to the innominates almost entirely by the sacroiliac ligaments. These are quite thin and weak anteriorly but very strong posteriorly and the sacrum is, in effect, slung from the iliac portion of the innominate by these ligaments. The short posterior sacroiliac ligaments are oriented transversely and form the major support for the sacrum. The more superficial long ligament is more vertical and blends inferiorly with the sacrotuberous ligament which, through the ischial tuberosity, is in line with, and indeed may be regarded as being, a continuation of the tendon of the long head of the biceps femoris. The line of bearing of the superincumbent weight on the sacrum falls in front of the likely position of the centre of rotation of the sacroiliac joint and, therefore, the weight tends to rotate the sacrum (into anterior nutation) about a transverse axis. This is resisted in particular by the sacrotuberous ligament and there is a cutaneous branch of S2–S3 which perforates the ligament giving the possibility that an entrapment might occur.

Recent research in Denmark[11] has shown that *in lower animals and many mammals parts of the biceps femoris and semitendinosus originate from the sacrum with a cutaneous nerve separating the two.* Perhaps its phylogenetic history helps to account for the importance of that ligament in certain pelvic dysfunctions.

MOTION OF THE JOINTS OF THE PELVIS

The function of the joints of the pelvic ring has been the subject of much research and argument. It is clear, however, that there is no longer any doubt that the sacroiliac joints are mobile, diarthrodial joints[12] and that they can be subject to dysfunction like other such joints in the axial skeleton. Motion analysis of walking indicates that the counterrotation of the innominates described by Pitkin and Pheasant[9] is an important part of the normal walking cycle (Greenman[13]). This counterrotation can only happen if the pubic symphysis is able to rotate about a transverse axis, a movement that tends to be lost if there is fixed distortion of the symphysis. When there is counterrotation of the innominates the sacrum is forced to rotate towards and to sidebend away from the side on which the innominate rotates posteriorly. Anything that interferes with the ability of the pelvis to perform these movements will render the walking cycle abnormal and for this reason dysfunctions of the pelvis are of primary importance in patients with back and leg pain, even if the complaint is higher in the back. There are other movements of the pelvic joints and, when any of these movements is restricted, the walking cycle will be affected.

Movements of the pubic symphysis

The first movement has already been described and is a rotation of one pubic bone on the other about a hypothetical transverse axis through the symphysis.

The other normal movement of the pubis is the 'vertical' shear (Fig. 2.1). In previous editions the shear movement of the pubic symphysis was described as abnormal. This is probably incorrect. Kapandji[14] describes a shear through the symphysis on one-legged standing as being abnormal but it seems that it can occur in normal joints if one-legged standing is prolonged[15,16]. The shear is parallel to the long axis of the symphysis and not truly vertical; it is produced by the innominate riding up on the side on which weight is borne, while that on the opposite side is dragged down by the weight of the lower limb. If the symphysis is mobile, correction will occur on standing on the other leg or on prolonged two-legged standing. Restriction of this movement is common and important as, if the symphysis is not mobile, all other movements of the pelvic girdle are affected.

Abnormal movements of the symphysis are separation and rarely an antero-posterior shear. These are almost only seen after ligament injury in childbirth or in association with pelvic disruption in accidents.

Movements of the innominates on the sacrum (iliosacral)

Normal movement involves counterrotation of the innominates on the sacrum and as described above is part of the normal walking cycle. Abnormal movements may happen when the sacral shape is unusual. They are the innominate shears and the flares. Diagnosis and treatment of innominate shear and flare dysfunctions are discussed in Chapters 4 and 7.

1. Innominate (iliac) shear movements
In sacroiliac joints of the most common shape the bevel changes usually at or near the junction of the second and third segments; above the change the dorsum of the sacrum is wider than the ventral aspect and below the change the opposite is true. Absence of the change in bevel reduces the resistance of the joint to translation of the innominate on the sacrum. This abnormality is thought to be required for innominate shears to occur. The innominate may shear superiorly, a dysfunction known often as an 'upslip', or, inferiorly, the 'down slip'. These are discussed in Chapters 4 and 7, but it is of interest to note that together they remain one of the six most common dysfunctions found in the 'failed back' patient. The superior shear is relatively common corresponding to the reported incidence of absence of bevel change in the SI joint of about

15 per cent (Greenman). Inferior shear is much less common, possibly because it tends to be self-correcting on weightbearing. Both are associated with symptoms that may be severe.

2. Innominate flares

These are abnormal movements in that they also only happen when the shape of the sacroiliac joint surfaces is abnormal. In the so called 'normal' the iliac surface of the SI joint is convex from front to back and the sacral surface correspondingly concave. When the curvature is reversed, with the iliac side concave and the sacrum convex, flares can occur with the ilium rotating about an axis roughly parallel to the long axis of the sacrum. The ilium can rotate in or out.

Movements of the sacrum between the innominates (sacroiliac)

These are all physiological and treatment is only required if they become restricted. The best studied movement of the sacrum was referred to above and is now commonly known as nutation[17], which may be anterior or posterior, sometimes called inferior and superior nutation or nutation and counternutation. In the fourth edition the terms used were superior and inferior sacral shear; in this edition nutation is preferred in order to avoid possible confusion with the innominate shears. The reason for these names is that the older terms of sacral flexion and extension had become unusable because they have come to mean the opposite movement in the context of cranio-sacral treatment. The other movements are called sacral torsions.

1. Anterior (or inferior) nutation is the movement inferiorly and anteriorly of the sacral base with respect to the innominate. It involves rotation of the sacrum about a horizontal transverse 'axis' and a translation of the sacrum caudally along the auricular surface of the innominate. This movement makes the sacral base less prominent from behind but makes the inferior lateral angle (the transverse process of S5) more prominent. Anterior nutation is the normal reaction of the sacrum to extension of the lumbar spine.

2. Posterior nutation is when the sacral base moves superiorly and posteriorly about the same hypothetical axis with a translation of the sacrum cranially along the auricular surface. The sacral base becomes prominent posteriorly and the inferior lateral angle is less prominent. Posterior nutation is the reaction of the sacrum to lumbar flexion. This is part of a general principle, *when not prevented from doing so the sacrum moves in the opposite direction to L5.* As with other normal movements, there is only a need for treatment if the movement becomes fixed and does not self-correct when the patient's position changes. Restriction of these movements on one side is common and often part of the cause of symptoms. Either side or both sides may be restricted.

3. Anterior or forward torsion is the sacral movement accompanying the counterrotation of the innominates in normal walking[18]. It may be to the left on the left oblique axis (left on left) or to the right on the

Fig. 2.4 Posterior view of sacrum to show the left oblique 'axis' and the inferior lateral angles (ILA).

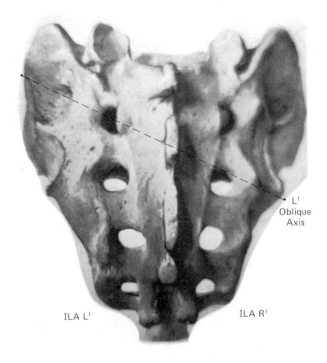

Lt Oblique Axis

ILA L^t   ILA R^t

right oblique axis (right on right) because in this movement the sacrum turns towards the side of the oblique axis (Fig. 2.4).

When standing the centre of motion of the hip joint is anterior to the vertical through the apparent centre of motion of the sacroiliac joint. Because of this, when the weight of the body is borne on the left leg, the left innominate is subjected to a turning moment and is rotated posteriorly by the weight of the trunk pushing the SI joint caudad and the supporting leg pushing the hip craniad. The weight of the right lower limb hanging on the hip will tend to rotate the right innominate anteriorly and complete the counterrotation. With reference to the effect on the walking cycle Greenman gives a 'theoretical construct . . . to describe all the movements found within the pelvic girdle and the potential dysfunctions therein'.

If the superior part of the left auricular surface of the sacrum is pushed posteriorly and that of the right auricular surface is pulled anteriorly by rotation of the innominates, it follows that the sacrum will be twisted. If the motion were antero-posterior only the axis would be parallel to the long axis of the sacrum but there is both rotatory and vertical motion, caudad on the left side and craniad on the right. The resulting sacral motion is usually described as torsion about an oblique axis; in this example, that on the left. The oblique axes are a convenient descriptive device without anatomical basis, there is one on each side starting from the upper pole of one SI joint and ending at the lower pole of the other. They are named for the side of the upper pole.

4. Posterior or backward torsion, is a physiological movement (although this was denied in the fourth edition) but it only happens when

the spine is operating in non-neutral mechanics and the movements of rotation and sidebending in the lumbar spine are coupled to the same side (see below).

If L5 is flexed the sacrum will go into posterior nutation, if the spine is now sidebent to the left, L5 rotates to the left because it is operating in non-neutral mechanics, a concept that is explained later in this chapter. The sacrum cannot rotate and sidebend to the same side and its reaction is to rotate in the sense opposite to the L5 rotation. Because the sacrum is already in posterior nutation, rotation to the right has the effect of pushing the right sacral base even further posterior. In this example the sacrum has rotated right and sidebent left and the right base is posterior; this is described as posterior or backward torsion, right on left (to the right on the left oblique axis). Right on left torsion is common and is another frequent finding in patients with a 'failed back'. Left on right (to the left on the right axis) torsion can also cause severe pain but is rather less common than right on left.

THE ANATOMY OF THE LUMBAR AND THORACIC SPINE

Muscles (Fig. 2.5a and b)

In order to find dysfunctions it is essential that the operator be familiar with the anatomy of the posterior spinal muscles.

The muscles of the upper back are arranged in three main groups[19]. The superficial group comprises the muscles connecting the shoulder girdle to the trunk. These are in two layers, trapezius and latissimus dorsi superficially and, deep to them, the rhomboids and levator scapulae. These muscles have all migrated caudally and are innervated by nerves from cervical segments. From the clinical point of view these two layers are separate and can be distinguished by palpation because of the different fibre orientation. In the lumbar spine the superficial layer is still the latissimus dorsi but in this region it is largely tendinous. The second layer is the serratus posterior superior and inferior which are small muscles of respiration and are difficult to feel. Fortunately they are of little importance in this connection.

The third layer are the muscles that are collectively known as the erector spinae or sacro-spinalis. These are of great importance clinically and are also divided into two main groups. Superficially there are three long muscles:

1. Medially, the spinalis which is relatively small and not easy to feel, being very close to the spinous processes.
2. Laterally, the iliocostalis is attached to the angles of the ribs and is important in the diagnosis and treatment of structural rib dysfunctions.
3. Intermediate, the longissimus which is the muscle that produces the long bulge visible under the skin of many patients centred about 2.5 cm (1 inch) lateral to the midline. It is separated from the spinalis by

Fig. 2.5 (a) Superficial (A) and intermediate (B) muscles connecting the back and upper limb (after Becker). (b) Deep muscles of the back (after Becker).

a

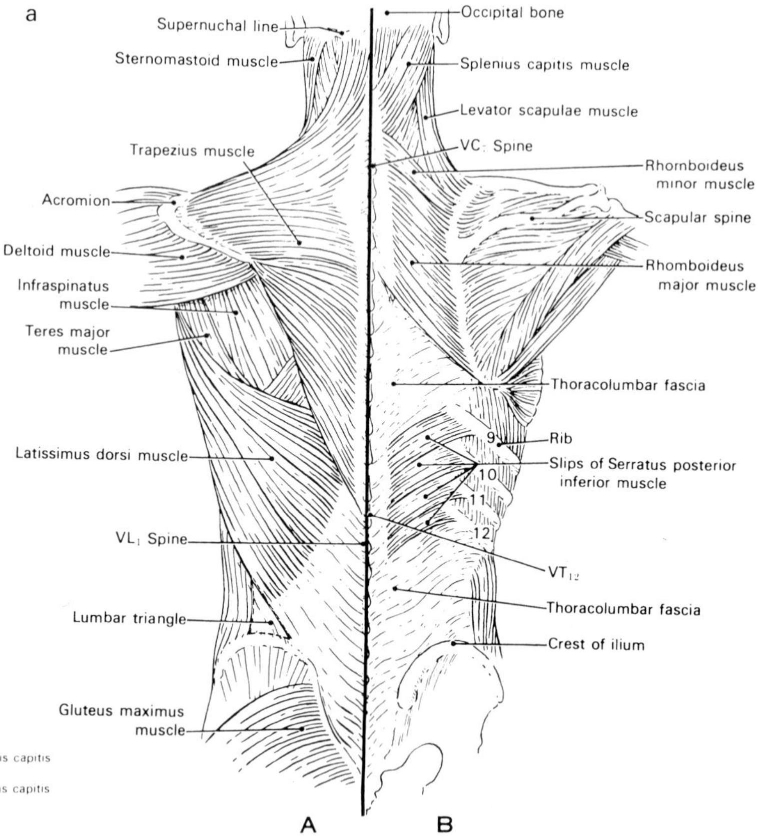

Supernuchal line
Sternomastoid muscle
Occipital bone
Splenius capitis muscle
Levator scapulae muscle
Trapezius muscle
VC$_7$ Spine
Rhomboideus minor muscle
Acromion
Scapular spine
Deltoid muscle
Rhomboideus major muscle
Infraspinatus muscle
Teres major muscle
Thoracolumbar fascia
Latissimus dorsi muscle
9
Rib
Slips of Serratus posterior inferior muscle
10
11
12
VL$_1$ Spine
VT$_{12}$
Thoracolumbar fascia
Lumbar triangle
Crest of ilium
Gluteus maximus muscle

A   B

b

Splenius capitis and splenius cervicis
Semispinalis capitis
Longissimus capitis
Serratus posterior superior
Iliocostalis cervicis
Longissimus cervicis
Semispinalis cervicis
Iliocostalis dorsi
Spinalis dorsi
Thoracolumbar fascia
Longissimus dorsi
Iliocostalis lumborum
Serratus posterior inferior
Quadratus lumborum
Erector spinae
External oblique
Multifidus

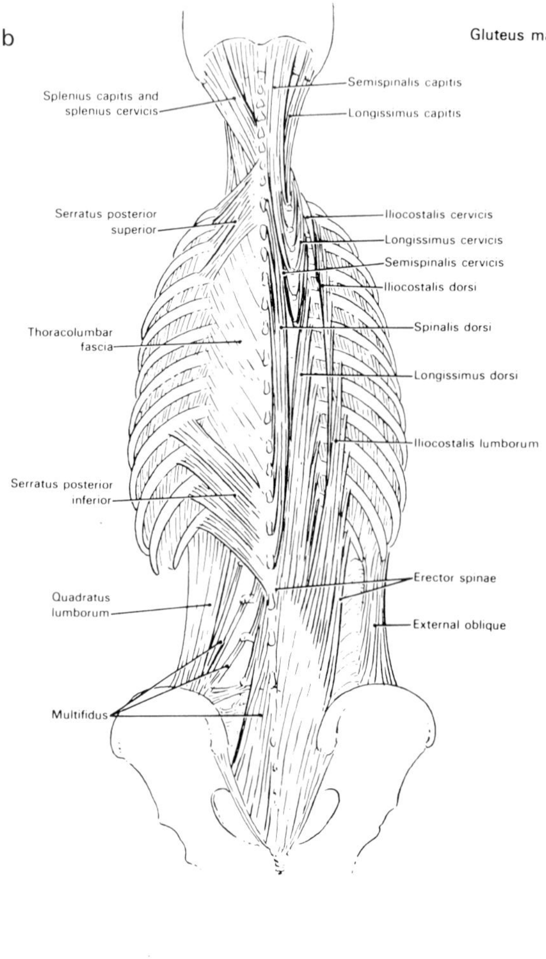

the medial intermuscular septum which can be felt as a longitudinal depression 0.5–1 cm ($\frac{1}{4}$–$\frac{1}{2}$ inch) lateral to the midline and is often known as the medial gutter. There is a similar intermuscular septum lateral to the longissimus, the lateral gutter, separating it from the third muscle in this layer, the iliocostalis.

The intermuscular septa are less well marked low down but in the thoracic region they are convenient routes for deep palpation in the area, it being easier to feel through the septum than through muscle, the more so if there is spasm in the third layer muscle as may happen in the early stages after injury.

The deep muscles are the multifidus which according to Gray[20] crosses from one to three (sometimes four) joints, the rotatores, the semispinales and the intertransversarii, which are divided into medial and lateral groups with different innervations, and the interspinales, both of which only cross one joint. Except for the lateral intertransversarii they are innervated by the dorsal rami of the spinal nerves. The lateral intertransversarii are innervated by the anterior primary divisions and their action is thought to be lateral bending with a tendency to produce forward flexion.

In a paper presented to the North American Academy of Musculoskeletal Medicine in October 1991, Willard[21] presented recent research into the posterior muscles. He showed that the multifidus is roughly confined to the lumbar region and consists of small bipinnate muscles, the parts of which are not equal in length, some crossing only one joint and others two or three joints. The deepest fibres are interesting in that they have tendons caudally which end as far down as the sacrotuberous ligament. The multifidus group is conical in shape narrowing from below; up and near the thoracolumbar junction it is replaced by the semispinalis superficially and the rotatores deeply. The semispinales are wider and cross several joints. The rotatores are more transverse and cross only one joint. In the cervical spine, at least, there is a higher concentration of spindles in the rotatores than has been found in other muscles but they are weak with relatively few contractile fibres.

Clinically the deep short muscles are of great importance in diagnosis and in assessing the result of treatment because the presence in them of tissue texture change is one of the best indications of the level of the dysfunction. The rotatores, the intertransversarii and the multifidus are all small muscles but they appear to be very important in spinal joint dysfunction and it has been suggested that they function as spindles for the larger more superficial muscles rather than as prime movers or restrictors[22]. Because of their small size they are difficult to palpate and because their ability to generate a forceful contraction is limited, it is important not to expect them to produce a major force during treatment.

From the clinical perspective the back muscles are usually described as forming four layers; first the trapezius and latissimus dorsi, second the rhomboids and the levator scapulae, third the spinalis, longissimus and iliocostalis and fourth the deep, short layer of multifidus, rotatores, interspinales and intertransversarii.

Lumbar bones and joints

In the lumbar spine the facet orientation is variable; according to Bogduk and Twomey[8], at birth the facets face forwards and backwards so that the joints are coronal. With growth the facets tend to rotate and the joints may become fully sagittal but, more commonly, they are curved either in a 'C' shape facing posteromedially or in a 'J' shape with the short limb projecting medially from the anterior end. Facets that are strictly sagittal provide little stability against forward displacement of the superior vertebra. Those that are curved provide better stability in the sagittal plane and both restrict rotation. Facets that are coronal provide excellent stability in the sagittal plane but allow free rotation, putting extra strain on the disc annulus. At the L5–S1 joint and sometimes at L4–5 the facets may be coronal and in that case there will be more rotation. It is not unusual to find coronal facing facets on one side and sagittal facing on the other. This is known as facet tropism. It leads to asymmetrical motion and puts more strain on the annulus.

Recent work by Guntzburg *et al*[23] showed that rotation was less when the spine was flexed than in neutral and that the amplitude of rotation was not influenced by articular tropism. For a description of how rotation takes place, and the strain involved in even the 3 degrees permitted, see Bogduk and Twomey[22]. Instantaneous centres of rotation were plotted by Cossette *et al*.[24] who found that the centres were anterior to the facet joints and that they tended to move towards the side to which rotation was forced. Farfan and Sullivan[25] found that rotatory injuries to the lumbar region are likely to damage the disc annulus and that when there is asymmetry rotation only occurs to the side of the more oblique (coronal) facet. He postulated as a result of his research[26] that disc degeneration is the result of torsional strains rather than compression.

In view of these findings it seems strange that several of the classical techniques for treating lumbar joint dysfunction use rotation as the corrective movement, whether it is introduced externally by the operator or intrinsically by the patient. These techniques have proved to be satisfactory for countless patients but sometimes may be contra-indicated. Other techniques not using rotation as the corrective force will also be described.

Atypical segmentation is often seen at the lumbosacral junction and, if there is asymmetrical sacralisation of L5 and facet tropism at L4–5 with a coronal facet on the side with the larger transverse process, a disc protrusion on that side at L4–5 is relatively common (Farfan *et al*.[34]).

For the purpose of treatment the lumbar spine can be thought of as not ending until T11 or even T10. Although the morphology of the joints is not the same as in the lumbar region, from the point of view of the type of symptoms produced T11 and T12 appear more related to the lumbar spine than to dysfunctions higher up. Treatment of the T11–12 and T12–L1 joints is commonly needed in patients with low back and leg pain, and even those with leg pain alone, and dysfunction of the 11th and 12th ribs can often be found in patients whose pain is entirely in the lower back. It is important to recognise that a full structural examination is necessary before the operator can satisfy himself that pain at one level is not a manifestation of dysfunction at another level which may be almost at the other end of the body.

The transverse processes of T12 and L5 present difficulties. That of L3 is easy to feel, being usually the longest of all TPs; it is usually possible to feel those of L1, L2 and L4. That of L5 is covered by the posterior ilium and cannot be felt; that of T12 is the shortest and failure to recognise this may lead to force being applied to the posterior aspect of the rib instead of to the vertebra. Repeated anterior force on the posterior shaft or angle of the ribs may lead to anterior subluxation, a dysfunction described in Chapter 10.

At the lumbosacral junction and at T12 the lamina of the vertebra is usually used in the assessment of rotation instead of the transverse process. The lamina is approached through the intermuscular septum between the longissimus and spinalis portions of the erector spinae muscle (the medial gutter). The transverse process is most easily approached via the septum between the longissimus and the iliocostalis muscles (the lateral gutter).

Thoracic spinal bones and joints

The transverse processes are the most convenient part of the vertebra for making the diagnosis and for one prone treatment technique it is very important to contact the TPs rather than the posterior parts of the ribs. In the thoracic region the TP can conveniently be found by using the thumbs (or fingers) to find the posterior rib shaft via the lateral gutter and then sliding medially along the rib until the tip of the TP is felt as a bony resistance.

The length of the TPs is not the same as one moves up and down the spine. Seen from behind they form two 'diamonds' of which the lower is widest at L3 and then narrows rapidly so than the shortest TPs are usually at T12. From there up the length increases slowly up to T1. It is relatively easy to feel the TPs in the upper thoracic region but very difficult at T12 (Fig. 2.6a).

The spinous processes are often used in the determination of the level of the joint being examined. The most prominent at the cervicothoracic junction is typically that of C7 but may sometimes be T1. The distinction can be made by placing the index finger on the spine which is thought to be C6 and passively extending the neck. In extension the spine of C6 is covered by C5 from above and by C7 from below so that it can no longer be felt. If the spinous process being contacted does not disappear on extension it is not C6.

The spinous processes of the thoracic vertebrae tend to slope downwards and backwards; that of T1 is horizontal and T2 and 3 have only a small slope. The 'rule of threes' says that the tips of the spinous processes of T4, 5 and 6 are half the depth of a segment below the corresponding transverse process, those of T7, 8 and 9 are a full segment lower but those of T10, 11 and 12 are at the same level as the transverse process. This is only an approximation; there is a gradual increase in the slope down to T7 or sometimes T6 and then a gradual decrease (Fig. 2.6b). For clinical purposes it is enough to remember that the tip of the spinous process of T7 is level with the transverse process of T8 and both above

Fig. 2.6 (a) Posterior view of spinal column to show variation in length of TPs (after Cunningham). (b) Side view of spinal column to show spinal process slope (after Cunningham).

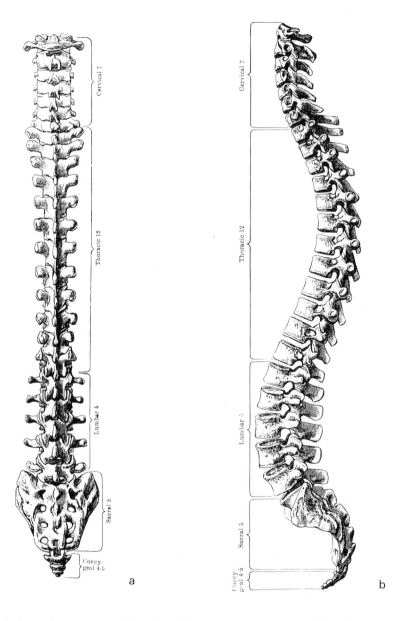

a

b

and below this segment the tip of the spinous process is less far below the transverse process.

In the thoracic spine the superior facets of the lower vertebra face posteriorly and superiorly. This would permit a free range of rotation were it not for the rib cage.

The anatomy of the ribs

The first rib is almost flat and has an inner and an outer margin. The inner margin is part of the boundary of the thoracic inlet (outlet) and dysfunction of the first rib is an important aspect of syndromes arising in this area[27,28]. The anterior end of the 1st costal cartilage can be found immediately inferior to the medial end of the clavicle. The lateral shaft can be palpated laterally in the anterior triangle of the neck but care is needed to avoid the neurovascular bundle to the arm. The first rib does not have an angle.

The second rib is also described as atypical largely because of its relation to the sternum with which it articulates at the angle of Louis. This junction between the manubrium and the body of the sternum is mobile at least into the early teens and retains some flexibility for much longer so that it is involved in the mechanics of the thoracic cage. The second rib can also be involved in the thoracic inlet syndrome and the space between it and the clavicle is narrow and contains the neurovascular bundle to the upper extremity. This can be a source of severe symptoms if the rib becomes restricted with the lateral part elevated (the laterally flexed rib described in Chapter 10).

Like the typical ribs, 3–9, the second has a head with two separate articular facets, one for the first thoracic vertebra and one for the second. It has a tubercle on which is the facet of the costotransverse joint, a curved shaft and a costal cartilage which articulates with the sternum at the junction of the manubrium and the body (the angle of Louis). By this attachment the second rib influences movement of the sternum. There is disagreement between anatomists as to the presence or absence of an angle in this rib (Fig. 2.7).

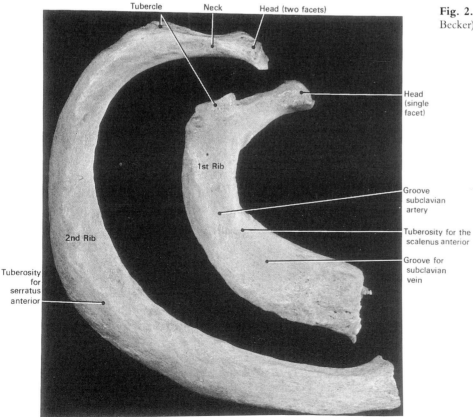

Fig. 2.7 Ribs 1 and 2 (after Becker).

The typical ribs have a sharp lower and a rounded upper border. They are attached at both ends and normally move together. They can be dysfunctional when they will not move fully on inhalation or on exhalation but they can also be dysfunctional if they have suffered subluxation, torsion or one of the other 'structural' dysfunctions described in Chapter 10. Rib dysfunctions are not uncommon in association with thoracic spinal joint problems and may resolve when the spinal joint is treated.

Ribs 11 and 12 have no anterior attachment and move in a manner somewhat different from those above. The motion is described as being like that of callipers, opening on inhalation and closing on exhalation.

The costovertebral and costotransverse joints

From the 1st to the 10th the ribs are linked to each other or to the sternum at the front end; this stabilises the thoracic spine and prevents too much rotation. Perhaps that is why the thoracic facet joints have not developed more restriction to rotation in themselves. The 11th and 12th ribs have no firm anterior attachment and it is at the T11–12 and T12–L1 intervertebral joints that most of the rotatory motion of the trunk takes place.

In addition to the intervertebral joints there are costovertebral and costotransverse joints which may also become dysfunctional. On the body of T1 is a single facet for the head of the first rib and, at the lower margin of the upper eight thoracic vertebrae, and sometimes at T9, is a demifacet for the upper aspect of the head of rib of the next lower level. The vertebrae from T2 to T10 also have a demifacet on the upper margin of the lateral aspect for the lower half of the corresponding rib head, sometimes at T10 a full facet for the whole of the rib head. The transverse processes of all thoracic vertebrae have a facet for the corresponding rib.

Rib motion

Rib movement is both up and down and in and out; the proportion of each changes as the rib number increases. The direction of the combined motion is determined by the orientation of the line joining the costotransverse to the costovertebral joints which is the axis of the motion. This orientation gradually changes from T1, where it is more coronal, to T12, where it is nearer to the sagittal plane. The corresponding rib motion is nearly sagittal in the upper ribs and more nearly coronal in the lower ribs. The former is known as pump handle motion by analogy with the old hand pump which used to be found in nineteenth century kitchens; the latter is known as bucket handle motion. In some ways this is an unfortunate term because bucket handles have fixed attachments at both ends while the rib does not. There is always an element of pump handle motion at the anterior end (Fig. 2.8a and b).

Restriction of rib motion may occur, either in inhalation or in exhalation and may need treatment. It may be necessary to treat specifically the pump or bucket handle element of the restriction; but it is of greater importance to treat the correct phase of respiration.

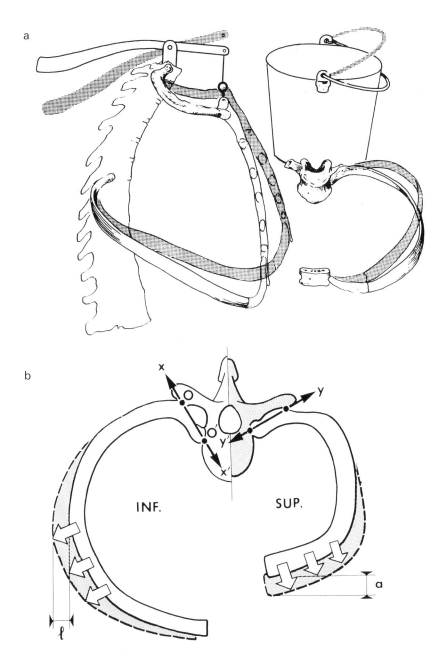

Fig. 2.8 (a) Rib motion diagram to show pump and bucket handle motion (after Becker). (b) Change in axis of rib motion, upper y, and lower x (after Kapandji).

THE ANATOMY OF THE CERVICAL SPINE

The vertebrae in the neck are different in many respects from those lower down. The upper two form a two joint complex with the occiput and there is a striking difference in structure between them and the typical cervical vertebrae which are more like those of the thoracic spine. The typical vertebrae are usually considered as from the lower half of C2 down to C7 but in some skeletons the C7–T1 joint is more cervical than thoracic in type. The complex of joints between the skull and C2 consists of the occipitoatlantal and atlantoaxial joints which each have their own motion characteristics but have complementary function, between them allowing motion in all directions.

Facet orientation

The facets of the typical vertebrae are set at an angle of about 45 degrees to the horizontal, with the superior facet facing posteriorly and superiorly (Fig. 2.9). They are weightbearing at all times and the 'neutral' type

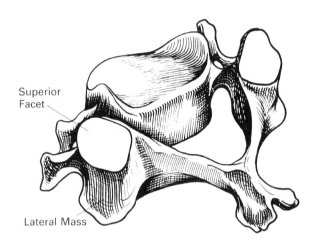

Fig. 2.9 Typical cervical vertebra showing facet facing and 'lateral mass' or interarticular pillar (after Kapandji).

Superior Facet

Lateral Mass

Fig. 2.10 (a) Superior aspect of C1. (b) Inferior aspect of C2.

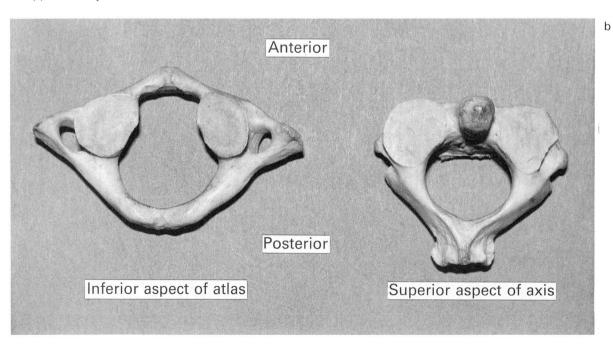

a

b

Anterior

Posterior

Inferior aspect of atlas

Superior aspect of axis

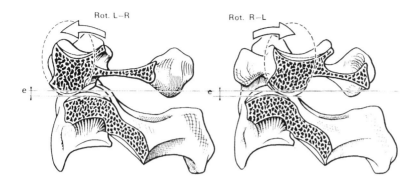

Fig. 2.11 Mechanism of vertical translation at C1–2 (after Kapandji).

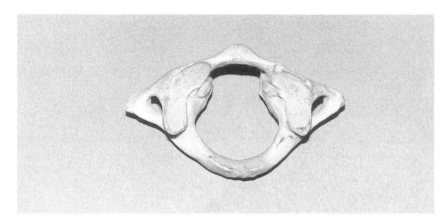

Fig. 2.12 Shape of superior facets of C1.

motion, and dysfunctions, do not happen at the joints between the typical vertebrae. The various types of motion are described under 'the physiological movements of the spine' later in this chapter.

The facets of the C1–2 joint may appear flat or concave in the skeleton (Fig. 2.10), but in life, when covered with cartilage, they are both convex[29]. This leads to a small amount of vertical translation of C1 on C2 when the head is turned to either side (Fig. 2.11). This elegant mechanism allows the ligaments which hold the odontoid process in place to remain tight even when the head is rotated fully to one side. The main movement at this joint is rotation but there is also a range of flexion and extension.

The facets of the occipitoatlantal joint are set at an angle of about 60 degrees to each other; at their anterior ends they are closer together than at the posterior end (Fig. 2.12). The superior facets of C1 are concave from side to side and from before backwards, the facets on the occipital bone are correspondingly convex. The plane of the facets is nearly horizontal in the anatomical position and, unlike all other joints in the spine, flexion (of the skull) causes the superior (occipital) facet to slide backwards on the inferior (C1) (Fig. 2.13). The shape of the facets and the angle between them cause the joint to 'bind' in extension by the impingement of the wider, more posterior part of the occipital facets on the narrow anterior part of the C1 facets. The same kind of bind does

Fig. 2.13 Flexion and extension at OA joint (after Kapandji).

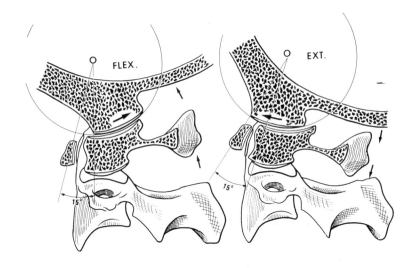

not appear to happen at the extreme of flexion. The main movement is flexion and extension but there is a small amount of sidebending, Kapandji[30] gives 3 degrees, and an even smaller amount of rotation coupled to the sidebend but with the rotation to the opposite side.

The transverse processes and articular pillars

The transverse processes of C2 and of the typical cervical vertebrae are small, they are placed anteriorly and are in close relation to the segmental nerves and vessels. They are often very tender and are not suitable as points for palpation if this can be avoided. Fortunately the typical vertebrae have large interarticular pillars or 'lateral masses' (shown in Fig. 2.9) which are convenient for that purpose. The cervical treatment techniques to be described in Chapter 10 make use of these parts of the vertebrae and it is important to recognise that they are some distance in front of and lateral to the spinous processes.

The transverse process of C1 is easily felt just in front of the tip of the mastoid process and is useful as a landmark in the upper neck. It should be handled with care because of the proximity of the vertebral artery as it arches over the top of the TP, on its way posteromedially, before perforating the occipitoatlantal membrane.

Spinous processes

Except at C7, the spinous processes of the cervical vertebrae are usually bifid, often with one side longer than the other and for this reason they are not good indicators of the midline. There is no spinous process at C1, only a small posterior tubercle which is very difficult to feel. That of C2 is long and easily felt but from there down to C7 they are covered by the nuchal ligament and may not be easy to feel accurately. The spinous process of C2 may be used as a landmark in the upper neck and that of C7 at the lower end. The spinous process of C7 is often, but not always, the most prominent. When there is doubt about which is C7, one method of ascertaining is described above.

THE INTERVERTEBRAL DISC

The intervertebral disc consists of three components, a vertebral end plate of which there is one above and one below, a nucleus pulposus and the surrounding annulus fibrosus. The vertebral end plates are sometimes considered part of the vertebral body and are composed of cartilage. They are bounded on all sides by the ring apophyses of the vertebrae so that they cover the nucleus completely but only part of the annulus. The layer next to the bone is hyaline cartilage but that next the nucleus is fibrous, the fibres of the inner layers of the annulus turning centrally when they reach the end plate and continuing across to the other side so that they completely surround the nucleus.

The annulus consists of 10–20 lamellae with the fibres in each lamella parallel to each other but the direction changes in alternate lamellae so that the fibres of one are set at an angle (of about 130–140°) to each other, the third having the same orientation as the first. The fibres of the outer lamellae are inserted into bone in the area of the ring apophysis.

The nucleus is a remnant of the notochord and is semifluid with a few cartilage cells and irregular collagen fibrils.

For further details see Taylor[31] and Bogduk and Twomey[3] who give a comprehensive bibliography.

The question as to how the disc gets its nutrition has not been settled. It is known that there is no major arterial supply to the disc except to the outermost layers of the annulus. Diffusion has been thought to be the most important method. The theory that motion helps by squeezing out fluid which then is regained by osmotic imbibition is an attractive one (it was suggested by Hendry[32] and Sylven[33]), but lacks experimental evidence. Colloid substances have the property of attracting fluid which is known as the imbibition pressure. In the intervertebral disc this tendency would be balanced by the action of the hydraulic pressure trying to squeeze out fluid from the disc substance. When the disc imbibes fluid, its size increases, the fibres of the fibrocartilaginous annulus become taut and, even if there were neither superincumbent weight nor muscle action, the imbibition process would reach a point of equilibrium. This is because of the hydrostatic pressure exerted on the disc substance by the end plates of the vertebral bodies above and below, and the fibro-cartilage of the annulus around the sides. That the process of imbibition could continue is shown by the fact that when a horizontal section is made through a normal disc and the cut surface is then immersed in saline, the nuclear material swells and rises above the level of the surrounding annulus. When the patient sits down or bends forwards, the hydrostatic pressure increases on the disc nucleus (Nachemson and Morris[34]) and it is probable that this increased pressure squeezes fluid out through the foramina in the vertebral end plate into the cancellous bone of the vertebral body. The rich blood supply of this bone is well equipped to remove metabolites and supply nutrients to the tissue fluid. When the posture is changed to one in which the hydraulic pressure is lower, a fresh supply of fluid containing nutrient would be sucked back into the disc by the imbibition pressure.

If this is a correct explanation of the process of disc nutrition, it is but a small step to assume that this imbibition pump is dependent for its function on the mobility of the intervertebral joint at that level. When one considers the structure of the intervertebral joint as a whole and the pressure to which the discs are subjected, it is probably unreasonable to say that the loss of movement would, except rarely, be so complete as to prevent the pump working at all. On the other hand, it seems certain that the efficiency of such a pump would be interfered with by stiffness such that no movement is detectable on X-ray examination in flexion and extension. That there can be this degree of loss of mobility in spinal joint injuries is established. The suggestion that the loss of nutrition is partial rather than absolute could be part of the explanation of the delay, so often observed, between the original injury and the appearance of any sign of a true disc protrusion.

THE RANGE OF MOTION IN SPINAL JOINTS

It is clear that before one can determine whether a joint is restricted in its motion, a knowledge of the expected range is needed. The variation between one person and another is wide, even if one does not include those who for reasons of profession, hobby or genetic makeup (e.g. dancers, acrobats and those with Marfan-like syndromes) have a wider range in their joints than most people.

Lumbar

Troup[35] reported fresh experimental work and reviewed the literature up to that time. By statistical analysis he showed that the method of radiographic measurement of range by successive superimpositions of individual vertebral outlines was significantly superior to other methods. It was originally described by Begg and Falconer[36] and was that used for the cervical spine by Penning.

Troup's figures are based on patients needing radiography for clinical purposes, his models all had lumbar symptoms and it is interesting to see from the tables that the results reported on supposedly normal subjects by Froning and Frohman[37] were greater at the L4–5 and L5–S1 levels.

Troup's and Froning and Frohman's results are reproduced in Tables 2.1 and 2.2. It is remarkable that there is very little loss of motion with advancing age in those who are apparently normal. A somewhat unexpected finding from Troup's figures is that there appears to be a similar reverse movement on flexion in the upper lumbar spine to that found by Penning at the occipitoatlantal joint.

Table 2.1 Range of sagittal motion in the lumbar spine (Troup)

Joint	Full flexion to extension		Full flexion to erect position	
	Mean	SD	Mean	SD
L1–2	7.5	2.3	8.6	1.7
L2–3	10.5	3.4	10.3	3.6
L3–4	11.1	2.8	11.2	2.5
L4–5	12.9	4.0	12.0	3.9
L5–S1	11.0	3.9	9.0	6.4

Table 2.2 Range of sagittal motion in the lumbar spine (Froning and Frohman)

Number of cases	Ages	L5	L4	L3	L2	L1
5	20–29	18	17	14	14	13
11	30–39	17	16	14	10	9
8	40–49	16	16	13	10	8
5	50–59	16	15	12	11	7
1	60–70	16	14	10	10	6
	Average	17	16	13	11	9

Radiographic analysis of motion in apparently normal males has been recorded by Pearcy *et al.*[38] and Pearcy and Tibrewal[39]. Their results show a remarkable uniformity in the overall range of flexion–extension of about 14 degrees (16 at L4–5) but the proportion of flexion–extension varied from 1 degree of extension and 13 of flexion at L3–4, to 5 degrees of extension and only 9 degrees of flexion at L1–2 and L5–S1. The mean figures for rotation were 2 degrees at L1–2 and 2–3 and L5–S1 and 3 degrees at L3–4 and 4–5.

In their tests the rotation was accompanied by lateral bending which was always to the opposite side at L1–2, 2–3 and 3–4 but varied at L4–5, some individuals showing rotation to the same side. At L5–S1, if sidebending occurred during rotation, it was always to the same side as the rotation.

In their results with abnormal spines Froning and Frohman found that there was a significant increase in the range of neighbouring joints adjacent to those showing restriction. This was confirmed by Jirout[40].

Thoracic

The authors are unaware of any experimental studies of the range of motion in the thoracic joints. In general their overall mobility is less than in the neck or the lumbar spine, partly because of the rib cage.

Table 2.3 Range of sagittal motion in the cervical spine (Penning)

Joint	Range in degrees	Average
C0–1	6–30	–
C1–2	3–35	–
C2–3	5–16	12½
C3–4	13–26	18
C4–5	15–29	20
C5–6	16–29	21½
C6–7	6–25	15½
C7–T1	4–12	8

There is an abrupt change in mobility between C5–6 and C7–T1, as will be seen from Table 2.3, but the major part of the change is between C5–6 and C6–7.

There is a relatively wide range of rotation at the lower end of the thoracic spine, T10–11, T11–12 and T12–L1 and there is a striking change in the morphology in this region between typical thoracic facets to the lumbar type. Davis[41] described the joint at which most change occurs as like a carpenter's mortice and said that, while it is most commonly the T11–12 joint, it may be either T12–L1 or less commonly T10–11. He described that at that joint there is little except flexion–extension motion and even that is restricted as compared to the joint on either side.

Cervical

Many workers have examined the range of motion in the cervical joints. One of the difficulties is that, in order to do so radiographically, the person must be exposed to radiation for other than clinical requirements. Penning[42] discusses figures given by several authors including himself and describes the method he used of drawing lines on X-ray films, taken in different positions when superimposed on each other. His figures are reproduced in Table 2.3 and his results are similar to those of other workers. He pointed out that there is difficulty in assessing the range of flexion at the occipitoatlantal joint. A lateral film must be taken with the head flexed on the neck and the neck itself less flexed because in full neck flexion the chin contacts the sternum and causes the O–A joint to extend.

THE PHYSIOLOGICAL MOVEMENTS OF THE SPINE

Coupling of rotation and sidebending

The first recorded observation of the coupling of rotation and sidebending in the spine was by Lovett[43] while working on the problem of scoliosis. He found that when an intact spine was sidebent from the neutral or flexed position, the vertebrae rotated to the side opposite to the sidebend as if trying to escape from under a load. If the spine was in extension when sidebent, the bodies rotated the other way. In looking for an explanation Lovett found that, if a column of vertebral bodies was separated from its posterior elements, on sidebending the bodies would rotate to the side of the convexity of the sidebend. He found, however, that the column of posterior elements always rotated to the same side as the sidebend. He further recorded his observation that, in extension, the facets were in close apposition but that this was not so in flexion and concluded that in extension the facets 'control' the movement but in flexion the vertebral bodies were not constrained in that manner.

Kapandji[44] describes automatic rotation of the intact vertebral column but does not mention the changes that occur if the spine is flexed or extended.

Fryette[45] confirmed Lovett's observations but showed that he had omitted to test the movement in the hyperflexed position. He found that, near the limit of flexion, the pattern once again follows the facet movement and the rotation is to the same side as the sidebend. He proposed two concepts, which he termed 'laws', of spinal motion arising from these observations and, for completeness, a third law was added. These concepts have become widely accepted, but there has been a recent change of opinion about the lumbar spine.

Fryette's concepts are:

I. With the spine in easy normal (neutral), the facets are 'idling' and the rotation is always towards the convexity of the sidebend (Fig. 2.14).

II. In extension and in nearly full flexion, the facets are in control and the rotation is towards the concavity of the sidebend (Fig. 2. 15).

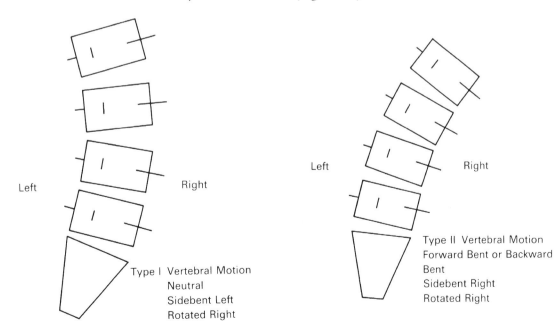

Left

Right

Type I Vertebral Motion
Neutral
Sidebent Left
Rotated Right

Left

Right

Type II Vertebral Motion
Forward Bent or Backward
Bent
Sidebent Right
Rotated Right

Fig. 2.14 Diagram to show 'neutral' coupling (after Greenman).

Fig. 2.15 Diagram to show 'non-neutral' coupling (after Greenman).

III. If movement is introduced into a spinal segment in any plane, the range of motion in the other two planes will be reduced.

Throughout the thoracic and lumbar spine the first concept has been confirmed by research. The second concept has been shown to be fully confirmed in the thoracic region but in the lumbar spine it has not been confirmed with respect to the extension end of the range of motion. In nearly full flexion the lumbar vertebrae have been shown to rotate into the concavity of the sidebend curve. Even although there is no research confirmation, clinical evidence does suggest that, in the lumbar spine, restrictions of flexion (ERS dysfunctions in which the joint is in extension) do occur with rotation into the concavity of the sidebend and that this happens particularly at the lumbo-sacral joint.

In the cervical spine the picture is different. The second concept always applies in the typical cervical joints where the facets are weightbearing and appear always to be 'in control'. At the atlantoaxial joint the motion is almost all rotatory and the concepts do not apply. At the occipito-atlantal joint the facets are set at an angle to each other in such a manner that what little sidebend there is must always be accompanied by (an even smaller amount of) rotation to the opposite side. This should not be confused with the type I (concept I) motion found in the spine in the thoracic and lumbar regions.

One of the points of clinical significance arising from these observations is that in moving from flexion to extension, there is a cross-over point where the rotation changes. This appears to correspond to the known danger of producing acute spinal joint dysfunction by bending down, turning to one side and coming up without first turning back to the straight position. It seems that the mechanism can become 'jammed' if one does this.

Concept III is important both for examination and treatment. During examination, if the spine is not in neutral, the range of motion may be reduced enough that the dysfunctions are not found. This is of particular importance when motion in the thoracic spine is being examined in the sitting position. Nearly all patients tend to slump and, if they are allowed to do this, the overall range may be so reduced that the dysfunctions are not detectable. The instruction must be to 'sit up tall' or some similar phrase. The concept is put to good use when positioning a patient in order to localise treatment to the precise level required. Details of the application of the concept will be given in the descriptions of the various techniques.

THE NATURE OF THE RESTRICTION

There has been extensive research into the detailed anatomy of the facet joints, some of which was referred to in previous editions[46,47,48,49,50]. The precise cause, or probably causes, of restriction is still not agreed. The fact that there is palpable tissue texture change at the level of any dysfunction in the spine indicates that the soft tissues are closely involved in whatever is the cause. Their close involvement does not prove that they are the cause and certainly not that they are the only cause. The disappearance of symptoms and of tissue texture changes that sometimes follows immediately after restoration of motion suggests that the soft tissues may be much involved in maintenance of a dysfunction. The fact that these changes can follow indirect treatment in which there is neither external application of force, nor patient effort, makes it likely that the role of soft tissues in maintaining a dysfunction is important. On the other hand, when in the course of a gentle 'muscle energy' treatment the joint suddenly lets go with a palpable (and often audible) movement, the concept of soft tissue being the sole cause becomes untenable.

The only constant findings in joint dysfunction are restriction of motion, asymmetry and tissue texture change, usually including hypertonus in muscle and other soft tissues. In some areas tissue changes may be difficult to feel, especially in the pelvis. In other areas asymmetry may be so common that it is of little value. As no one has found a convincing mechanical basis for joint restriction that can be instantly relieved by treatment, the question comes back to the soft tissues. Why should they remain tight? The immediate nature of the release which often happens in treatment might be likened to the release of a locked knee and thought to be due to entrapment of a (damaged) intra-articular meniscoid but there has been much research to confirm that theory without success. The immediate release strongly suggests that there is no structural change in the muscle or other soft tissues. The most likely answer appears to be a change in the mechanism by which the central nervous system controls muscle tone. The principal effect of the muscle energy techniques described here appears to be to stretch muscles (and their associated soft tissues) that will not relax to their normal resting length. When thrusting treatment is used the soft tissues are of necessity stretched before motion can be restored. From the point of view of what is described here, it is reasonable to make the simplification that what is mainly required is to restore soft tissues to their normal resting length. The achievement and maintenance of increased soft tissue length can be assisted by individually prescribed exercises as described in Chapters 14 and 15. However, there are other approaches to treatment which are beyond the scope of this volume.

TYPES OF SPINAL JOINT DYSFUNCTION

Corresponding to the first two of Fryette's concepts, there are two different types of dysfunction which may need treatment in the spine. Type I or neutral dysfunctions occur when the spine is neither flexed nor extended, that is when concept I mechanics are operative with rotation and sidebending to opposite sides. These dysfunctions always occur in groups of three or more vertebrae and often begin as a compensation to bring the upper spine vertical when there is sidebending due to another lesion. Many will resolve when the cause is removed and for this reason they are second in priority for treatment. If, as is common, the cause is a type II dysfunction it will often be found at one or both ends of the neutral curve.

The second is known as type II or non-neutral dysfunction and occurs when the spine is operating in non-neutral mechanics with sidebending and rotation to the same side. Type II dysfunctions are nearly always traumatic in origin, and the trauma will have occurred with the spine either in extension or in nearly full flexion. Correspondingly, one will have restriction of flexion if it occurs in extension, or of extension if the causative trauma happened in flexion. They are frequently painful and should be treated first because they are often the cause of the neutral curves, which only need treatment if they persist after the cause has been corrected.

In most instances type II dysfunctions are single (in a directional sense) in any one joint, but sometimes one finds that both flexion and extension are limited in the same joint, or the joint may have restriction on both sides. Type II dysfunctions are individual entities needing individual treatment but may occur stacked one on another. This makes precise diagnosis more difficult and it is emphasised that the position of a vertebra is always assessed with reference to the one below.

While both type I and type II dysfunctions can occur in the thoracic and lumbar regions, in the cervical spine the picture is not the same. In the typical cervical joints there is only type II motion and therefore all dysfunctions are of the type II, non-neutral variety. At the atlantoaxial joint the dysfunction is in rotation only and at the occipitoatlantal joint there is a small amount of rotation in the opposite direction to the sidebending. This however is an isolated joint and the mechanics are not the same as in a neutral (type I) group. The amount of rotation at the occipitoatlantal joint is small and for treatment purposes it can be neglected, so long as it is not blocked.

THE INNERVATION OF THE INTERVERTEBRAL JOINTS

The innervation of the intervertebral joints was described by Pedersen *et al.*[51]. and more recently by Wyke[52,53]. Wyke's findings were essentially similar to Pedersen's, he described:

(a) branches of the posterior primary rami supplying the apophyseal joints, the periosteum and the related fasciae of the surfaces of the vertebral bodies and their arches, the interspinous ligaments and the blood vessels;

(b) pain afferents in the sinuvertebral nerves having endings in the posterior longitudinal and flaval ligaments, the dura mater and the surrounding fatty tissue, the epidural veins and the periosteum of the spinal canal;

(c) a plexus of nerve fibres which surrounds the paravertebral venous system.

He reported that receptors supplied by these nerves are found throughout the same area as those supplied by the sinuvertebral nerve. All the pain afferent fibres are small, either thinly or not at all myelinated.

Wyke makes many interesting observations, some of which are opposed to classical neuroanatomical teaching. Nociceptor afferent innervation of dermatomes is not unisegmental. The sinuvertebral nerves have branches that extend over at least four segments, and the innervation in the lumbar region is by branches of from three to five posterior primary divisions of the spinal nerves. No joint in the lumbar region has monosegmental innervation.

THE AUTONOMIC NERVOUS SYSTEM

Knowledge of the anatomy of the autonomic system is important in manual medicine partly because of the frequent involvement of the spinal musculature as a secondary effect of visceral disease (viscero-somatic reflexes), and partly because in clinical practice cases are seen in which there is no apparent reason for a symptom unless the autonomic pathways are involved. Chronic constipation relieved by treatment of upper lumbar or low thoracic joint dysfunction and the relief of bronchospasm by treating upper thoracic dysfunctions are examples.

Barnes[54] concluded that it was unlikely that pain actually travelled in sympathetic afferent fibres on the following grounds.

1. No sensory change of any kind has ever been demonstrated in a sympathectomised limb.

2. In cord lesions where the cord is damaged below the lowest sympathetic outflow, the sympathetic innervation of the lower limbs is intact but there is a total insensibility of the area supplied by somatic nerves arising in segments below the damage.

3. A low spinal anaesthetic will relieve the pain of causalgia before there is any effect on the sympathetic fibres.

Table 2.4, based on Mitchell[55], gives his description of the anatomy of the sympathetic system. He states that the afferent pain fibres from the

Table 2.4 Sympathetic innervation of more important structures (based on Mitchell)

Structure	Location of pre-ganglionic cells	Chief efferent pathways
Eyes	T1–2	Internal carotid plexus to ciliary nerves or along vessels
Vessels of head	T1–2 (and 3)	Vascular plexuses
Upper limbs	T2(3) to T6(7)	Rami communicates to roots of brachial plexus
Heart	T1–4(5)	Cardiac sympathetic nerves to cardiac plexus
Stomach	T6–9(10)	Via coeliac plexus
Kidneys	T12(11) to L1(2)	Via coeliac plexus
Bladder and uterus	T12(11) to L1(2)	Lumbar splanchnic nerves
Lower limbs	T11(10) to L2	Rami communicates to lumbar and sacral nerves

Fig. 2.16 Autonomic nervous system (after Carpenter).

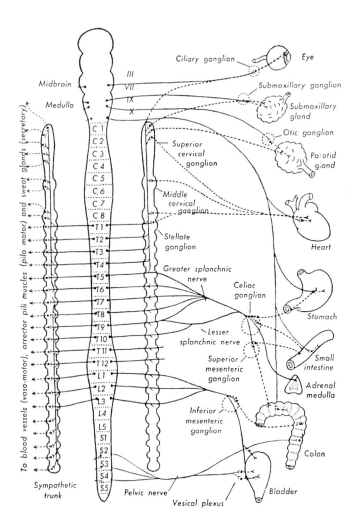

cervix uteri, the base of the bladder, the prostate and the rectum are carried in the pelvic splanchnic nerves with cell bodies located in the dorsal root ganglia of the 2nd, 3rd and 4th sacral nerves.

Figure 2.16 is a diagram of the autonomic nervous system showing how the various parts of the body are innervated. It is included because it shows the fundamental difference between the innervation of the soma and that of the organ systems. The internal organs have innervation from both parts of the autonomic system but the soma receives sympathetic fibres only, even for the skin viscera.

The sympathetic chain ganglia, which contain many cell stations for that part of the autonomic system, are in close anatomical relation to the sides of the vertebral bodies and the costovertebral joints. This introduces the possibility that oedema or inflammatory reaction around those joints could affect the function of the ganglia.

SENSORY DISTRIBUTION OF THE SPINAL NERVE ROOTS

It has been known for many years that the distribution of sensory fibres to the skin from the various spinal nerve roots does not correspond to the distribution of any of the cutaneous nerves except over the trunk where the correspondence is fair. Head[56] studied the distribution of the cutaneous hyperalgesia and the vesicles in cases of herpes zoster. His results allowed him to draw a map showing the distribution of the various spinal nerves to the skin and he also drew a chart of the points where the sensation appeared to be maximum from each nerve. His charts were reproduced in the fourth and earlier editions. Also in 1893 Sherrington[57], working with experimental nerve sectioning in the rhesus monkey, drew a similar chart. There was some difference in the lumbar and sacral nerves, possibly because the rhesus monkey has a different configuration of the lumbar spine. Sherrington found significant overlap of neighbouring areas, while Head's were discrete. Both Head's and Sherrington's results appeared to show a gap in innervation of some of the nerves in the proximal part of the limbs. The concept (the loop theory) that the growing limb bud drew away all the fibres to the periphery has not been confirmed by subsequent workers but the general distribution is considered to be very similar to that described by Head and Sherrington.

Keegan and Garrett[58] using patients with sensory nerve damage from disc protrusion, showed a similar chart although differing in some details (Fig. 2.17). They were also able to demonstrate a fainter overlap distribution often

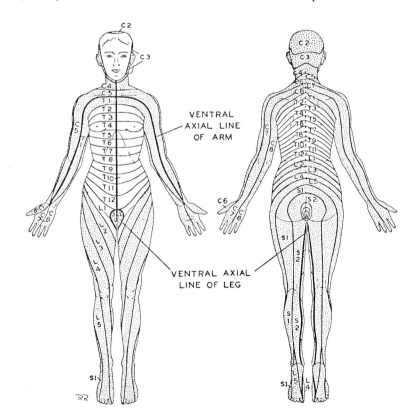

Fig. 2.17 Dermatome chart of the human body drawn by Keegan and Garrett.

extending 2.5–5 cm (1–2 inches) on either side of the main distribution. This may well explain the difference between Head's and Sherrington's charts. Sutherland[59] gives a chart for the anterior distribution that is in all respects similar to Keegan's and Garrett's. He does not show a posterior chart but he does say that the dorsal root of T12 'descends through muscle to pierce the lumbo-dorsal fascia . . . to innervate the skin of the buttock as far down as the greater trochanter'. This is shown by Head but not by Keegan. Clinically there appears to be evidence that T11 dorsal ramus also has a distribution in the buttock.

While it may be helpful to recognise the distribution of sensory fibres from each level, it must be remembered that referred pain does not always follow anatomical nerve pathways.

REFERENCES

1. Mixter W.J., Barr J.S. (1934). Rupture of the intervertebral disc. *New Eng. J. Med.*; **211**:210–215.
2. Armstrong J.R. (1965). *Lumbar Disc Lesions*, 3rd edn. London: Livingstone.
3. Bogduk N., Twomey L. (1987). *Clinical Anatomy of the Lumbar Spine*. London: Churchill Livingstone.
4. Kapandji I.A. (1978). *The Physiology of the Joints*, Vol. 3, p.70. London: Churchill Livingstone.
5. Fryette H.H. (1954). *The Principles of Osteopathic Technique*. Carmel: Academy of Applied Osteopathy.
6. Greenman P.E. Personal communication.
7. Brooke R. (1934). The sacro-iliac joint. *J. Anat.*; **58**:299–305.
8. Weisl H. (1955). Movement of the sacroiliac joint. *Acta Anat.*; **23**:80–91
9. Pitkin H.C., Pheasant H.C. (1936). Sacrarthrogenic telalgia. *J. Bone Jt Surg.*; **18**:111–133, 365–374.
10. Bowen V., Cassidy J.D. (1981). Macroscopic and microscopic anatomy of the sacroiliac joint until the eighth decade. *Spine*; **6**:620–628.
11. Midttun M., Midttun A., Bojsen–Møller F. (1989). The N. Cutaneous Perforans S2–S3. Abstracted in *Laboratory for functional anatomy*, University of Copenhagen Activity Report. Copenhagen.
12. Vleeming A., Stoeckart R., Snijders Ch.J., van Wingerden J.-P., Dijkstra P.F. (1990). The sacro-iliac joint – anatomical, biomechanical and radiological aspects. *J. Manual Medicine*; **5**:100–102.
13. Greenman P.E. (1990). Clinical aspects of sacroiliac function in walking. *J. Manual Medicine*; **5**:125–130.
14. Kapandji I.A. *loc. cit.* p.70.
15. Chamberlain W.E. (1930). The symphysis pubis in the roentgen examination of the sacroiliac joint. *Amer. J. Roentgenology*; **24**, 621.
16. Dihlmann Wolfgang (1980). *Diagnostic Radiology of the Sacroiliac Joint*. Yearbook Medical Publishers Inc.: Chicago and London.
17. Kapandji I.A. (1974). loc. cit. p.64.
18. Mitchell F.L. (1948). The balanced pelvis and its relationship to reflexes. *Yearbook, Academy Applied Osteopathy*; **48**:146–151.
19. *Grant's Method of Anatomy*, 7th edn. (1965). Baltimore: Williams and Wilkins.
20. *Gray's Anatomy*, 22nd English edition, p.460. London: Longmans Green.

21. Willard F.H., Associate Professor of Anatomy, University of New England, Biddeford, ME.

22. Bogduk and Twomey *loc. cit.*

23. Guntzburg R., Hutton W., Fraser R. (1991). Axial rotation of the lumbar spine and the effect of flexion. *Spine*; **16**:22–28.

24. Cossette J.W., Farfan H.F., Robertson G.H., Wells R.V. (1971). The instantaneous center of rotation of the third lumbar intervertebral joint. *J. Biomechanics;* **4**:149–153.

25. Farfan H.F., Sullivan J.D. (1967). The relation of facet orientation to intervertebral disc failure. *Can. J. Surg.*; **10**:179–185.

26. Farfan H.F. (1970). The effects of torsion on the lumbar intervertebral joints. *J. Bone Jt Surg.,* **52a**:468–497.

27. Lee R., Farquharson T., Domleo S. Subluxation and locking of the first rib: a cause of thoracic outlet syndrome. *Australian Association of Manual Medicine Bulletin*; **6(2)** p:50–51.

28. Lindgren K-A., Leino E. (1988). Subluxation of the first rib: a possible thoracic outlet syndrome mechanism. *Arch. Phys. Med. Rehab.*; **68**:692–695.

29. Kapandji I.A. *loc. cit.* p.174.

30. Kapandji I.A. *loc. cit.* p.184.

31. Taylor J.R. (1990). The development and adult structure of lumbar intervertebral discs: *J. Manual Medicine*; **5**:43–47.

32. Hendry N.G.C. (1958). The hydration of the nucleus pulposus. *J. Bone Jt Surg.*; **40B**:132–144.

33. Sylven B. (1951). On the biology of the nucleus pulposus. *Acta Orthopaed. Scand*; **20**:275–279.

34. Nachemson A., Morris J.H. (1964). In vivo measurements of intradiscal pressure. *J. Bone Jt. Surg.*; **46a**:1977.

35. Troup J.D. (1968). PhD thesis, London University.

36. Begg C., Falconer M.A. (1949). Plain radiography in intraspinal protrusions of intervertebral discs. *J. Bone Jt Surg.*; **36**:225.

37. Froning E.C., Frohman B. (1968). Motion of the lumbar spine after laminectomy and spine fusion. *J. Bone Jt Surg.*; **50A**:897–918.

38. Pearcy M.J., Portek I., Shepherd J. (1984). Three dimensional x-ray analysis of normal movement in the lumbar spine. *Spine*;**9**:294–297

39. Pearcy M.J., Tibrewal S.B. (1984). Axial rotation and lateral bending in the normal lumbar spine. *Spine*; **9**:582–587.

40. Jirout J. (1955). Studies in the dynamics of the spine. *Excerpta Acta Radiol.*;**46**:Fasc.

41. Davis P.R. (1935). The thoraco-lumbar mortice joint. *J. Anat.*; **89**:370–371.

42. Penning L. (1968). *Functional Pathology of the Cervical Spine.* Amsterdam:Excerpta Medica.

43. Lovett R.W. (1902). The mechanics of lateral curvature of the spine. *Boston M.S.J.;* **142**:622–627; Lovett R.W. (1902). The study of the mechanics of the spine. *Am. J. Anat.*; **2**:457–462.

44. Kapandji I.A. *loc. cit. p. 42.*

45. Fryette H.H. (1954). *loc. cit.*

46. Schmincke A., Santo E. (1932). Zur normalen und pathologischen Anatomie der Halswirbelsaule. *Zbl. Path.*; **55**:369–372.

47. Santo E. (1935). Zur Entwicklungsgeschichte und Histologie der Zwischenscheiben in den kleinen Gelenken. *Zeitschr. f. Anat. u. Entwicklungsgesch*; **104**:623–634.

48. Tondury G. (1940). Beitrag zur Kentniss der kleinen Wirbelgelenke. *Zeitschr. f. Anat. u. Entwicklungsgesch.*; **110**:568–575.

49. Dorr W.M. (1958). Uber die Anatomie der Wirbelgelenke. *Arch. f. Orthop. u. Unfall-Chir.*; **50**:222–234.

50. Lewin T., Moffett B.,Viidik A. (1961). The morphology of the lumbar synovial intervertebral joints. *Acta Morphologica Neerlando-Scandinavica*; **4**:299–319.

51. Pedersen H.E., Blunk G.F.J., Gardner E. (1956). Anatomy of lumbo-sacral posterior rami. *J. Bone Jt. Surg.*; **38A**:377–391.

52. Wyke B. (1970). The neurological basis of thoracic spinal pain. *Rheumatol. Phys. Med.*; **10**:356–366.

53. Wyke B. (1980). The neurology of low back pain. In *The Lumbar Spine and Back Pain*, 2nd edn. (Jayson M., ed.): pp. 265–339. Tunbridge Wells: Pitman Medical.

54. Barnes R. (1954). Causalgia in peripheral nerve injuries. *MRC Special Reports* Series 282. London: HMSO.

55. Mitchell G. (1963). *The Anatomy of the Autonomic Nervous System.* Edinburgh: Livingstone.

56. Head H. (1893). Disturbances of sensation with special reference to the pain of visceral disease. *Brain*; **16**:1–33, 339–480.

57. Sherrington C.S. (1893). Experiments in the examination of the peripheral distribution of the fibres of the posterior roots of some spinal nerves. *Phil.Trans.*; **B184**:641–763; **B190**:45–187.

58. Keegan J.J., Garrett F.D. (1948). Segmental sensory nerve distribution. *Anat. Rec.*; **102**:409–437.

59. Sutherland S. (1978). *Nerves and Nerve Injuries.* London: Churchill Livingstone.

Chapter 3

Examination, general considerations

TERMINOLOGY AND NOMENCLATURE

In order to simplify description of techniques of examination and treatment in this book the patient will be designated by the female gender and the examiner by the male.

There is a troublesome diversity of names for many of the dysfunctions of the pelvic ring. Members of the osteopathic profession are those who have worked out the details which will be presented but even among themselves there are differences. The terms used in this edition are only slightly different from those adopted for the 4th edition.

The distinction of Sacroiliac from Iliosacral is based on the clinical observation that dysfunction of the sacrum as it moves between the ilia needs different treatment from that required by dysfunction in the motion of one innominate on the sacrum. At the sacroiliac joint the position may be described as that of the sacrum with respect to one (or both) innominates or the other way round.

The need for a revision of nomenclature is illustrated by the fact that one sacral position was referred to in one context as flexion and in another context as extension. Unfortunately there are still a number of different names in use for some of the dysfunctions and, for these, the alternative names in most common use will be given in parentheses.

To avoid any misunderstanding the following terms are defined.

1. *Flexion* is used to mean forward tilting of the superior surface of the vertebra.

2. *Extension* means backward tilting of the same surface.

3. *Rotation* of both vertebrae and sacrum is named for the side to which the anterior surface turns.

4. *Sidebending* is named for the side to which the superior surface of the vertebra tilts.

5. *Translation* is used to describe motion in a plane, most often referring to the horizontal (transverse) plane with respect to the body in the anatomical position.

The use of translation to achieve sagittal or coronal plane overturning motion will be mentioned in many technique descriptions, Fig. 9.2a shows sidebending to the left produced by translation of the 3rd thoracic vertebra to the right.

6. *Motion of a vertebra*, or of the skull, will always be related to the structure immediately below. For instance, if L4 is said to be flexed and sidebent to the right, the joint involved is that between L4 and L5.

7. *Neutral* refers to the range of flexion/extension in which rotation of lumbar and thoracic vertebrae is coupled to opposite sides, Fryette type I motion; in most joints this is a wide range.

8. *Non-neutral* refers to the range near to the end of flexion or extension where the coupling is of rotation and sidebending to the same side, Fryette type II motion.

9. *TP* singular or plural will be used as a shortening for Transverse Process(es).

10. *TrP(s)* refers to myofascial trigger point(s), as defined by Dr Janet Travell which are the characteristic finding in the myofascial pain syndrome *(MPS)*.

11. *TeP* refers to the tender points found in the fibromyalgia syndrome *(FMS)*.

12. *Sulcus* is used for the interval between the medial aspect of the posterior superior iliac spine (PSIS) and the lamina of the first sacral vertebra unless otherwise specifically stated.

13. *Caudad*, which is of Latin derivation, is in general use and needs no explanation.

14. *Craniad* is the corresponding term of Latin parentage for the opposite direction. This will be used rather than cephalad which means the same but is of Greek derivation.

15. *Innominate bone* is a long established term and will be used for what some anatomists now like to call the 'hip' bone.

SOMATIC DYSFUNCTION

This term, coined by the osteopathic profession, is now widely used for what has had many names in the past, spinal joint lesion, osteopathic lesion, chiropractic subluxation etc. It has the advantage that it emphasises the concept of dysfunction rather than pathology. The concept, in a somewhat less inclusive form, can be conveyed by joint dysfunction, if that is preferred. In Europe joint blockage is the most common term and this also suggests the absence of pathology. However, both joint blockage and joint dysfunction could be understood to imply that the fault is primarily of a mechanical nature in the joint, a concept now widely disputed. It is also known as the 'manipulable lesion'. In the USA the term somatic dysfunction is useful because it is the diagnosis which insurance carriers will accept if they are paying for treatment. It is defined as:

> Impaired or altered function of related components of the somatic (body framework) system; skeletal, arthrodial, and myofascial structures; and related vascular, lymphatic and neural elements.

The inclusive nature of the definition is important if only to remind us that the human body is a whole, not simply a number of separate systems. The separate organ systems may need their own specific treatment, but the patient is not well unless they all work together in harmony. Of these systems the musculoskeletal is the largest, consumes by far the most energy and is that by which we communicate and express ourselves in any way whatever. It is strange that the musculoskeletal system has, in the past, been so neglected by orthodox medicine.

The characteristic signs of somatic dysfunction for which treatment by manipulation may be appropriate are:

1. asymmetry,
2. restricted movement,
3. change in tissue texture, primarily hypertonus in muscle.

Because it is not possible for a patient to produce asymmetry at will, to restrict motion voluntarily at one spinal joint only or to cause tissues to tighten at one individual level, these signs are truly objective. The subjective sign of tenderness may also be useful but it should not be forgotten that the points to which pain is referred may be as tender as the points of origin of the referred pain. Tenderness is helpful to the operator as a confirmation of objective findings at the same level. It is also helpful to the patient when, for instance, the point of origin of a referred pain is found in an area of which the patient is not complaining. If it were not for the tenderness some patients might regard as meddlesome the treatment of such primary areas.

In teaching, the acronym ART, *A*symmetry, *R*estriction of motion and *T*issue texture change is often used. Some use TART (*T*enderness ART). These serve as a reminder of the signs to be sought.

Asymmetry is common in the axial skeleton and structural asymmetry must be distinguished from that due to dysfunction. This is especially true of the pelvis. It has been said with some justification that no two sacroiliac joints are alike even from right to left in the same patient. Asymmetry of structural origin can be distinguished from that due to dysfunction by the fact that, while a dysfunctional joint will always have some restriction of motion, in the absence of dysfunction (or of some additional congenital anomaly) in a case of structural asymmetry the joint will have normal mobility.

Restriction of motion is often a consequence of joint injury. This happens in peripheral as well as spinal joints and, if untreated, may be persistent. Stiff joints are not necessarily painful, but in the event of a further injury, they may easily become so. At least in the spine there are other factors that can cause silent dysfunctional joints to become painful and it seems that 'tension' is one of these factors. Stiff joints around which there is no detectable tissue texture change are probably not often the immediate cause of symptoms but treatment may be important in the management of the patient. This is because defective segmental motion at any spinal level does tend to cause other levels to become dysfunctional and to make such dysfunctions tend to recur even after successful treatment. In this context it should be recognised that the tissue texture change associated with dysfunction at the sacroiliac joint is easily missed.

In the presence of old injury with degenerative changes, and in some without such mechanical obstructions, it may be impossible to restore a full range of motion. For the relief of symptoms, however, it is usually enough to restore some motion and, as far as possible, correct the asymmetry. If this is done the tissue texture abnormality will usually become less severe. In this connection it is important to address asymmetry of muscle length and strength as well as of joint motion (see Chapter 14).

It is appropriate, at this point to emphasise that this treatment is not dealing with dislocations, there is not 'a little bone out of place' nor is it designed to reduce a 'slipped disc', although if motion is restored by manual methods some patients with disc protrusions confirmed by CT, MRI scan or myelogram, may show significant reduction of the protrusions on repeat imaging. Some of the pelvic and rib dysfunctions do involve unphysiological movements and can therefore be described as subluxations but, in the large majority of spinal joints, the problem is of restriction within the normal range of motion.

There are a number of different tissue texture changes, some or all of which may be present at a dysfunctional level. One of the most important is localised hypertonus in muscle at that joint. This is most significantly found in the fourth (deepest) layer muscles close to the laminae and transverse processes. The fourth layer muscles are quite small, they can only be felt when they are hypertonic and, of importance when muscle energy treatment is used, the force which they can generate is also small. There are other changes which can be helpful in localising the dysfunction and some of these appear to be due to altered tone in the autonomic nervous system. These include:

1. Localised skin changes such as 'skin drag' probably due to increased water content in the epidermis.
2. Changes in the skin and subcutaneous tissues leading to a positive skin-rolling test.
3. Actual oedema which may be superficial or deep.
4. Circulatory changes; the area may have a different temperature when compared to neighbouring skin and it is common to find a 'red reaction' after touching the area.

In patients who show a red reaction it can be of diagnostic value as an indication of altered sympathetic activity at that level. If the operator slides his index and middle fingers down the spine from above while using an even, moderately firm pressure, a red reaction at any level strongly suggests local dysfunction.

In those who have a positive skin rolling test a 'pop' can sometimes be produced by lifting the skin and subcutaneous tissues off the deeper layers at the dysfunctional level which suggests that there may be actual adhesions. A technique for the skin rolling test is described under 'scanning examination' below.

Tenderness can be from deep or superficial tissues. Skin that gives a positive rolling test is usually tender and hypertonic muscle is probably always so. As mentioned above, tenderness is also found at the point to which pain is referred and it is most important that the point of origin and the reference point are not confused. Treatment of the reference point may reduce the pain for a short time but unless the point of origin is also treated it is unlikely to give any lasting relief.

PALPATORY SKILL

One of the difficulties which people have in understanding and applying techniques of manual medicine is that both diagnosis and treatment require a degree of palpatory skill that is different from, and in some ways greater than, that used in other branches of medicine. The difficulty can be likened to that of an untrained person trying to read the dots of Braille writing. To those who have not practised, such as the authors, this seems impossible but, as is well known, it can be learned.

In addition to its variation in thickness, subcutaneous tissue is different in its density from one person to another. Some will be found with tissue through which it is easy to feel and the beginner needs to look for these and be encouraged by what he can feel in them. There are others in whom the tissue is dense and through which it is difficult to feel even when not very thick. Practice helps but the skill takes time to develop and perseverance is needed. A most important point is that palpatory pressure should be as light as possible. Excess pressure renders proprioceptors less sensitive. This change in sensitivity is a natural phenomenon, any balance used in weighing is much more sensitive to small changes in weight when the load is small.

Palpation is used to find asymmetry of position or structure, changes in tissue texture, and range and quality of motion. Rough or irregular movement may signify dysfunction even in the presence of a full range in the plane being examined (there will often be restriction in one of the other planes of motion). There is also a difference in the 'end feel', that is the feel of the increasing resistance to motion as the limit is reached, depending on the cause of the motion restriction. In designing treatment it is helpful to be able to distinguish between different end feels as the various causes of restriction do not necessarily respond equally to any particular form of treatment.

THE BARRIER CONCEPT

The point beyond which a joint will not move is referred to as the barrier. There is no joint in the body in which motion is unlimited and all joints have barriers. A normal joint will move through a certain range of active motion. Beyond the end of what the muscles can do actively, there is a small additional passive range. The limit of active motion is called the 'physiological' barrier, that of passive motion the 'anatomical' barrier. If the anatomical barrier is exceeded there will be disruption of tissue, either subluxation, dislocation or fracture.

In manual medicine we are particularly interested in what is called the restrictive barrier, in some texts it is called 'pathological' but in manual medicine we are concerned with dysfunction rather than pathology. A truly pathological barrier is unlikely to be caused by something that would respond to manual treatment. A restrictive barrier is abnormal and may be due to a variety of causes.

Restrictions may be major or minor; the barriers for these are illustrated diagrammatically in Fig. 3.1 (after Kimberly)[1]. In a normal joint, motion between the physiological barriers is free and should be smooth. As passive motion is introduced after the end of the active range the tension increases steadily but slowly until the slack has been taken out and then much more rapidly until motion ceases as the barrier is reached. The point when the slack has been taken out is described by some as an elastic barrier.

Fig. 3.1 The barrier concept. (a) Represents a normal joint. The range of physiological movement is represented as the distance between B and B_1. The total possible movement is that between A and A_1. The ranges A,B and A_1,B_1 are the passive ranges at either end. D represents the 'point of maximum ease'. (b) Represents a joint with a minor and (c) a major motion restriction; the available active range is from B to C and the total range A to C. Note the change in location of D, the point of maximum ease.

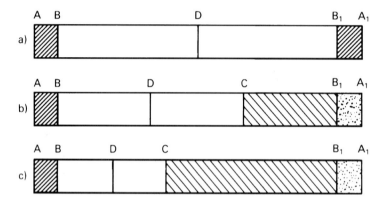

In a diagram the barrier is shown as existing in one plane but in the spine the joints are all multiplanar and the barrier must be found in each direction of motion. For descriptive purposes the three cardinal planes of the body in the anatomical position are used but it must be noted that the barrier is not strictly a point but rather a continuum. The precise position of the barrier in any plane will depend in part on whether the movement first introduced was in that plane or in one of the others.

The operator's ability to sense the position of the barrier is of great importance in treatment. Before either a thrusting or a muscle energy procedure, it is most important to take the joint up to, but only just up to, the barrier in all three planes. Each time that the 'slack is taken out' after the patient effort when giving a muscle energy treatment, it is essential that the new barrier be found and the movement stopped just before it is reached. If the movement is taken too far so that the barrier is 'mashed into' the procedure is likely to fail. This is the most common fault of those starting to use manual treatment.

In medico-legal work, the barrier assumes importance because it is an objective sign which can be found, and if necessary even demonstrated, and which after treatment can be shown to have moved. The ability of the witness to claim that he/she can say where the barrier is or was is much appreciated in legal circles.

END FEEL

There are a variety of different 'end feels' at or near the restrictive barrier, corresponding to a variety of different causes of restriction. The most important are probably:

1. Oedema; the end feel is 'boggy'.
2. Myofascial shortening; there is a similar restriction at each end. It is this that athletes try to remove by their warm-up routines and is relatively common with advancing age.
3. Fibrosis; the build up of tension tends to be earlier than in the normal and the curve is steeper.
4. Hypermobility; there is very little resistance until close to the end (the anatomical barrier) when the tension builds rapidly, and there may be an overall increase in range.

The importance of the end feel is that it gives some indication of what is likely to be the most efficient treatment. For instance joints with an oedematous barrier are better treated by muscle energy than by high velocity thrusting. Fibrosis, on the other hand is better treated by thrusting. Myofascial shortening may need exercises and will probably respond better to muscle energy than to thrusting treatment. Hypermobility is one of the few real contraindications to manipulation, certainly to thrusting, but only at that level. Often *there will be a hypomobile joint nearby which can be treated*; indeed the hypomobile joint is frequently the cause of the symptoms and the hypermobile joint little more than a reaction to the neighbouring stiffness.

POINT OF EASE

In every joint there is a point of maximum ease; it is the point from which movement in either direction causes the soft tissues to become more tense. In a normal joint it is usually near the midpoint of the range. When there is a restrictive barrier the point of ease will be found to have moved, usually to about the midpoint of the remaining range. When there is a major restriction the point of ease may be close to the physiological barrier at the normal end. As with the barrier, the point of ease exists in each plane of motion but in this case also around each axis. It becomes of great importance when so-called 'indirect' treatment is contemplated. The term 'loose packed' is used for a joint that has been positioned, at least in the available planes of motion, at the point of maximum ease. The converse is 'close packed' when a joint is positioned so that it will move no further in a particular direction.

GENERAL EXAMINATION

Even in a practice entirely made up of patients referred by other physicians, it is important to recognise that the pain may be coming from other than a musculo-skeletal source or from other than the axial skeleton. Even when there is in the axial skeleton a source of pain for which manual treatment may be appropriate, it is important to find if that is the main cause of the symptoms or only a secondary cause. An example of this, common in the practice of one of the authors, is back and leg pain associated with a degenerative hip arthritis. These patients will often also have spinal dysfunction because restricted hip joint movement will cause more than normal strain to be put on the pelvic and lumbar joints. In such cases it is not uncommon to find that treatment of the spinal dysfunction will relieve the symptoms sufficiently to permit treatment of the hip to be delayed. Even so, the spinal dysfunction will tend to recur because of the alteration to the mechanics caused by the hip arthritis. If this happens too frequently there is reason to suggest that treatment of the hip condition is required. Besides the mechanical cause, there is another factor for the association which has a much more general importance; *in the presence of pain, the segmental spinal muscles react by becoming hypertonic,* and if the pain is long lasting, the hypertonus may become self perpetuating, causing a dysfunction. Possibly, for this reason, it is common to find dysfunction at the L3–4 level when it is associated with an osteoarthritic hip. See also Mellin[2] and Ellison et al.[3].

Anterior chest pain, with or without neck and arm radiation, may be due to cardiac ischaemia. Pain indistinguishable to the patient[4] may be due to dysfunction in the cervicothoracic region of the spine. Clearly, such pain could be due to both causes operating at the same time. The experience of the authors is that very often both causes are operating and both may need treatment. It is said that about 60 per cent of anterior chest pain seen in emergency rooms is skeletal in origin. Awareness of the possibility of a cardiac cause is essential but it is of economic importance to try to find and treat the skeletal ones before a full cardiac investigation is performed. It is worthy of note that treatment of the skeletal dysfunctions that are often associated with cardiac ischaemia can be helpful in the management of these patients.

Abdominal pain may arise in a viscus or be referred. One cause of referred pain is spinal joint dysfunction and it is just as important for the gastroenterologist to recognise this as it is for the practitioner of manual medicine to be aware of the possible visceral aspect of the condition[5].

Low back pain can be caused by a growth in the pelvis and, as many of those patients may also have spinal joint dysfunctions, it is necessary to maintain a high index of suspicion. Rectal examination will usually help.

Herpes zoster is a cause of segmental pain and, when seen before the vesicles appear, can be difficult to distinguish from joint dysfunction. The patient, however, is sick while the dysfunctional patient is not and the pain of shingles is usually more localised and more severe. Part of the common post herpetic pain is in some cases caused by spinal joint dysfunctions which may have been there before or may result from the reflex hypertonus referred to above.

Generalised back ache is more often due to a virus infection than to joint dysfunction. Treatment during the course of a viral infection is unlikely to be very helpful and it is wiser to encourage such patients to stay away until the infection is over, for their own health as well as that of the practitioner.

At least a local neurological examination is advisable on the first visit. In most patients it will be normal and, if the abnormality is nothing more than a depressed reflex, there is no contraindication to manual treatment, if this is otherwise appropriate. The examination, or at least any abnormal parts of it, can be repeated at subsequent visits, the more so if there is deterioration. *An increasing neurological deficit is one of the indications to consider urgent surgery.*

THE DOMINANT EYE

The differences that have to be appreciated when one is examining for minor changes of level, rotation etc. are small enough that it is essential that one's dominant eye is located so that it is equidistant from the two sides. In other words the dominant eye should be over or directly behind the midline of the patient being examined. This advice is confirmed every time a teacher is monitoring a pupil's examination; the teacher, standing a little to one side sees things differently.

The dominant eye is found most easily by making a circle with index finger and thumb of one hand or between the index fingers and thumbs of both hands (Fig. 3.2). The hand(s) are held out in front at arm's length and, with both eyes open, a specific object is looked at through the hole. Without moving the hand(s) the left eye is closed. If the object remains visible through the hole, the right is the dominant eye. If the object is no longer seen in the hole, the left is the dominant eye. This can be

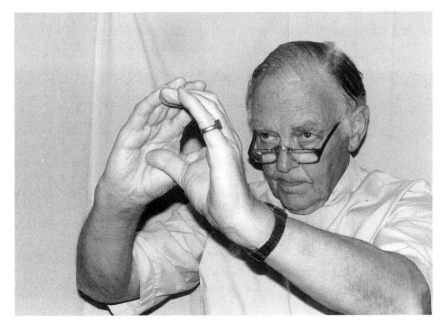

Fig. 3.2 Method of finding one's dominant eye.

confirmed by doing the same thing again only, this time, closing the right eye. The dominant eye is fixed in most people but there are those in whom it may change from time to time. Those who tend to switch dominance from one eye to the other are advised to shut one eye when faced with any problem in this field.

PROPRIOCEPTORS

For many operators the eye is the most sensitive means of finding asymmetry. In patients with even moderately long hair examination of the cervicothoracic junction in extension is obscured unless something is done about the hair. With practice it is not difficult to assess relative position and motion by means of the proprioceptors in one's upper limbs. The practice required is no more than taking the trouble to notice what the proprioceptors are feeling when one is examining a patient in the ordinary way. With this ability to feel as well as see, the operator will find that the perception of asymmetry is easier than when using vision alone, even when that is not obscured.

THE MUSCULOSKELETAL SYSTEM

The concept that it is possible to predict the site of origin of a pain by its nature and location is often not correct in this field. Travell[6], Mennell[7] and more recently Travell and Simons[8] have mapped pain reference patterns from 'trigger' points in muscle and have shown that the pain does not necessarily follow the pattern of the dermatome, myotome or sclerotome. They were working with Travell trigger points, but it seems that the same is true of other myogenic pain. Travell triggers are a relatively common complication of spinal joint dysfunction and the picture is made more complex by the superimposition of their pain reference patterns on those of the primary joint dysfunction. Dr Philip Greenman puts it bluntly: 'It is no use chasing the pain.'

In order to make a structural diagnosis it is necessary to examine each joint and the segmental muscles. In the same way, in order to perform a treatment properly, it is necessary to treat each abnormal segment. Constraints of time and consideration of the patient's general condition may make a less thorough treatment necessary on any one occasion. Considerations of time when in practice make it essential to have some means by which abnormal segments can be located rapidly for detailed examination. It would take far too long to put every joint through the full examination procedure. This is the reason for the screening tests to identify abnormal regions and, in some areas, scanning to pin-point the actual segment.

The examination should not be restricted to the axial skeleton, even if one includes the pelvis. A short lower limb will have a marked effect on both pelvis and spine as they adapt to keep the eyes and balance organs level. This applies no less to those with a congenital leg length difference than to those whose legs are unequal from injury or disease. Lack of symmetry of length and/or strength of the lower limb muscles may be very important in the maintenance of axial joint dysfunction (see Chapter 14). Although the effect is less striking, the upper limbs can also affect the spine especially if their mobility or strength is not symmetrical.

Structural examination can then be divided into:

1. The overall screen.
2. A scan of areas indicated by the screen.
3. Segmental definition.

When the examination is complete it should be possible to say which joints need treatment, where the barrier is in all three planes and what treatment is advisable.

It will be seen that, in order to save time and patient movement, some of the tests done during the overall screen really are part of the scan or even of the segmental definition.

THE OVERALL SCREENING EXAMINATION

This is done walking, standing with and without movement, sitting, supine and prone. The whole examination should be complete in a few minutes.

1. Walking

The examination is best done from front, back and at least one side. Attention is directed to gait, including length and symmetry of stride, heel and toe strike, reaction of the pelvis to change in side of weight-bearing, swing of the arms and behaviour of the shoulder girdle. Rotation of the lumbar vertebrae is looked for and whether it is to the same side as the sidebend at that moment or to the opposite side.

2. Standing, static

(a) From in front, observe the placement of the feet, the general posture, the relative shoulder height, tilting of the head and any rotation of the face.

(b) From the side, look for flattening or exaggeration of the spinal curves, and for the 'gravity line' – is the head 'poked'?

(c) From behind, observe the relative levels of the gluteal folds, the posterior superior iliac spines judging by the ledge underneath (Fig. 3.3), the iliac crests (Fig. 3.4), the scapulae and the shoulders, look for tilting of the head, for any difference in the gap between the elbow and the trunk on the two sides as an indicator of scoliosis (Fig. 3.5), for asymmetry of muscle tension in the feet, legs or thighs. It is as well to remember that in the lumbar spine a scoliosis may not be seen if one looks at the spinous processes because, with the vertebrae rotating towards the

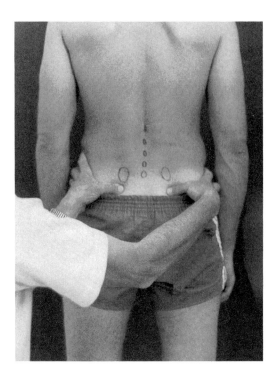

Fig. 3.3 Examination for the height of the PSIS, standing.

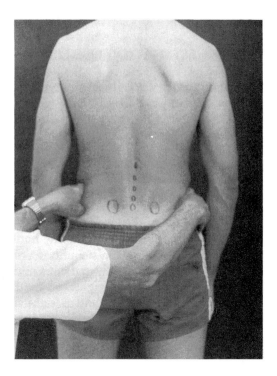

Fig. 3.4 Examination for the heights of the iliac crests standing.

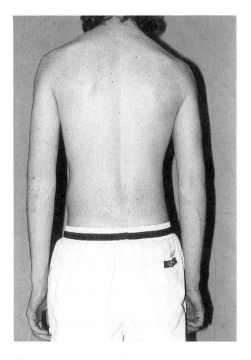

Fig. 3.5 Asymmetry of the gap between the elbow and the trunk.

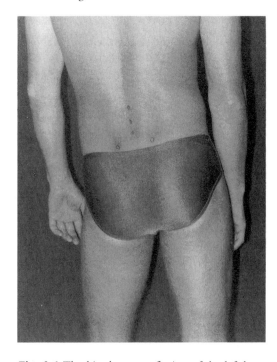

Fig. 3.6 The hip drop test, flexion of the left knee allows the left hip to drop, sidebending primarily at L5–S1.

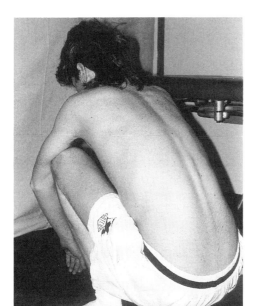

Fig. 3.7 The squat test.

convexity of the scoliotic curve, the spinous processes may be in a straight line, although the bodies are not. Fullness on one side produced by the rotation of the transverse processes is easier to see.

3. Standing with motion

Observe from behind the smoothness of the curve on flexion, extension and sidebending to each side. Are there 'flat spots' or segments which do not move with the rest? Are there segments which on sidebending rotate to the side of the sidebend? In unrestricted motion in the upright position ('neutral' or 'easy normal'), rotation occurs to the opposite side to the sidebend in the thoracic and lumbar regions.

An alternative to sidebending is the 'hip drop' test in which the patient allows one knee to flex while keeping the other leg straight (Fig. 3.6). The amount of lumbar sidebend produced and the corresponding rotation of the lumbar vertebrae are compared with the other side.

A general test for mobility of the lower limb joints may be done by having the patient attempt a full knees bend (squat) keeping the heels flat on the floor (Fig. 3.7).

The standing forward flexion test (standing FFT)
In a clinical situation it saves time if the standing forward flexion test is performed at this stage, and for that reason it will be described now although it is not a screening test. It is a scanning test for loss of normal

Fig. 3.8 The operator's foot as a gauge for the patient's foot position.

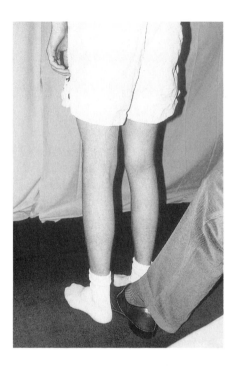

motion in the pelvic mechanism, it does not indicate which dysfunction is present, but it does give an indication as to the affected side.

(a) The patient stands evenly on both legs with the heels about 15 cm (6 inches) apart and the operator sits or kneels behind her with his eyes roughly at the level of her pelvis. An easy way to have the feet at the correct separation is for the operator to put one of his feet between the patient's heels and have her bring her feet as close together as his shoe will permit (Fig. 3.8).

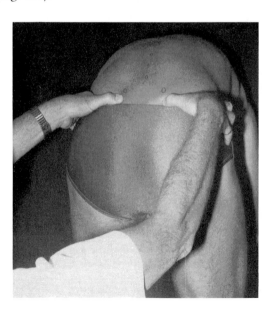

Fig. 3.9 Position at the end of the standing forward flexion test (FFT).

(b) The operator finds the ledge *under* her posterior superior iliac spine (PSIS) on each side with his thumbs by coming up to the PSIS from below and observing their relative heights with the dominant eye behind the midline of the patient (Fig. 3.3). (The posterior aspect of that piece of bone is rounded and impossible to compare accurately for position against the horizontal plane.)

(c) The patient is then asked to bend forwards as far as possible without bending her knees. The operator observes whether the motion of the PSIS on the two sides is symmetrical (Fig. 3.9).

(d) If one side rises or goes forward more than the other the test is positive; *the side that moves first or furthest is the restricted side* because the sacrum has picked up the ilium more quickly owing to the loss of motion in the sacroiliac joint.

4. Clinical estimation of relative leg length difference

This is conveniently performed at this stage because the patient starts standing and sits as part of the examination.

The importance of a structural difference in the length of the legs is often overlooked. Even more common is failure to recognise that estimation of relative leg length is difficult by any clinical test. The standard measurement from the anterior superior spine to the tip of the medial malleolus is open to gross errors if the pelvis is twisted, as is so common. Measurement from the greater trochanter to the lateral malleolus is incomplete and tends to be inaccurate, especially in the obese. The clinical methods of estimation which are most helpful are as follows.

1. Comparison of the levels of the PSISs from behind with the patient standing as in 3(b) above, then either:

(a) Turn the patient round and examine the levels of the anterior superior iliac spines (ASISs), again coming up from below to find the ledge underneath. If the ASIS is high on the same side as the PSIS the probability is that the leg is long (or the pelvis is asymmetrical). Or:

(b) Keep the thumbs in position under the PSISs and have the patient sit down on a level seat (Fig. 3.10). If they are now level the probability is that the legs are unequal, their influence having been removed. If the PSISs remain unlevel the likelihood is that the pelvis is twisted with restricted mobility.

2. Comparison of the levels of the PSISs by having the patient flex fully and then sighting from either behind or in front along the index fingers placed over the PSISs on each side (Fig. 3.11).

3. Comparison of the levels of the gluteal folds from behind with the patient erect.

4. Comparison of the iliac crest height by placing the index fingers along the crest on each side (see Fig. 3.4). Note that it is easy to include an asymmetrical amount of soft tissue under the fingers in this examination. It is most accurate if the fingers approach the crest by contacting the lateral aspect first and slide over the top close to the bone.

In all these examinations it is well to be aware of the possibility of observer error, even in operators with long experience. It is helpful to

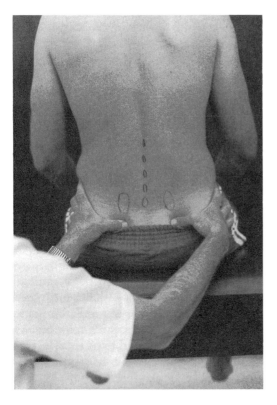

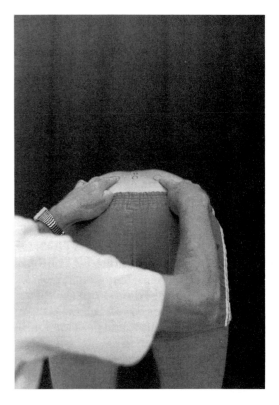

Fig. 3.10 Finding the ledge under the PSIS in sitting.

Fig. 3.11 Examination for the heights of PSISs as a guide to relative leg length.

use proprioception as well as sight when making these level estimations. Accurate measurement requires special X-rays and is described at the end of this chapter.

Dr James Fisk has pointed out that an error can be introduced in these estimations if the patient stands with her feet together. The error will be small unless there is marked unilateral muscle spasm causing her to lean to one side. As shown in Fig. 3.12, if the feet are together, the leg away from which the patient leans appears longer; if they are separated by about the distance apart of the hip joints the error is removed. A useful approximation can be achieved by putting a shoe between her feet and having her bring them as close together as is then possible as in Fig. 3.8 above.

5. Seated

The patient should be sitting with the weight equally on the two sides. If her feet do not reach the floor they should be supported on a stool as otherwise she might lose balance on forward bending. In this position the spinal motion tests are done again to find if there is a difference when the weight is not being taken by the lower extremities. It is useful to check for flat spots on flexion and extension and for areas with limited sidebend. The rotation associated with sidebending is also noted. It is

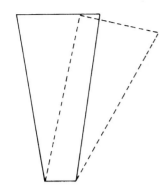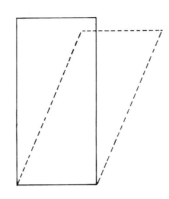

Fig. 3.12 Diagram to show the possible error in leg length estimation if the feet are close together.

important that the patient sits up and does not slump; any tendency to slump will reduce the available motion in the other planes.

While the patient is 'sitting up tall' rotation can be checked for range and symmetry, both actively by having her rotate her upper trunk as far as she can, and passively by the operator performing the movement with her relaxed. This movement takes place maximally in the area of the thoraco-lumbar junction.

Also in this position an overall evaluation of function of the upper limbs can be made by having the patient fully abduct her arms and put the backs of her hands together above her head. If she can do this symmetrically there is no major dysfunction in shoulders, elbows, wrists or hands (Fig. 3.13).

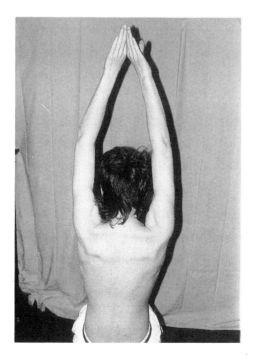

Fig. 3.13 Screen for upper limb function, note the minor failures of abduction and pronation on the left.

Still in the sitting position, the active and passive movements of the head can be tested. Passively extension is normally about 90 degrees and flexion about 45 degrees. Rotation and sidebending are also tested and here note is made more of asymmetry than of range.

The most important tests at this point are again not strictly screening. They are the sitting forward flexion test and the examination for vertebral rotation in the flexed position which is most conveniently done at this stage.

The sitting forward flexion test (sitting FFT)

Part 1. This is performed in a similar manner to the standing test except that the patient is sitting with her knees apart. The operator finds the ledge under the PSIS on each side with his thumbs (see Fig. 3.3) and watches the motion of the PSISs as the patient bends between her knees as far forward as she can. As in the standing test, the side that moves first is the abnormal side. The operator should be sitting or kneeling to bring his eyes to about the level of the PSISs. This test is most conveniently performed with the patient sitting on a stool with her feet on the floor. If she is sitting on the treatment table and cannot reach the floor with her legs there is the possibility that she might fall forward and it is wise to have her feet supported in some manner. If it is necessary to have her sitting on a chair and the chair seat is tilted from before backwards, the examination can be done with her sitting near the front of the seat and the operator observing from behind the chair back (Fig. 3.14). If the seat is level it is easier to have her sitting sideways.

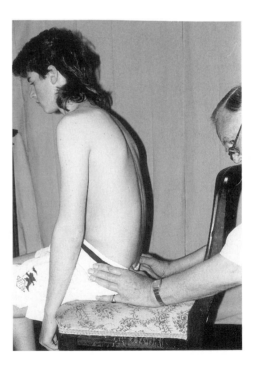

Fig. 3.14 The sitting FFT on a chair with a sloping seat.

Part 2. This part is important for the full assessment of sacral motion asymmetry. The test is similar to part 1 but the operator has his thumbs on the inferior lateral angles (ILAs) of the sacrum, rather than under the PSIS, and monitors their motion to find if their relative position changes with respect to the coronal plane (anteriority), or the transverse plane (superiority) in the move from the erect position to forward flexion (Fig. 3.15).

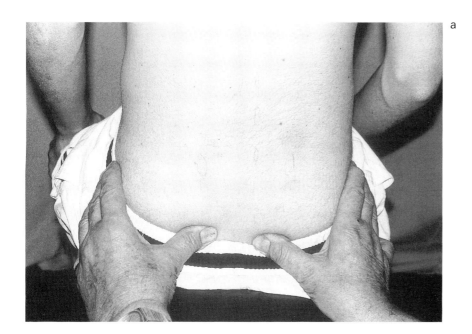

a

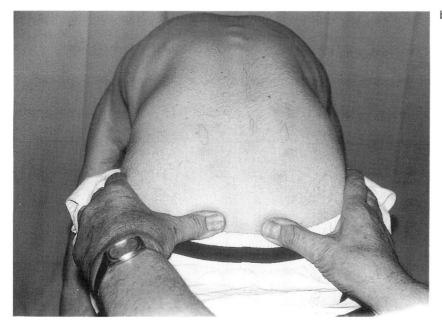

b

Fig. 3.15 The sitting FFT at the inferior lateral angles (ILAs). (a) Upright; (b) forward bent.

The inferior lateral angles of the sacrum are developmentally the modified transverse processes of the fifth sacral vertebra. They can be found by placing the tip of one index finger in the sacral hiatus and the tips of the index and middle fingers of the other hand about 2 cm (¾ inch) away on each side (Fig. 3.16); this is more conveniently done in the prone position. They are flat pieces of bone with a posterior surface and inferior and lateral margins. The observation of anteriority is made from the posterior surface but for that of superiority the finger tips should slide, on bone, down under the inferior margin.

Fig. 3.16 To find the ILAs.

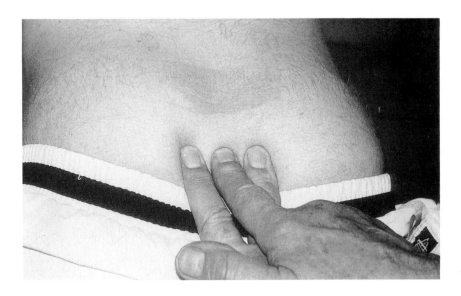

Examining for vertebral rotation and sacral position
In making a structural diagnosis, part of the information required is the relative rotation of the vertebrae in the flexed position. This examination could be done with the patient standing, but for most patients it is more comfortable to do it sitting. The information required is the relative rotation of the vertebra being examined with respect to the one below. This is best estimated by the thumbs which, from L4 up, are placed over the transverse processes and it may be necessary to lean down and sight along the spine to appreciate small differences (Fig. 3.17). If there is much superficial muscle spasm the best route to the tip of the transverse process is through the intermuscular septum lateral to the longissimus muscle. The transverse process of L5 is not palpable, it is covered by the posterior ilium so that at that level the rotation is assessed from the position of the lamina. In forward flexion this is not easy to feel because of the thick lumbosacral fascia which is tight in that position. It is found by placing the thumbs on the most posterior part of the posterior superior iliac spine and moving medially and *craniad* at an angle of about 30° (Fig. 3.18a).

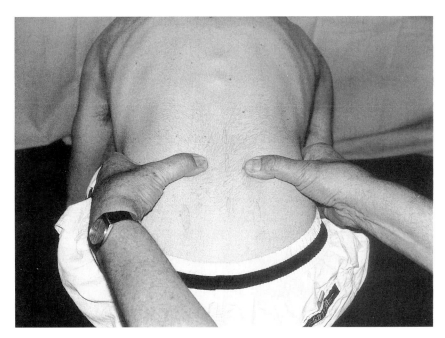

Fig. 3.17 Examining for lumbar rotation in flexion.

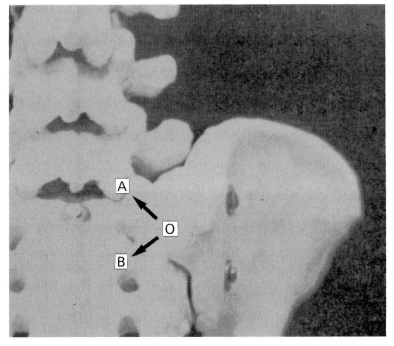

Fig. 3.18 To find the laminae of L5 (A), and S1 (B). (O) is the most posterior part of the PSIS.

The rotation of L5 is always to be assessed as compared to the position of the sacral base. The latter is found by moving the thumbs from the most posterior part of the PSIS medially and *caudad* about 30° (Fig. 3.18b). The rotation of the sacral base with reference to the coronal plane is examined and the ILA position is also noted in this position.

6. Supine

The first priority in this position is the estimation of the relative superiority of the pubic ramus on each side. The examination is done by placing the flexed terminal phalanges of the two index fingers over the top of the pubic tubercle on each side and, with the dominant eye over the patient's midline, sighting down the terminal phalanges to see which is superior or if they are level (Fig. 3.19a). The ramus of the pubis may be used instead of the tubercle but it is important that the corresponding part of the bone is used on each side. The tubercle is found about 2 cm (3/4 inch) lateral to the symphysis and is preferred because, being the site of insertion of the inguinal ligament, it will often be tender and sometimes swollen when there is pubic dysfunction. The superior pubic rami can be found without the examination appearing to be threatening if the hand is first laid on the anterior abdominal wall, fingers pointing craniad, and then moved distally until the pubis is felt (Fig. 3.19b). If there is asymmetry of the pubes it is the first **STOP** sign, the pubic dysfunction should be treated before proceeding (see Chapter 7).

The relative superiority of the iliac crests is the next test (Fig. 3.20). If they are unlevel the patient should be examined prone and, if the same crest remains superior, prone and supine, that is the second **STOP** sign. An innominate shear dysfunction should be suspected, examined for and treated, if present, before proceeding (see Chapter 7).

The position of the anterior superior spine can be estimated in this position but it is of greater importance after the sacroiliac dysfunctions have been treated.

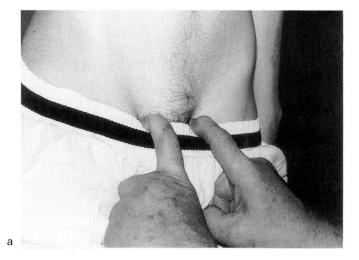

a

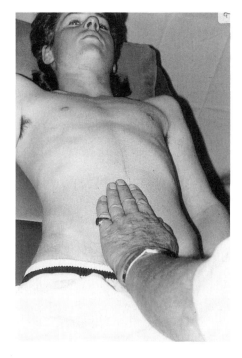

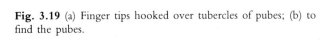

Fig. 3.19 (a) Finger tips hooked over tubercles of pubes; (b) to find the pubes.

b

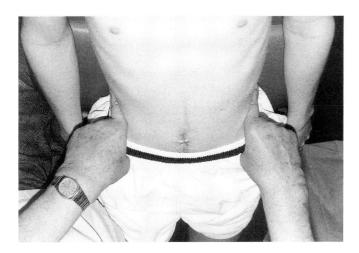

Fig. 3.20 Supine examination for iliac crest height.

Confirmatory tests for restriction of motion in the SI joints in this position are described at the end of Chapter 4.

The position of the medial malleoli with respect to relative superiority is examined in this position and will reflect the rotatory position of the innominate bones. With the patient supine the innominates are free to rotate because the weight of the body is resting on the sacrum. Anterior rotation of the innominate will make the leg on that side appear longer; posterior rotation will make it appear shorter.

The motion of the thoracic cage is tested in this position and asymmetry may give useful indication of dysfunction of thoracic intervertebral joints as well as of rib joints. It is important to evaluate both inhalation and exhalation movement; the examination starts in the upper ribs and proceeds down. The operator's finger contact must be light or the movement will be affected and he should to stand with his dominant eye over the patient's midline and observe, with his peripheral vision, on which side the movement continues longer. The examination is described in detail in Chapter 10.

Also in the supine position, the mobility and strength of the lower limbs may be tested. This is especially indicated if the 'squat' test proved positive. The examination should include the range of motion in the joints, especially the hips, and the relative length and strength of the muscles, especially the long muscles of the hip and thigh.

7. Prone

At this point the screening examination merges with segmental definition in a way that makes it difficult to describe them separately. The prone position is very important for the assessment of pelvic dysfunction but for details of the examination of the pelvic mechanism see Chapter 4.

The importance of the relative height of the iliac crests in this position has been referred to in the section on supine examination. If the crest is higher on one side both in the prone and in the supine position suspect an innominate shear dysfunction, check for its presence and if present treat it before proceeding (see Chapter 7).

The rotation of the lumbar vertebrae is estimated, always with reference to the lower member of the motion segment (e.g. L3 with reference to L4 and L5 with reference to S1). This is done both with the patient flat and with her spine extended in the so-called 'sphinx' position. The sphinx position is with the patient prone and with her upper trunk raised up on her elbows. She should hold her chin in her hands to allow the extensors to relax (Fig. 3.21a and b). The elbows should be close together and almost directly under the chin so that good extension is obtained. The abdominal muscles must be allowed to relax. It is not always easy to be sure of the rotation of L5 but the estima-

a

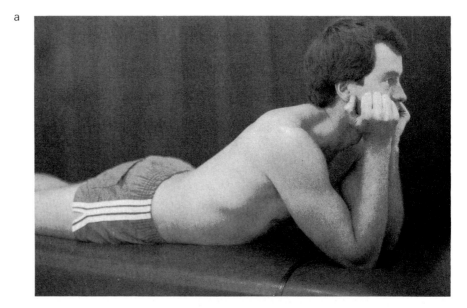

b

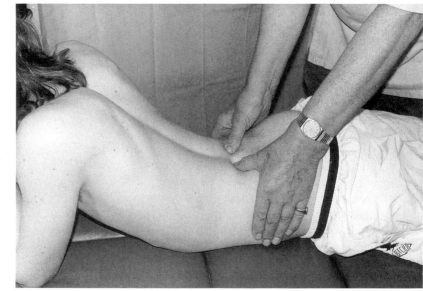

Fig. 3.21 (a) The sphinx position. (b) Examination for lumbar rotation in extension.

tion is very important both for pelvic and lumbar diagnosis. It is also important to find whether the asymmetry is more marked in flexion or in extension.

The relative superiority of the medial malleoli in the prone position is estimated and is a reflection of the lumbar scoliosis, the innominates are not free to rotate because the weight is being borne on the pubis and the ASIS on each side. On the side of the lumbar convexity the leg will appear longer because of the tilt produced in the pelvis.

THE SCANNING EXAMINATION

If the screening tests show an abnormality in a region it may be worth using scanning procedures to narrow the possible levels that will require segmental definition or, in other words, the detailed diagnosis.

The most valuable of these tests are examination of the soft tissues for texture abnormalities, and segmental motion testing. Examination of tissue texture is most frequently done with the index fingers alone or the index and middle. The finger tips are usually thought to be more sensitive to tissue texture changes while the thumbs are better for depth perception. Examination for tissue texture changes can be done in many ways, either directly or by a technique known as 'skin rolling'.

Lumbar

With the patient lying first on one side then on the other, tissue texture and motion testing can be done at the same time in the lumbar region. The operator uses one hand to examine both for tissue texture, on the side away from the table, and for motion as the spine is gently flexed and extended by his other hand controlling the flexed upper leg. The fingers are best placed so that they palpate in the 'gutter' between the longissimus and spinalis muscle. Alternatively the operator can control the upper leg with his abdomen or hip which allows him to use his second hand to assist in palpation (Fig. 3.22a and b).

The scanning examination can also be done prone and the two sides can then be compared for tissue texture. This position is the same as for part of the assessment for vertebral rotation (for segmental definition) but does not permit motion testing at the same time.

Thoracic

In the thoracic spine tissue texture examination can be done prone, sitting or even supine, but it is difficult to do motion testing at the same time even with the patient sitting. For the prone examination the fingers are, once again, in the medial gutter and in this region the tension in the deep structures is often most easily felt by moving the finger tips gently up and down in the gutter. In the sitting position the fingers can be used in the same manner.

Fig. 3.22 Scanning the lumbar spine sidelying. (a) Using hand control; (b) Using abdomen to control motion.

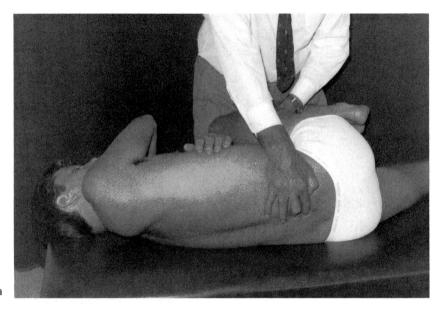

a

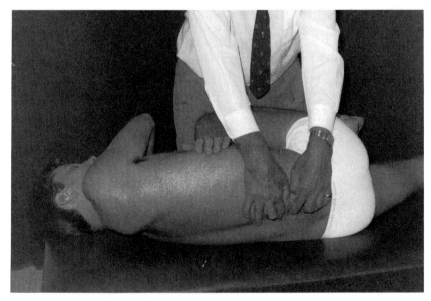

b

A variation of this can be helpful to the patient who has been seen by other physicians and led to believe that there is nothing structurally wrong and that 'it is all in her head'. If the examination of the upper thoracic region for levels of excess muscle tone in the medial gutter is done from the front, with the patient's head resting against the opera- tor's chest, she will usually be able to relax (Fig. 3.23). Tissue texture change can often be located very quickly and the patient is likely to recognise that the operator has found something by the fact that it will be tender. This can be of great value by instilling the beginnings of

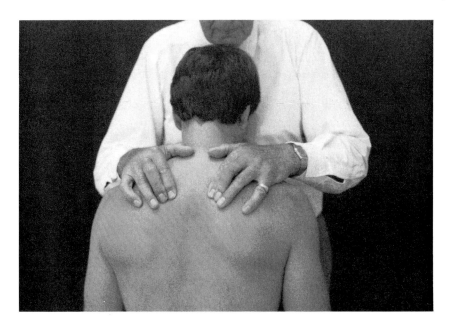

Fig. 3.23 Sitting test for hypertonus in upper thoracic 4th layer muscles.

confidence and it sometimes helps to make a remark like 'that's a funny place to keep your head'. It also helps by pin-pointing a level of dysfunction even if it is still necessary to find the precise position of the barrier by other tests.

Motion testing of the thoracic intervertebral joints can be done, with the patient sitting, by sidebending or by flexion-extension or rotation. When examining for motion it is essential that the patient sits up 'tall'; any slump will restrict the available range. For the sidebending examination the operator stands to one side behind her; if to her right he uses his right forearm and hand to control motion as in Fig. 3.24[9]. His index

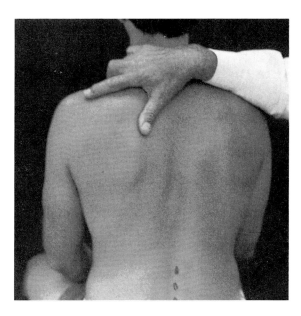

Fig. 3.24 Dr. Stiles's grip for upper thoracic screening.

finger is extended over her left shoulder, his thumb points down her back and his other fingers curl over her trapezius with his forearm resting on her right shoulder. This position gives surprisingly good control of sidebending to either side and leaves his left hand free to localise the motion by lateral pressure on the spinous process at each level to be examined. If desired or when in doubt about a finding, the test may be repeated from the other side. For flexion/extension and rotation the patient sits with her fingers laced together behind her neck and her elbows together in front. The operator controls motion through her elbows, in either direction and his other hand is used to assess where there is loss of normal range (Fig. 3.25).

Fig. 3.25 Upper thoracic motion test, sitting.

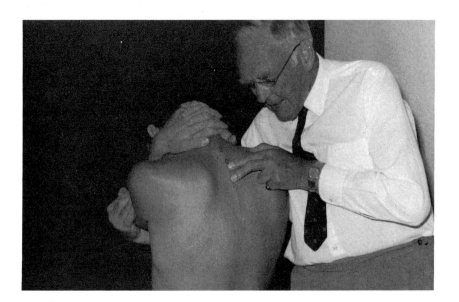

Cervical

Scanning in the cervical spine is best done by finding the levels of tissue texture change. This can be done sitting when it is easiest for the operator to be in front of the patient with her head resting against his chest and his fingers examining both sides of the cervical muscles at the same time. The same thing can be done supine when it serves conveniently as a start to the segmental definition in this region.

SKIN ROLLING

In both lumbar and thoracic spine skin rolling is most easily done with the patient prone. To perform the test from below upwards the operator should stand to one side of the patient facing her head. The test may be used either across the midline or to one or both sides. It is performed by picking up a fold of skin between index (or index and middle) finger and thumb of each hand. The digits of one hand are moved while those of the other, holding the same skin fold, are still (Fig. 3.26). In this way the skin can be rolled so that the fingers advance up the back and the skin texture is palpated. The movements, which should be smooth, should maintain the lifted roll of skin as it is advanced up the back. The process can be done from above down if more convenient.

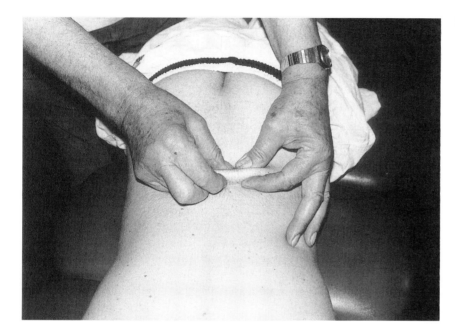

Fig. 3.26 Skin rolling.

Normal skin is easily rolled although the roll will vary in thickness between patients. When it is abnormal the skin will feel thicker, it will not roll so easily, it is likely to cause pain provocation and in some patients will even have an appearance similar to 'peau d'orange'. There will almost always be tenderness in the positive area and the middle of the area will give an indication of the level of the associated spinal dysfunction.

In a clinical setting, all that needs to be completed in a few minutes!

X-RAYS

Films taken in standard positions

The lesion known as somatic or joint dysfunction does not show on any ordinary X-ray. The abnormalities so often seen in patients who present with back pain are commonly the result of injury some years before and may bear little relation to the problem with which the patient presents.

The one abnormal finding in standard films that seems to be of significance that might not be expected is unilateral sacralisation of L5 with a 'bat wing' transverse process and joints between that and the ilium laterally and the sacrum below. When this anatomical variant is present the disc above is statistically more at risk than in the usual configuration.

If reliance is to be put on X-ray pictures it is essential that they are of good quality. Poor quality films are a serious danger. The appearances that can warn the operator to be more careful, or not to proceed, can be subtle and may well be missed in poor films. Even normal films of good quality do not guarantee that there is no condition that would be better not manipulated.

While it is wise for the inexperienced operator to see good films before treating patients by thrusting manipulation, there is reason to consider that the muscle energy, myofascial and indirect treatments are such that if a diagnosis of somatic dysfunction has been made, it is proper to proceed before seeing films. For the experienced operator with well trained fingers the necessity for radiography is much less. The fingers will tell so much more than the X-ray that in these circumstances it is reasonable to treat a patient without ever having films, if recovery is occurring satisfactorily. On the other hand, if films already exist, there is an argument that failure to see them could amount to malpractice. If old films are available there may be no need to obtain new ones unless to exclude the development of some other pathology.

It is important that any manipulator should maintain a high index of suspicion for contraindications. Of these the most important are hypermobility, osteoporosis, infection and tumours. These are dealt with in more detail in Chapter 12.

Demonstration of altered mobility

In most spinal joints loss of mobility, and occasionally hypermobility, can be demonstrated by X-ray but special projections may be needed. For the typical cervical joints lateral views in flexion and extension will provide evidence which is usually sufficient. At the occipitoatlantal joint a special film is needed to demonstrate flexion. When the head and neck are fully flexed in the usual way the chin soon comes up against the manubrium and from then on, with continued flexion effort, the O–A joint will extend[10]. In order to see full flexion of the O–A joint a lateral film must be taken with the neck extended and the head fully flexed on it. A similar loss of induced motion has been shown to occur at the thoraco-lumbar junction[11] and a similar motion is thought to occur at the cervicothoracic junction. For the remaining thoracic and lumbar joints plain lateral films in flexion and extension should suffice for simple mobility but films taken with stressed motion are needed to exclude hypermobility.

A radiological technique for demonstrating sacroiliac motion was devised by Chamberlain in 1932 and might be useful for those who still do not believe![12]

Lordosis

The concept that a deep lordosis is associated with dysfunctional spinal joints is an old one. Hansson *et al.*[13] tested this hypothesis and showed that there was no difference in the distribution and range of lordosis between three groups of men. The first were those who had pre-employment films and claimed to have had no back pain at any time. The second were those who had films during what they claimed to be their first episode of back pain and the third were chronic back pain patients.

Pope *et al.*[14] had similar findings with respect to lordosis but they also recorded that 'LBP (low-back pain) patients had less flexor and extensor strength and were flexor overpowered, had diminished range of motion for spinal extension and axial rotation and diminished straight leg raising capacity'. This fits well with the clinical observation that more lumbar joint dysfunctions have extension restriction than flexion restriction.

Demonstration of evidence of dysfunction

Except when motion loss can be demonstrated, the only evidence is positional because there is no associated change in bone structure. If in the AP projection a short scoliotic curve can be seen in which one or more vertebrae are rotated towards the concavity of the curve, there is a strong suggestion that there is a type II dysfunction at that level.

Films taken in flexion and extension and in sidebending right and left can demonstrate dysfunction and the more so if the positions are stressed.

Degenerative changes and spondylosis

Regrettably the spurring on the edges of the vertebral bodies is still sometimes called osteoarthritis. Osteoarthritis is a disease of diarthrodial joints and the term should not be applied to changes on the margins of the disc. It is the opinion of the authors that these degenerative changes represent the adaptation of the body to the absence of a normally resilient disc structure and that they usually occur slowly over many years, nearly always being the result of trauma to the joint. These changes of spondylosis are not a contra-indication to treatment by manipulation but it is as well to remember that the symptoms may well arise from another joint.

Torgerson and Dotter[15] at the Lahey Clinic showed that 'spondylosis (osteophyte formation) did not appear to have any direct relationship to low-back pain. Degenerative disc disease appeared to be a major cause of low-back pain'. It is possible that their findings would more correctly be interpreted as showing that degenerative disc disease and back pain are closely associated rather than that degenerative discs are necessarily causative.

Measuring leg length difference

For the accurate determination of leg length difference X-ray examination is essential. There are many ways of doing this and the subject is dealt with by Greenman[16] in detail. The measurement which he prefers is to the sacral base line because this takes into account asymmetry of the pelvis as well as structural leg length difference. He makes the measurement at a vertical through the hip joint up to a line drawn across the sacral base. This measurement can then be converted directly into a heel lift if required. One of the authors has, for years, used a radio-opaque level suspended in front of the film when the X-ray of the pelvis was taken in the upright position. This was because of experience with older X-ray apparatus in which the film did not necessarily lie horizontally. With modern apparatus this may no longer be necessary but can be used to ensure accuracy. When this film is taken it is important that the X-ray table is vertical, the feet are about 15 cm (6 inches) apart, the backs of the heels against the table top and the knees straight.

The difference in the length of the legs themselves is easily measured by the difference in the height of the head of the femur above the base of the film (Fig. 3.27). The tilt of the sacral base is not as easy to measure accurately, an X-ray film is needed which shows comparable parts of the upper margin of S1. A line is then drawn across S1 and extended on either side at least as far as the verticals through the weightbearing area of the hip joints. In this way the difference in effective leg length can be measured by comparing the distance between the lower edge of the film and the point where the line crosses the vertical through the hip joint on each side.

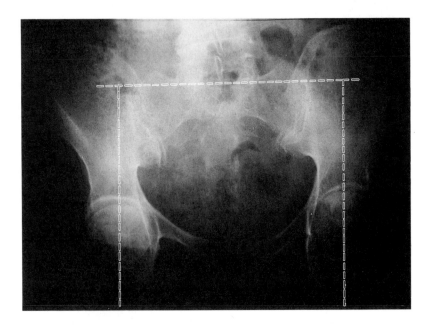

Fig. 3.27 Method of measuring leg length and sacral base unlevelling by standing pelvis X-ray.

The difficulty is to find strictly comparable points on the outline of the superior surface of S1. This problem is discussed by Irvin[17], from whose paper Fig. 3.28 is reproduced. In a personal communication he says

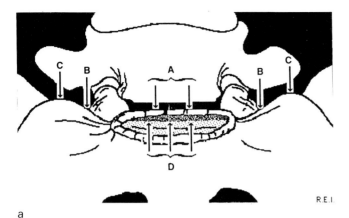

a

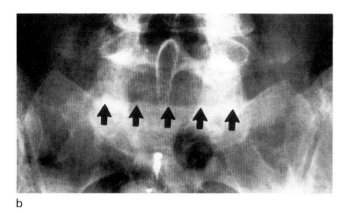

b

Fig. 3.28 Assessment of sacral base plane by X-ray (after Irvin). (a) Bony references for delineation of the sacral base. Those used by previous investigators are A, the most posterior superior margin of the sacral base; B, the lateral junction of the superior articular process with the sacral ala; C, the most superior aspect of the sacral alae. D is the radio-opaque stratum of eburnation used by Irvin. (b) The radio-opaque stratum of eburnation (arrowed) used by Irvin to delineate the weightbearing plane of the sacral base.

For the patient who is radiographically normal, but for the unlevelness of the sacral base, this visualised reference for the sacral base can be described as the transverse line of greatest radio-opacity that represents condensing change within subarticular bone of the superior sacral surface, and where these changes are extreme, this radio-opacity is called eburnation.

Irvin[18] considers that unlevelling of the sacral base is of primary importance in handling chronic somatic dysfunction and recommends that even a difference of 1.5 mm ($\frac{1}{16}$th inch) should be corrected.

REFERENCES

1. Kimberly P.E. (1980). Formulating a prescription for osteopathic manipulative treatment. *JAOA*; **79**:506–513.
2. Mellin G. (1988). Correlations of hip mobility with degree of back pain and lumbar spinal mobility in chronic low-back pain patients. *Spine*; **13**:668–670.
3. Ellison J.B., Rose S.J., Sahrmann S.A. (1990). Patterns of hip rotation range of motion: a comparison between healthy subjects and patients with low back pain. *Physical Therapy*; **70**:537–541.
4. Lewis T., Kellgren J.H. (1939). Observations relating to referred pain. *Clin. Sci.*; **4**:47–71.

5. MacDonald G., Hargrave–Wilson W. (1935). *The Osteopathic Lesion*. London: Heinemann Medical.
6. Travell J., Rinzler S.H. (1952). The myofascial genesis of pain. *Postgrad. Med*; **11**:425–434 and many other papers.
7. Mennell J. McM. (1975). The therapeutic use of cold. *JAOA*; **74**:1146–1158.
8. Travell J., Simons D.G. (1982). *Myofascial Pain and Dysfunction*. Baltimore: Williams and Wilkins.
9. As demonstrated by Dr Edward G. Stiles DO, FAAO.
10. Penning L. (1968). *Functional Pathology of the Cervical Spine*. Amsterdam: Excerpta Medica.
11. Troup Duncan, (1968). PHD thesis London University (unpublished).
12. Chamberlain W.E. (1932). The X-ray examination of the sacro-iliac joint. *Delaware State Med. J.*; **4**:195–201.
13. Hansson T., Bigos S., Beecher P., Wortley M. (1985). The lumbar lordosis in acute and chronic low back pain. *Spine*; **10**:154–155.
14. Pope M.H., Bevins T., Wilder D.G., Frymoyer J.W. (1985). The relation between anthropometric, postural, muscular and mobility characteristics of males ages 18–25. *Spine*; **10**:644–648.
15. Torgerson W.R., Dotter W.E. (1976). Comparative roentgenographic study of the asymptomatic and symptomatic lumbar spine. *J. Bone Jt Surg.*; **58a**:850–853.
16. Greenman P.E. (1978). Lift therapy: use and abuse. *JAOA*; **79**:238–250.
17. Irvin R.E. Reduction of lumbar scoliosis by use of a heel lift to level the sacral base. *JAOA*; **91**:36–44.
18. Irvin Robert E. (1986). Postural balancing: a protocol for the routine reversal of chronic somatic dysfunction (abstr). *JAOA*; **86**;608.

Chapter 4

Detailed examination: the pelvis

FUNCTIONAL ANATOMY OF THE PELVIS

Both the inguinal and sacrotuberous ligaments are important in pelvic diagnosis. In the common dysfunctions of the pubic symphysis the insertion of the inguinal ligament at the pubic tubercle on the dysfunctional side is often the site of tissue texture abnormality and tenderness; in the less common shear dysfunctions of the innominate, tension and tenderness in the sacrotuberous ligaments are important.

The complexities of dysfunctions at the sacroiliac joints defy simple mechanical explanation. It seems impossible, for instance, that on the same side, in the same patient there should be an inferior pubis and a posterior rotation of the innominate. Such a combination is uncommon but the fact that it can occur indicates that some other explanation must be sought. The answer appears to be that the positional deformity results from tightness of soft tissues, especially muscle, and that if something has caused different groups of muscle to fail to relax properly, when the first group has been persuaded to relax, the antagonistic group may be found to be hypertonic.

Movements of the ilia on the sacrum are not always the same when the patient is sitting as when standing. In the standing position the ilia are much influenced by the long thigh muscles, especially the hamstrings, the adductors, the gluteals and the ilio-psoas. In the sitting position the long thigh muscles are usually inactive and the influence is more from the anterior abdominal muscles (especially rectus), the quadratus lumborum and the ilio-costalis. In both sitting and standing the sacrum will respond to the tensions in the trunk. The standing forward flexion test (FFT) is considered to give a better indication of restriction of motion of the ilium on the sacrum while the sitting test gives more information about the motion of the sacrum between the ilia.

The effect of muscle hypertonus on SI position is not the same when the patient is supine as when prone. When the patient is supine the weight is being borne largely on the sacrum and the innominates are free to rotate in response to tensions from below. When the patient is prone the innominates are stabilised by the weight resting on the two anterior superior spines and the pubic symphysis so that the sacrum can respond to the influence of the lumbar spine.

The absence of readily palpable muscle crossing the SI joint makes the detection of tissue texture abnormalities more difficult than with intervertebral joints. Diagnosis, therefore, depends primarily on asymmetry of position and of motion. Tender areas around the sacroiliac joint

Fig. 4.1 Posterior view of the pelvic bones. See text for figures.

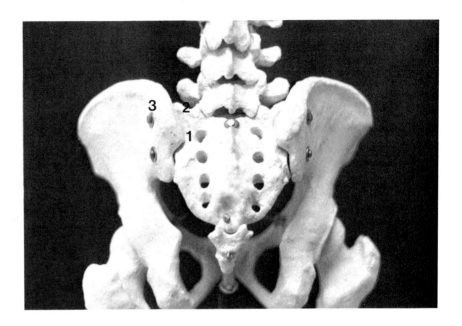

do not necessarily mean dysfunction of that joint. In Fig. 4.1 the numbers refer to common areas of tenderness; 1, over the posterior SI ligament, is likely to be connected with actual SI dysfunction. 2 is more likely to be caused by trouble at the L5–S1 joint and 3, in the origin of the gluteal muscles, may be found in association with dysfunction several joints higher.

The distinction between iliosacral movement (that of one ilium on the sacrum) and sacroiliac movement (that of the sacrum between the ilia) will be made in this edition and the approach which considers the sacrum as an atypical lumbar vertebra is only mentioned as a possibility. In that approach after dealing with the sacrum as if it were L6, the treatment of the SI joint is restricted to what is described otherwise as iliosacral.

Landmarks

In making a diagnosis of pelvic dysfunction, the most important landmarks are as follows.

1. The iliac crests
These are assessed against the transverse (horizontal) plane for vertical height with the patient standing and for relative superiority (referred to the anatomical position), both prone and supine.

2. The greater trochanters
Also assessed for vertical height against the transverse plane.

3. The pubic tubercles
Assessed supine for superiority and also for tissue texture change.

4. The anterior superior iliac spines (ASIS)
Assessed supine for anteriority, inferiority and, after correction of other pelvic dysfunctions, for relative distance from the midline. The reference point is the ledge under the ASIS for superiority, the anterior aspect for anteriority and the medial aspect for laterality.

5. The posterior superior iliac spines (PSIS)
Assessed for superiority and posteriority and for motion in forward flexion, both standing and seated for which the reference point is the ledge under the PSIS. Also used as a guide to find the sacral base and the lamina of L5 when the patient is prone. For this and for the one-legged standing or 'stork' test, the most posterior part of the PSIS is used.

6. The sacral base
Assessed for relative posteriority on the two sides, that is the position of the sacral base with respect to the coronal plane, which indicates the rotation of the sacrum. Also for the depth of the sulcus, that is the position of the sacrum with respect to the posterior superior iliac spine on each side.

7. The inferior lateral angle of the sacrum (ILA) on either side of the sacral apex (Fig. 2.4)
Assessed for relative posteriority against the coronal plane and/or inferiority, sitting, both upright and forward bent, prone and prone in extension (sphinx position).

8. The ischial tuberosities
These are large rounded pieces of bone and it is essential to find the most inferior (caudal) part. This is then assessed prone for relative inferiority against the transverse plane.

9. The sacrotuberous ligaments
These are found from the ischial tuberosities by sliding the thumbs round the medial edge of the tuberosity, without losing contact with the bone. The thumbs are advanced craniad deep to the edge of the gluteal muscles and then a little posteriorly. The curved edge of the ligament can be felt and is assessed for relative tightness and tenderness.

10. The medial malleoli
Assessed prone and supine, for relative inferiority to determine apparent leg length discrepancy.

Sacral motion

The possible movements of the sacrum are as follows.
   1. *Anterior and posterior nutation,* otherwise known as inferior and superior nutation respectively, or as inferior and superior sacral shear and formerly called sacral flexion and extension.

In this movement the sacrum rotates about a transverse axis forwards and downwards (anterior) or backwards and upwards (posterior) but there is a also translation of the sacrum on the innominate. Owing to the shape of the auricular surface, anterior nutation must be associated with inferior translation of the sacrum and posterior nutation with superior translation. There is still discussion about the mechanics of this motion and diagrams of the various theories are given by Kapandji[1]. The nature of the short, deep fibres of the posterior sacroiliac ligament would appear to make the mechanism ascribed to Farabeuf (Fig. 4.2) to be the most likely. In that mechanism the centre of motion is considered to be in the area of the short posterior fibres but because there is translation as well as rotation, the centre itself must move as the nutation occurs.

Fig. 4.2 Farabeuf's axis of rotation of sacrum (after Kapandji).

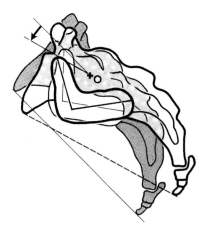

Anterior and posterior nutation are physiological movements and are the reaction of the sacrum respectively to backward and forward bending of the lumbar spine. When motion is normal, the sacrum always nutates and rotates in the opposite direction to the movement of the lumbar spine. When there is restriction of nutational movement it may be bilateral but is much more commonly seen on one side and it is correct to prefix the description with unilateral. The one sided restriction is so much more common that, if bilateral is not specified, the dysfunction is assumed to be unilateral.

2. *Anterior or forward sacral torsion* (or simply forward torsion). The torsional movements occur about a line from the superior pole of one sacroiliac joint to the inferior pole of the other (Fig. 2.4). This line is known as the 'oblique axis' and is named for the side of the superior pole. In anterior torsion the sacrum rotates to the side of the axis — the side of the superior pole. It is a physiological movement and is part of the normal cycle of pelvic motion in walking. It only requires treatment if the motion becomes restricted in the twisted position. Rotation of the sacrum to one side is always accompanied by sidebending to the other side.

Anterior or forward torsion may be to the left on the left oblique axis, often known as 'left on left' or simply L on L. It may also be to the right on the right oblique axis (R on R). As a dysfunction left on left torsion is more common than right on right.

3. *Posterior or backward sacral torsion* is when the sacrum rotates to the side opposite to the oblique axis around which it is moving. It is a physiological movement but does not occur in normal walking. For posterior torsion to occur the lumbar spine must be forward bent far enough to introduce non-neutral mechanics and for this reason it is often considered as the 'non-neutral' mechanics of the sacrum. Restriction of motion in this position is usually the result of trauma and is one of the common causes of the 'well man bends over, cripple stands up' syndrome.

Posterior torsion can be to the right on the left oblique axis (right on left or R on L) or to the left on the right oblique axis (left on right or L on R). Restriction of the former is the more common. Posterior torsion is always associated with non-neutral dysfunction(s) in the lumbar spine and may be difficult to correct unless the lumbar dysfunction has first been treated.

As in the case of anterior torsion, treatment is required, and indeed the positional diagnosis can only be made if the sacrum becomes restricted in this position.

Innominate motion

In normal walking the innominates perform an alternating counterrotation about a transverse axis through the pubic symphysis. This movement must involve anterior rotation against the sacrum on one side and posterior rotation on the other side. This innominate motion is a necessary counterpart to sacral torsion, but does not necessarily become restricted. These movements are physiological but they may become restricted at either end of the range causing dysfunctions known as the anterior and the posterior innominate.

The other movements which can occur are only possible in the presence of unusual anatomy and are properly regarded as subluxations.

Dysfunctions of physiological motion are as follows.

1. *Posterior innominate*, sometimes known as anterior sacrum. This is common, more so on the left than the right, and will often be associated with other pelvic or lumbar dysfunctions. It can be a cause of either local or referred pain and, as in other dysfunctions of the SI joint, the pain will often be felt on the opposite side. When one innominate is in the posterior position the opposite side will usually be in the anterior position, but will often not be restricted.

2. *Anterior innominate* (posterior sacrum). This can also be the cause of symptoms and is common more on the right than the left, often associated with other dysfunctions.

Dysfunctions of abnormal motion are as follows.

3. *Superior innominate (iliac) shear*, also known as 'upslip'. This is the most common of the abnormal movements; it is probable that it can only happen if there is no bevel change in the SI joint so that there is less

than normal up and down stability of the sacrum on the innominate. It can result from a single traumatic incident such as a fall on one buttock, but may also be produced by repeated minor trauma as when stepping down from a height always on to the same foot.

When the innominate on one side slips up on the sacrum all the landmarks on the innominate are high on the affected side in both prone and supine positions. *When standing, however, the height of the innominate is a function of relative leg length and is not altered by an innominate shear.*

The superior innominate shear is a subluxation, the SI joint is hypermobile and weightbearing tends to predispose to recurrence. Many practitioners use a sacroiliac belt after reduction to make recurrence less likely and this will certainly be required if the condition recurs.

4. *Inferior innominate (iliac) shear* (down slip). This is much less common, being caused almost solely by a fall forwards with the foot trapped. It is reported to be more common in areas where horse riding is widespread, the mechanism being a fall leaving one foot caught in the stirrup and the rider being dragged by the horse. Weightbearing tends to reduce the deformity and it may be that many are reduced by standing and walking before they are ever seen. They are stable after reduction.

5. *Inflare and outflare.* These dysfunctions involve a rotation of the ilium around a descriptive axis roughly parallel to the length of the sacrum but for which there is no anatomical basis. For this motion to occur the auricular surface of the sacrum must be convex laterally about this axis whereas the usual shape has a concavity (see Fig. 2.3). The authors find these dysfunctions rare but they will be described; they should not be diagnosed until all sacroiliac and other iliosacral problems have been treated because anterior rotation of the ilium does result in some outflare and posterior rotation some inflare. The flare dysfunctions are said to be found at times in association with superior innominate (iliac) shears. If this is found it is important to support the unstable pelvis with a belt after treatment. A similar appearance may occur as a result of imbalance of length and strength of the hip rotator muscles.

Pubic motion

There are two basic physiological movement patterns at the pubic symphysis. In common with many pelvic dysfunctions, when asymmetry is found, the appearance will be very similar whether one side is restricted in one direction or the other side in the opposite direction. It is important to treat the correct side but most of the tests except those for motion will look the same. The first and most important lateralising sign for dysfunctions of the pubis is the standing forward flexion test (FFT). When this is positive bilaterally, or otherwise equivocal the next most valuable finding is tissue texture change and tenderness at the pubic tubercle. If these are not present lateralisation depends on secondary tests of pelvic motion, on direct motion testing of the pubis itself or on the success of trial treatment. Other motion tests are described at the end of this chapter.

The movement patterns are as follows.

1. The motion which is an essential component of the normal walking cycle. This is an antagonistic rotation about an axis that is roughly transverse through the symphysis. If this motion is lost, as it may be if there is restriction in an asymmetrical position, the remaining movements of the pelvic bones are altered and, for this reason, treatment of unlevelling of the pubis is considered as the first priority.

2. The second movement is a vertical shear (see Fig. 2.1). It was described in previous editions as abnormal. The results of research do suggest that, like many other movements in the pelvis, it should only be regarded as abnormal when it becomes restricted in an asymmetrical position. It has been shown that there is often a small amount of vertical shear at the pubis in prolonged one-legged standing (Kapandji[1]). In this movement one side of the pubis rises higher than the other and that, when restricted, is the superior pubis. If the one that is restricted is that which is depressed caudally it is an inferior pubis. The asymmetry can be seen on X-rays when it has become fixed (Fig. 4.3).

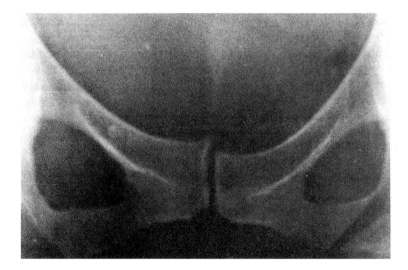

Fig. 4.3 X-ray showing unlevelling of pubic symphysis.

3. Much less common abnormal movements found occasionally are a simple separation and an antero-posterior displacement usually of slight extent. These may also interfere with the rotation at the symphysis.

Common patterns of pelvic dysfunction

Pelvic dysfunctions are commonly multiple and some patterns are much more common than others. The less common patterns are indications to check that the results of the examination have been correctly interpreted. The less common patterns seem to be associated with more severe symptoms than the common patterns.

The more common patterns include:

1. Right inferior pubis, left on left sacral torsion and right anterior innominate.
2. Left superior pubis, left anterior sacral nutation and left posterior innominate.
3. Right posterior sacral nutation and right anterior innominate.

Among the less common findings are:

1. Right superior pubis.
2. Left inferior pubis.
3. Left posterior sacral nutation.
4. Right anterior sacral nutation.

DETAILED EXAMINATION

It is clear that more than just the pelvis is being examined during these tests. They are arranged in this manner because this is how they are usually performed in order to save time in a clinical situation.

1. Standing, static examination, illustrated in Chapter 3, Figs 3.3, 3.4 and 3.5.
   (a) The relative height of the iliac crest on each side.
   (b) The relative height of the greater trochanters.
   (c) The relative height of the inferior ledge of the PSIS on each side.
   (d) The relative height of the inferior ledge of the ASIS on each side.

Standing with motion.
   (e) The range and symmetry of sidebending to each side and whether the vertebral rotation occurring with the sidebend is in neutral or non-neutral mechanics; that is, do the vertebrae rotate to the opposite or to the same side as the sidebend. Either the 'hip drop' or simple sidebending, or both may be used. Of the two the hip drop test probably gives a better indication of the range and coupling of sidebending at the lumbosacral joint[2].
   (f) The overall range of forward flexion and of extension.
   (g) The standing forward flexion test (standing FFT), as described in Chapter 3.
   (h) The 'stork' or one-legged standing test[3]. This test is in two parts, of which the first is of general importance; the second is a means of assessing the motion at the lower pole of the SI joint. The starting position is the same for both. The patient stands with her feet together and should be close enough to a table or other object so that if necessary she can steady herself with the tips of her fingers. The operator sits or kneels behind her to get his eyes down close to the level of her posterior superior iliac spines. For both tests the patient is asked to raise her knee first on one side then on the other. The knee must be lifted at least as high as the hip joint for the test to be reliable. The patient is instructed to lift the knee on the side on which the operator's thumb is on the

ilium. The test is then repeated on the other side. For both part 1 and part 2 Kirkaldy-Willis uses slightly different points in his description.

Part 1 for upper pole motion: the operator places one of his thumbs on *the most posterior part* of the patient's PSIS on the side to be examined while his other thumb contacts the upper part of the sacral crest, preferably the spinous process of S1, if present (Fig. 4.4a–c). Normal sacroiliac motion is shown by the PSIS dropping (caudad) with respect to the sacrum. Restriction is shown by the PSIS rising or remaining at the starting level.

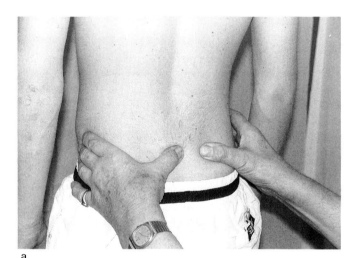

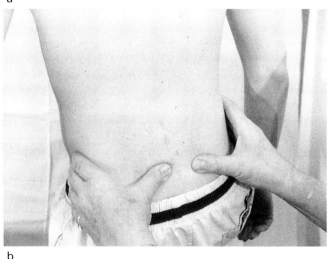

a

b

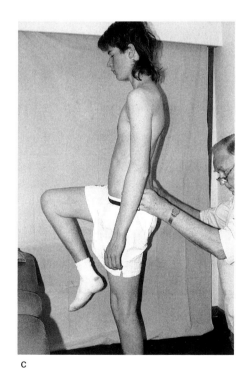

c

Fig. 4.4 Upper pole stork test for restriction of sacroiliac motion. (a) Placement of thumbs, upper pole test; (b) positive test, the right thumb has not dropped; (c) patient position.

Part 2 for lower pole motion: the operator places his thumbs on the ilium in the region of the posterior inferior iliac spine (PIIS) and on the lowest part of the median sacral crest. Normal motion of the lower pole is shown by the PIIS moving laterally and caudad (Fig. 4.5a and b).

Fig. 4.5 Lower pole stork test. (a) Placement of thumbs; (b) negative test, thumbs have separated.

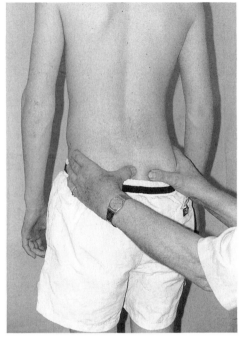

a

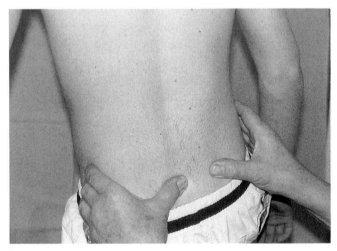

b

2. Sitting.

(a) Sidebending; is the motion the same as when standing?

(b) Sitting forward flexion test (sitting FFT). See Chapter 3.

(c) From the forward bent position in (b) note any rotation of the lumbar vertebrae (see Fig. 3.17). The lamina of L5 is found as in Fig. 3.18; the TPs are used above that level. Assessment of rotation could be done standing but that would put more strain on the spine.

(d) The ILA position when erect and when in maximum forward bending. Does one ILA either become more posterior or more inferior than the other in flexion? (see Fig. 3.15).

The ILA is the transverse process of S5 and is found by placing one index finger in the sacral hiatus and the index and middle fingers of the other hand on either side at the same level but about 2 cm (¾ inch) away. It is usually a flat piece of bone and has a posterior surface and an inferior margin (see Fig. 3.16).

3. Supine.

(a) Because of the number of patients that one of the authors has seen with hip abnormalities in addition to, or in place of, the back problem for which the patient had been referred, it is his rule to examine the hip joint movement in every patient. The most sensitive indicators of abnormality are abduction and rotation in the 90 degree flexed position and this can conveniently be tested at this point in the examination. The possibility that any restriction of motion may be due to tight muscle must not be forgotten. Recent studies have reported a correlation between loss of internal rotation and the presence of low back pain[4,5].

(b) The straight leg raising test may also be performed at this stage. Greenman[6] has pointed out that, if the test is being used as a measure of hamstring length, the end point is indicated by the first palpable motion of the opposite ASIS, not the limit of pain-free motion.

(c) The relative superiority of the pubic ramus on each side. Either the ramus or the pubic tubercle may be used but it should be the same point on each side. There is an advantage in using the tubercle because, in patients with pubic dysfunction, there is often tissue texture change that can be felt in the inguinal ligament where it inserts at the pubic tubercle (see Fig. 3.19a).

Unlevelling of the pubes is the first stop sign. If the pubes are unlevel all other diagnostic signs in the pelvis may be unreliable. When unlevelling is found it should be treated and the examination started again at the standing FFT.

The signs of a superior pubis on the left are very similar to those of an inferior pubis on the right. If the standing FFT is equivocal, or bilaterally positive, and other motion tests for the SI joint are inconclusive, a direct motion test may be performed by moving each ramus up and down between the operator's finger and thumb; the side that moves less easily is the one to treat. It is important that the operator does not grip the ramus tightly because that can be very painful. When it is impossible to be sure on which side is the main restriction, treatment may be given by the 'blunderbuss' method, or first to one side and then if needed to the other also.

(d) The relative height of the iliac crest on each side. If there is a difference suspect an innominate shear (see Fig. 3.20). *This is the second stop sign.* To check for the presence of a shear dysfunction go to 'prone examination a, g, and h' below, and, if there is a shear, it should be treated before returning to the examination.

(e) The position of the ASIS on each side. At this stage in the examination the relative superiority of the ASIS, estimated from the position of the inferior ledge, is all that need be examined. After treatment of the sacroiliac dysfunctions the relative anteriority and laterality will be examined, if the sacroiliac motion tests remain positive.

(f) The relative position of the medial malleolus on each side. Is one superior to the other? If the legs are structurally equal, apparent inequality of leg length in the supine position is a function of innominate rotation, the weight being supported by the sacrum leaving the innominates free to rotate (see also 4.(i). below).

4. Prone.

(a) The relative height of the iliac crest on each side.

(b) The relative position of the PSIS on each side with respect to superiority and anteriority.

(c) The position of the sacral base relative to the coronal plane (see note 3 below).

(d) The relative position of the ILA on each side with respect to posteriority and inferiority (Fig. 4.6).

Fig. 4.6 Testing for asymmetry at the ILAs prone.

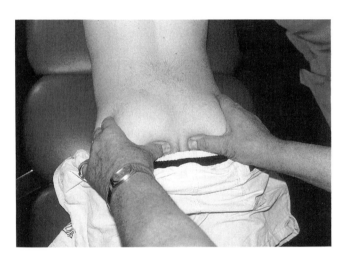

(e) The depth of the lumbar lordosis.

(f) The lumbar spring test. This is performed by a springing force, directed anteriorly, on the spine of L5 and will be negative (i.e. it will spring) when there is a lordosis but positive when the sacrum is extended and L5 flexed.

(g) The relative position of the ischial tuberosity on each side against the transverse plane (Fig. 4.7). If on one side the tuberosity is not less than 7 mm ($\frac{1}{4}$ inch) superior to the other, suspect an innominate shear.

(h) The relative tightness of the sacrotuberous ligament on each side.

(i) The relative position of the medial malleolus on each side. In the prone position rotation of the innominates is prevented by contact of the ASIS and the pubes on the table, difference in apparent leg length is then a function of the lumbar scoliosis.

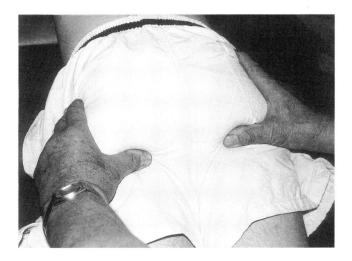

Fig. 4.7 Test for asymmetry of ischial tuberosity position.

(j) Lumbar rotation in the neutral position, assessed as when sitting 2(c) above.

5. Prone in hyperextension.

The 'sphinx' position is used. The patient supports herself on her elbows, holding her chin in her hands. To maximise extension the elbows need to be almost directly under the chin and should be close together and it is essential that the patient allows her abdominal muscles to relax (see Fig. 3.21).

In each case the question is whether any asymmetry is increased or decreased.

(a) The relative position of the ILAs.

(b) The sacral base position.

(c) Lumbar rotation in extension (see 4(j) above).

6. After treatment of all pubic, innominate shear and sacroiliac dysfunctions, there may still be iliosacral dysfunctions and the following tests are recommended to exclude the presence of flares or incomplete treatment of other dysfunctions:

(a) One or more of the tests for sacroiliac mobility.

(b) Supine: repeat tests 3(e) for superiority, anteriority and laterality, and 3(f) above.

(c) Prone: repeat test 4(b) above.

Notes

1. In the forward flexion tests the innominate on the restricted side is picked up by the moving sacrum more easily than that on the mobile side. The more severe the restriction the sooner the movement begins. The one which moves first or furthest is the positive (restricted) side. Bilaterally positive tests are common and are easily mistaken for normal motion. The 'stork' or one of the other tests for SI mobility will help to make the distinction.

2. When the FFT is more strongly positive standing, suspect that the dysfunction is iliosacral or pubic or from below. If the sitting test is the more positive the problem is likely to be sacroiliac or from above. Asymmetrical hamstring tightness may cause a false positive standing test on the opposite side, asymmetrical quadratus lumborum tightness may cause a false positive test on the same side.

3. When examining the position of the sacral base it is best to apply a constant pressure with the thumbs for a few moments before making the observation. The tissue in this area often contains excess fluid and this needs to be dispersed.

4. In any sacroiliac dysfunction look for maladaptive lumbar lesions and, if present, treat these first. Indeed many operators always treat the lumbar spine before the pelvis, except for pubic unlevelling and innominate (iliac) shears. It is very important to look at and treat the lumbar spine before attempting to correct a posterior sacral torsion since there will always be at least one type II lumbar dysfunction which, if untreated, may make treatment of the torsion difficult or impossible.

5. Normal adaptation to an asymmetrical sacral position is a neutral (group) curve to bring the superincumbent spine vertical in order to compensate for sacral base unlevelling. Non-neutral dysfunctions in the lumbar spine would prevent that adaptation and if present they need to be treated first or the sacral problem may be very difficult to correct. The non-neutral dysfunction which prevents normal adaptation may be at L5 or higher; up to L3 is common. It should be remembered that the normal motion of the lumbosacral junction is such that, in flexion/extension and in rotation, L5 moves in directions opposite to the sacrum. If the sacrum is in anterior nutation, L5 extends and if the sacrum is rotated to the right, L5 rotates to the left. In the forward flexion tests the sacrum begins to move in the same direction as L5 after the range of antagonistic motion is exceeded.

Some practitioners treat the lower and some even the upper thoracic dysfunctions before returning to the pelvis. It is more usual to treat the remaining pelvic dysfunctions after the lumbar spine, or at least the non-adaptive lumbar dysfunctions, have been treated.

6. Pelvic dysfunctions are commonly multiple.

7. If iliosacral dysfunctions are recurrent, always check the legs. Look for structural difference in leg length and for imbalance of muscle length and strength, especially in the long thigh muscles and the piriformis.

DIAGNOSIS

Fourteen different dysfunctions are described in the pelvis[7]. In earlier editions of this book a simpler approach was also described but further experience with teaching suggests that this is not necessary and may be confusing. It is fair to say, however, that there are experienced manipulators who do use a different approach, usually one in which the sacrum is considered as an abnormal extra lumbar vertebra and treated accordingly. That approach still has to recognise the pubic dysfunctions and the innominate shears as well as the anterior and posterior innominate dysfunctions and the much less common 'flare' dysfunctions of the innominates.

The diagnostic method which will be presented is that used and taught at the courses in manual medicine offered at Michigan State University College of Osteopathic Medicine and in its present form is due in large part to the expertise and energy of Dr Philip E. Greenman DO, FAAO and Dr Paul E. Kimberly DO, FAAO who have played a very large part in the development of this facility.

Types of dysfunction of the pelvis

The pelvic dysfunctions that need to be recognised are as follows.

1. Pubis

(a) Unlevelling at the symphysis. This may be due to one pubic bone being superior or to the other being inferior. This dysfunction is very common and important because when present it prevents the normal motion of the pelvis in the walking cycle. This dysfunction is often missed and is one of the six common findings in the 'failed back'.

(b) The much less common separation of the symphysis.

2. Sacroiliac dysfunctions

(a) Anterior torsion of the sacrum about the hypothetical oblique axis, torsion to the left (anterior surface of the sacrum turning to the left) on the left axis which is very common, or to the right on the right axis which is much less common. According to Greenman the ratio is usually about 4 : 1. Anterior torsional movements occur in normal walking; it is only when the motion becomes restricted that treatment is needed. Symptoms are usually minor and consist mostly of back pain but correction of the dysfunction may be important because the function of other joints is compromised.

(b) Posterior torsion about the oblique axis. Torsion to the right on the left axis which is common or to the left on the right axis which is rather less common. Posterior torsion is a physiological movement but it only occurs when the lumbar spine is operating in non-neutral mechanics. It is one of the common causes of the 'well man bent over, cripple stood up' syndrome and is always associated with some strain, often happening when an unguarded sidebend is made while the spine is flexed. Symptoms are often severe.

(c) Unilateral anterior (or inferior) nutation of the sacrum (unilateral inferior sacral shear or unilateral sacral flexion). Common on the left and often associated with a posterior innominate on that side. Rare on the right. Difficult to get to stay corrected. May be bilateral. This dysfunction is commonly found in those with chronic symptoms, especially those that get worse with standing and later in the day. The pain is commonly in the back and buttock.

(d) Unilateral posterior (or superior) sacral nutation (unilateral superior sacral shear or unilateral sacral extension). Common on the right but rare on the left (ratio about 20 : 1). May be associated with an anterior innominate on the same side. This also may be bilateral and is usually produced by trauma. It is not uncommon in those injured in rear-end collisions.

The right sided dysfunction is easily confused with right on left posterior torsion. Like posterior torsion it may cause severe symptoms. The pain will be in the back and leg and there may be 'soft' signs suggesting S1 root involvement. There will often be an FRS dysfunction on the same side at the L4–5 level.

3. Iliosacral dysfunctions
   (a) Anterior innominate. Common; more so on the right than the left.
   (b) Posterior innominate. Common; more on the left than the right.
   (c) Superior innominate shear (upslip). Not rare; important because usually associated with relatively severe symptoms and often missed. One of the important dysfunctions found in the 'failed back'.
   (d) Inferior innominate shear (downslip). Much less common; requires an unusual type of injury for its production and will often be self-correcting on weightbearing.
   (e) Outflare, and
   (f) Inflare. Both uncommon; they can only happen if the sacral auricular surface is convex laterally instead of the usual concavity.

Diagnostic findings

These will be described for one side only because in each case the findings for the other side will be found by reversing the side labels. In most cases the more common side is described.

   1. Superior pubis on the left.
   (a) Standing forward flexion test (FFT), positive left.
   (b) Pubic tubercle and superior ramus, superior left.
   (c) Inguinal ligament, tender and may be tense left.
   (d) The left pubis does not move down easily on direct motion testing.

   2. Inferior pubis on the right.
   (a) Standing forward flexion test (FFT), positive right.
   (b) Pubic tubercle and superior ramus, inferior right.
   (c) Inguinal ligament, tender and may be tense right.
   (d) The right pubis does not move up easily on direct motion testing.
   Note that the main difference between 1 and 2 is in the side of the standing FFT.

   3. Separated symphysis.
   A gap may be felt, the pubic rami and tubercles will be level and the FFT probably negative.

   4. Anterior or forward sacral torsion, to the left on the left oblique axis (L on L). The main restriction is the inability of the right sacral base to move into posterior nutation.
   (a) Sitting FFT, positive right (usually).
   (b) Left inferior lateral angle of the sacrum (ILA), posterior and slightly inferior, worse when forward bent (sitting test), often level in extension.

The asymmetry becomes more marked on further flexion because the right sacral base is unable to nutate posteriorly.

(c) Base of sacrum, anterior right, less so or level on extension because the left side goes into anterior nutation when the lumbar spine is extended.

(d) Lumbar lordosis, increased and springing test negative.

(e) Medial malleolus prone, superior left.

(f) Lumbar scoliosis, convex right.

(g) Normal lumbar adaptation when in neutral, L5 rotated right.

(h) The piriformis will be tight on the same side.

5. Posterior or backward sacral torsion, to the right on the left oblique axis (R on L). Note that the main difference between this and forward torsion (on the opposite oblique axis) is the change in the signs on alteration of the flexion and extension position. The main restriction is the inability of the right sacral base to move into anterior nutation.

(a) Sitting, FFT positive right.

(b) Right inferior lateral angle of the sacrum (ILA), posterior and slightly inferior, nearly level when forward bent (sitting test), worse in extension.

(c) Base of sacrum, posterior right, worse on extension.

(d) Lumbar lordosis, absent and springing test positive.

(e) Medial malleolus prone, superior right.

(f) Lumbar scoliosis, convex left.

(g) Normal lumbar adaptation when in neutral, L5 rotated left.

6. Unilateral anterior (or inferior) sacral nutation on the left (unilateral inferior sacral shear). The main restriction is inability of the left sacral base to go into posterior nutation.

(a) Sitting FFT, positive left.

(b) Inferior lateral angle of sacrum, inferior and slightly posterior, left, worse in flexion. The asymmetry does not disappear in extension because of the translation which is present as well as the overturning motion.

(c) Base of sacrum, anterior left.

(d) Lumbar lordosis, normal or increased and spring test negative.

(e) Medial malleolus prone, inferior left.

(f) Lumbar scoliosis, convex left.

(g) Normal lumbar adaptation when in neutral, L5 rotated left.

7. Unilateral posterior (or superior) sacral nutation on the right, (unilateral superior sacral shear). The main restriction is the inability of the right sacral base to go into anterior nutation. The asymmetry does not disappear in flexion because there is a translation as well as the overturning movement.

(a) Sitting FFT, positive right.

(b) Inferior lateral angle of sacrum, superior and slightly anterior, right.

(c) Base of sacrum, posterior right.

(d) Lumbar lordosis, reduced and spring test positive.

(e) Medial malleolus prone, superior right.

(f) Lumbar scoliosis, convex left.

(g) Normal lumbar adaptation when in neutral, L5 rotated left.

8. Bilateral sacral nutation, anterior or posterior (bilateral sacral shear, inferior or superior).

(a) Sitting FFT, bilaterally positive (suspect if both PSIS begin to move almost at once). Check with stork test which will be bilaterally positive.

(b) Lumbar lordosis, increased with negative spring test in anterior nutation and decreased with positive spring test in posterior nutation.

All other signs are negative being the same on each side.

9. Anterior innominate, right.

(a) Standing FFT, positive right.

(b) ASIS supine, inferior right.

(c) Medial malleolus supine, inferior right.

(d) PSIS, slightly superior right.

(e) Sacral sulcus, shallow right.

10. Posterior innominate, left.

(a) Standing FFT, positive left.

(b) ASIS supine, superior left.

(c) Medial malleolus supine, superior left.

(d) PSIS, inferior left.

(e) Sacral sulcus, deep left.

11. Superior innominate shear (upslip), left.

(a) Standing FFT, positive left.

(b) Iliac crest superior, prone and supine, left.

(c) Medial malleolus, prone and supine, superior left.

(d) PSIS and ASIS, superior left.

(e) Ischial tuberosity, superior left by at least 7 mm (¼ inch).

(f) Sacro-tuberous ligament, lax left.

12. Inferior innominate shear (down slip), right.

(a) Standing FFT positive, right.

(b) Iliac crest inferior, prone and supine, right.

(c) Medial malleolus, prone and supine, inferior right.

(d) PSIS and ASIS, inferior right.

(e) Ischial tuberosity, inferior right by at least 7 mm (¼ inch).

(f) Sacro-tuberous ligament, tight right.

13. Inflare right.

(a) Standing FFT, positive right.

(b) ASIS, medial right.

(c) PSIS, lateral right.

(d) Sacral sulcus, wide right.

14. Outflare left.

(a) Standing FFT, positive left.

(b) ASIS, lateral left.
(c) PSIS, medial left.
(d) Sacral sulcus, narrow left.

Notes

1. It will be clear from the above that the signs of, for instance, an anterior innominate on the right are very similar to those of a posterior innominate on the left. The most important difference is in the side of the positive forward flexion test.

2. Sometimes it is difficult to be certain which is the positive side and many patients have positive tests on both sides. In such cases the other tests for sacroiliac motion may be helpful; the stork test and one or more of the prone springing tests are among the most useful.

3. In torsions the sacral base and the ILA are posterior on the same side. In nutations the base and ILA go in opposite directions.

ADDITIONAL TESTS FOR MOBILITY OF THE SACROILIAC JOINTS

1. The prone springing test (Fig. 4.8)

(a) The patient lies prone.

(b) The operator uses the index and middle fingers of one hand in the sulcus on the side being examined, in such a way that he can sense the position of the sacral base with the finger tips and that of the PSIS with the pads.

(c) The heel of the other hand is used to apply springing pressure to the sacral apex, preferably on the ILA on one or other side. If the hands are on the same side of the sacrum the motion about the transverse axis is tested, if on opposite sides the oblique axis mobility is being examined.

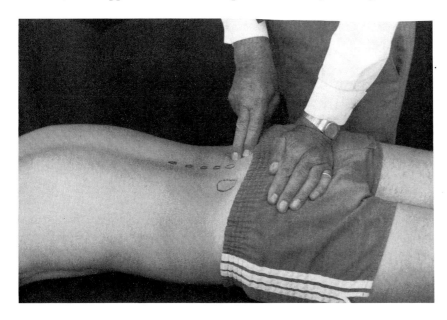

Fig. 4.8 The prone springing test for sacroiliac mobility.

Fig. 4.9 The two thumb springing test for sacroiliac mobility.

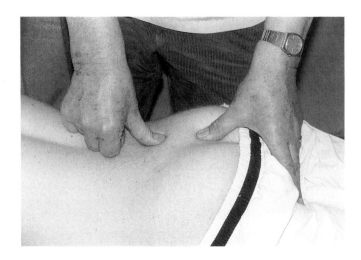

2. The two thumb spring test (Fig. 4.9).

This is very similar to the above. The patient is prone but this time the operator uses his two thumbs to perform the springing, one on the ILA and the other on the sacral base on the same or the opposite side. The springing pressure can be applied either from above or from below while the other thumb monitors the motion.

Fig. 4.10 The four point springing test.

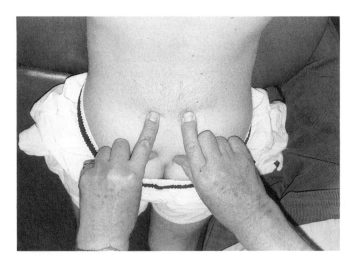

3. The four point spring test (Fig. 4.10).

This test is again similar. Instead of just his thumbs, the operator uses both index fingers as well. The thumbs are at the sacral base on each side, the index fingers are on the ILAs or vice versa; by these contacts it is possible to spring either SI joint in either direction across both transverse and oblique axes.

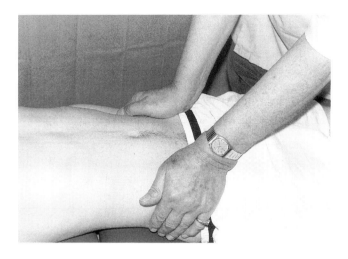

Fig. 4.11 The supine iliac springing (bounce) test.

4. The supine iliac 'bounce' test (Fig. 4.11).

(a) The patient lies supine.

(b) The operator stands to either side and with the palms of his hands applies light downward (posterior) pressure to her ASIS on each side.

(c) While maintaining the light pressure on the opposite side he presses more firmly on first one side and then the other to detect resilience.

When this test is performed, the patient will often be able to appreciate the difference between one side and the other.

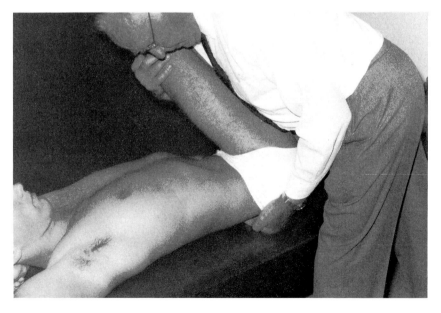

Fig. 4.12 The supine femoral leverage springing test.

5. The supine femoral spring test (Fig. 4.12).

(a) The patient lies supine.

(b) The operator stands on the side on which the joint is to be tested and fully flexes her hip and knee on that side. If needed, stability can be increased by dropping her other lower leg over the table edge.

(c) For her right SI joint the operator slides his left hand under her right buttock until his index and middle finger tips reach the sulcus and he can feel the sacral base with the tips and the PSIS with the pads.

(d) The operator takes up the slack in her hip joint by adduction and, using his trunk and free hand, alternately rocks the ilium on the sacrum by adduction and abduction using his left fingers to assess motion.

In previous editions a leg lengthening test was also described. This test is omitted as being more difficult to interpret and less easy to perform than those described above.

REFERENCES

1. Kapandji I.A. (1978). *The Physiology of the Joints.* Vol. 3, p.67. London: Churchill Livingstone.
2. Mitchell F.L., Moran P.S., Pruzzo N.A. (1979). *An Evaluation and Treatment Manual of Osteopathic Muscle Energy Procedures.* p.239; Valley Park, Mo., U.S.A.: Mitchell, Moran and Pruzzo Associates.
3. Kirkaldy-Willis W.H. (1988). *Managing Low Back Pain.* 2nd ed., p.135: New York: Churchill Livingstone.
4. Mellin G. (1909). Correlations of hip mobility with degrees of back pain and lumbar spinal mobility in chronic low back pain patients. *Spine;* **13**:668–670.
5. Ellison J.B., Rose S.J., Sahrmann S.A. (1990). *Physical Therapy;* **70**:537–541.
6. Greenman P.E. (1989). *Principles of Manual Medicine,* p.26. Baltimore: Williams and Wilkins.
7. Greenman P.E. (1990). Clinical aspects of sacroiliac function in walking. *J. of Manual Medicine;* **5**:125–130.

Chapter 5

Detailed examination: the spine

In recent editions a semispecific approach has been described as well as the fully specific one. Experience with teaching suggests that it is better to go straight to the fully specific approach and that is all that will be described in this edition.

The spinal joints are examined to determine their mobility, the location of any restriction, and the presence or absence of abnormalities of tissue texture. In the first three editions of this book the tissue texture changes were related to hypertonic muscle. It is becoming clear, however, that other tissues are also involved and the most important is probably fascia. Whatever the precise tissue, the changes that occur are palpable and consist of thickening, tightness of muscle and sometimes a feeling of bogginess probably due to local oedema. At first people find these tissue texture changes difficult to feel. Like learning to read the dots of Braille, which at first seems impossible, nearly anyone can learn to feel them well enough if they will persevere with practice.

In order to make a fully specific diagnosis it is necessary to find the precise point in the range of motion where there is restriction. The motion of all spinal joints is universal in type, even if a few have little range in some planes. For this reason the point at which motion is restricted must be found in all three planes. This applies to every dysfunctional joint, each of which must be treated as a separate entity, except in group dysfunctions.

When performing this examination it will be found that a position is reached from which no further movement is possible in that direction; this is known as the barrier. The barrier is not truly a point as its precise position will change depending on in which plane the motion is first introduced. The amount of sidebending needed to reach the barrier will be different if the positioning starts, for instance, with the patient slumped rather than sitting erect in the so called 'neutral' position.

At this point it is appropriate to give a warning. It is not uncommon to find that there is a major restriction, for instance of extension in the upper thoracic spine. If the motion examination is started on the extension side of neutral the restriction may be missed and it may sometimes be necessary to start from almost full flexion.

LESION DESCRIPTION AND NOTATION

When the dysfunction in a joint is described in records or in a report it should be in sufficient detail that someone else would know what treatment to give. The level must be specified and, by convention, the structure mentioned (vertebra or skull) is the upper component of the joint, thus L4 would refer to the L4–5 joint and C1 to the atlantoaxial. Sacroiliac is used to signify dysfunction of the sacrum between the ilia, iliosacral the dysfunction of one ilium on the sacrum.

In some schools the motion restriction is specified, in others the position of the joint as found at examination. Unfortunately these two are exact opposites and care must be taken that one *or* other is used or confusion will follow.

In this, as in previous editions, the position of the joint as found at examination will be used and will be emphasised by the past tense (e.g. flexed, rotated and sidebent). When restrictions are described the imperfect tense will be used (restriction of extension or of sidebending or rotation). The actual notation will consist of capitals to indicate the position in the three planes followed by small letters, rt or lt, to designate right or left. Thus FRSrt means that on examination the upper component of the motion segment specified is found to be rotated and sidebent to the right and is flexed. (The corresponding restriction would be of rotation and sidebending to the left and of extension.) This is a slight simplification from the original which would have been FRrtSrt, the simplification is possible because if either *F*lexed or *E*xtended the joint must have a non-neutral dysfunction and, as has been described in Chapter 2, in these the rotation and the sidebending are always to the same side (except only at the occipitoatlantal joint).

For neutral dysfunctions (type I) the letter *N* may be used followed by rt or lt to designate the side to which the group is rotated. For clarity this may be expanded slightly to *NR*, followed by rt or lt, and that is the notation used in this edition. In older texts the longer NRrtSlt may still be found and indicates the same dysfunction. In some texts the notation used may be *EN* rather than the simple N; it stands for 'easy normal'.

At the occipitoatlantal joint there is a small amount of rotation to the side opposite to the sidebend. For this reason the notation, in full, is FRltSrt or FRrtSlt for flexed joints with restriction of extension, and ERltSrt or ERrtSlt for extended joints with restriction of flexion. The sidebend is more important than the rotation and the notation may be shortened to *FSrt* (or lt) and *ESlt* (or rt). The shorter notation will be used here.

SPINAL MOTION CHARACTERISTICS AND TYPES OF DYSFUNCTION

As has been said earlier (Chapter 2), sidebending and rotation are coupled movements at all levels in the spine except at the upper two cervical joints. The only significant motion at C1–2 is rotation and the smallness of the range at the occipitoatlantal joint makes the coupling unimportant but it is still there. In the thoracic and lumbar spinal joints the coupling changes between the upright (neutral or easy normal) and the flexed or, in the thoracic spine at least, the extended position.

In the neutral, 'sit-up-tall' position the joints in both thoracic and lumbar spine follow Fryette's 1st concept of spinal motion[1]. Sidebending to the right is always accompanied by rotation to the left. The vertebrae can be thought of as 'crawling out from under the load'.

In the flexed position both thoracic and lumbar joints follow Fryette's 2nd concept and rotate to the same side as the sidebend. That this happens in the fully flexed spine is certain but it does not seem to require the limit of full flexion for the second concept to be operative. On the other hand there is a fairly wide range of neutral in which the first concept operates. It is probable that the precise amount of flexion at which the motion characteristics change varies from patient to patient.

In the extended position the thoracic joints also show coupling in accord with Fryette's 2nd concept. It used to be taught that coupling of motion in the lumbar spine in extension also followed in the same way. This has not stood up to experimental investigation although it is true in the thoracic spine.

Because the motion coupling in the neutral range of the antero-posterior plane follows Fryette's 1st concept, dysfunctions occurring in neutral have come to be known as type I, while those occurring in a non-neutral situation are known as type II as they are associated with Fryette's concept 2. This applies equally to dysfunctions with restriction of flexion and those with restriction of extension.

Type II dysfunctions in both flexion and extension occur in the thoracic spine. In spite of the absence of experimental evidence, it is found clinically that type II dysfunctions of the lumbar spine do occur in extension, although not commonly except at the lumbo-sacral joint. From the point of view of treatment of the patient the type of dysfunction that would be expected to accompany changed coupling in extension does occur and may need to be treated. The recent research is noted, but it will be disregarded from the point of view of this chapter and that on treatment of the lumbar spine.

In the cervical spine the situation is not the same. In the typical cervical joints, C2 to T1, there is no neutral, probably because the shape and orientation of the articular facets is such that they are always 'engaged' and therefore control movement. For this reason, type I dysfunctions do not occur in these joints. Type II dysfunctions in flexion and in extension do occur. At the atlantoaxial joint the only movement with a range of more than a very few degrees is rotation so that there is neither a flexion nor an extension component to dysfunctions at this level.

The occipitoatlantal joint is also unusual. Here the main movement is flexion/extension but there is enough sidebend and just enough rotation for there to be a coupling. The coupling is determined by the shape of the articular facets and is such that rotation is always to the side opposite to that of the sidebend. This should not be confused with the neutral mechanics of the thoracic and lumbar spine; it is not a neutral mechanism and treatment will always need to be either in flexion or in extension.

Facet and transverse process motion

While this is simple anatomy, it is important that it is well understood in order to interpret the findings that will be described and to convert them into a diagnosis.

When the superior vertebra flexes on the one below, the inferior facets of the upper vertebra slide upwards. They also slide forwards by an amount which depends on the facing of the facets and therefore varies from one region to another. When examining a patient it may be found that in some areas it will be easier to determine which facet is anterior (or posterior); in other areas it may be easier to determine which becomes superior on flexion or inferior on extension. It is important to recognise that the anterior facet is always superior and the posterior facet is always inferior.

In most patients the facets in the thoracic and lumbar regions are difficult to feel. The transverse processes (TPs) are easier to palpate and are used to determine the position of each vertebra with respect to the one next below. The transverse process of T12 is very short and it is usually necessary to use the lamina for palpation. At L5 the lamina is used because the TP cannot be reached.

In the cervical spine the articular pillars, which carry the facets above and below, are the most important landmark in the typical joints and can easily be felt. The transverse processes are small, and in close relation to both nerves and vessels which makes them very tender, for this reason they are avoided although that of C1 is a useful landmark.

The interpretation of the findings depends on these facts:

1. On flexion the facet joints 'open' (the inferior facet of the superior vertebra slides up on the superior facet of the inferior vertebra). Similarly the TPs rise, and because of the obliquity of the joints, they become less easy to palpate as they are more anterior.

2. On extension the facets 'close' (the inferior facet of the superior vertebra slides down on the superior facet of the inferior vertebra) and the TPs drop and become more posterior.

3. On sidebending left the left facet closes and the right facet opens. The left TP drops and becomes more posterior and the right one rises and moves anteriorly.

4. On sidebending right the right facet closes and the left facet opens. The right TP drops and becomes more posterior while the left one rises and becomes more anterior.

It is possible to make a definitive diagnosis either dynamically or statically. In the dynamic method the operator observes the movement of the vertebra while it is happening, in the static method observations are made in three positions, flexed, neutral and extended. Either method gives the required information, the dynamic method is usually easier in the upper thoracic spine and the static method in the lower thoracic and lumbar regions. In any of these examinations sighting with the eyes can, with advantage, be reinforced by the proprioceptors of the operator's upper limbs. It is not difficult to train oneself to feel position and movement in this way and that ability is useful, for instance, when examining the upper thoracic area in a patient with long hair.

The argument for conversion of these data into a diagnosis is as follows:

1. If in extension the TPs of, say T4, are level but in flexion that on the left is lower and more prominent (inferior and posterior) than that on the right, the indication is that the left facet will not open, in the sense of the facet sliding up on that of T5. In other words there is restriction of flexion and of right sidebending, both of which require that the left facet joint should open. The joint therefore is found left sidebent and extended. Left rotation can be assumed because we already know that in dysfunctions in either flexion or extension, the sidebending and rotation are to the same side. In the most commonly used notation the naming of dysfunctions specifies the starting position in which the joint is found on examination. In this example that would be *Extended, Rotated* and *Sidebent* left, or in short, *ER*Slt.

2. If the TPs are level in flexion but that on the right remains superior and anterior (less prominent) in extension, the fault is that the right facet joint will not close. The restriction of sidebending is again to the right but, this time, the joint will not extend and therefore is thought of as being found flexed. Once again, the rotation follows the sidebend and the full description of the restriction is of extension and of sidebending and rotation to the right. The position in which the joint is found is *Flexed, Rotated* and *Sidebent* left, or in the common notation *FR*Slt.

3. If in neutral the transverse processes of say T5, 6 and 7 are all rotated to the left and on flexion and extension the rotation remains, even if it changes somewhat in amount, there is a neutral group dysfunction for which the notation would be *NR*lt, neutral, rotated to the left.

Note that in this notation, which will be used throughout, both the non-neutral examples are recorded as left (for rotation and sidebending) in spite of the fact that in one the left facet joint is dysfunctional and in the other it is the right side that is not moving properly.

In type I (neutral) dysfunctions the asymmetry is present throughout the range of flexion and extension but will usually be maximal in neutral. The other main difference between type I and type II (non-neutral) dysfunctions is that the former always occur in groups of three or more vertebrae all rotated in the direction opposite to the sidebend. While the group are all rotated in the same direction in space, the uppermost, when compared with the one below, is rotated slightly to the side of the sidebend.

POSITIONAL DIAGNOSIS TECHNIQUES

Thoracic and lumbar

1. Static examination
This usually begins immediately after the sitting forward flexion test. In those patients for whom forward bending while standing is not

uncomfortable it can be done standing. For most patients with back trouble, the sitting position is preferable.

For this examination, as for most, it would require a prohibitive amount of time to check each joint in turn all the way up. This is the reason for the examination process being divided first into an overall screen to demonstrate which areas need further attention; second, if desired, by a scan to pin-point joints for detailed assessment; and third by segmental definition to find the precise position of the barrier at each of the joints shown by the scan. The following description refers to the segmental definition.

As the transverse processes (TPs) will be used as the main indicator of vertebral position in these tests, it is important that they can be found with some accuracy. In this connection it must be remembered that they vary in length (see Fig. 2.7). The longest are usually at L3 and the shortest at T12. The TPs are most easily found by palpating deeply in the lateral gutter between the longissimus and iliocostalis muscles. In the thoracic region the tip of the TP is easily found by palpating in the lateral gutter to find the posterior part of the rib; the rib is then followed medially until a resistance is felt which is the tip of the transverse process. It is important at that point to lighten one's pressure until the TP can only just be felt, because the lighter the contact, the more one can feel. It is possible to feel through a relaxed longissimus but this is less accurate and, when it is hypertonic it can be impossible to feel the deeper layers.

The most important part of the examination at this stage is the determination of the position of the vertebra as compared to the one below.

The rotation, if any, of the lumbar and lower thoracic vertebrae is estimated by finding the relative posteriority of the transverse processes. It is generally accepted that the thumbs are more sensitive for perception of depth and they are used in preference for this examination. Note that when there is a major restriction in either flexion or extension, there will be asymmetry in the neutral position. When the restriction is relatively minor, the appearance in neutral will probably be symmetrical.

1.1　Flexed.

In the fully flexed position of the lumbar spine the tightness of the lumbosacral fascia makes the examination more difficult and occasionally it is necessary to examine in the other two positions and to extrapolate from those results the probable position in flexion. As noted above, at L5 it is the lamina which is palpated as the TP is hidden by the ilium. This makes it a little more difficult.

(a) The patient sits with her knees apart and her feet on the floor or supported on a stool. She should bend forwards as far as possible with her arms hanging between her knees. For the examination of the lumbar spine, if she has full knee and hip flexion, the 'knee chest' position on the table may be used or she may lie across the table with legs hanging down on one side and arms on the other. Neither of the latter alternatives gives good flexion of the thoracic region.

(b) The thumbs are placed one on either side of the same vertebra to find the tips of the TPs from L4 up. At L5 the laminae are found by starting from the most posterior part of the PSIS and moving medially and craniad at an angle of about 30° (see Fig. 3.18).

(c) With moderate pressure, equal on the two sides, the depth (anteriority) of the thumbs is noted, and compared with the level below. For determination of the rotation of S1, when examining L5, the lamina is used (the sacral base) and is found from the most posterior part of the PSIS by moving medially and 30° caudad. If there is doubt about the rotation it may help if the operator bends forwards and sights tangentially along the back. The determination of rotation of the sacral base is often difficult and it may help to confirm it by deduction from the relative position of the ILAs in flexion and neutral.

(d) The examination is repeated at each of the levels indicated by the scan up to the mid thoracic spine.

The observations are described in the order in which they are often done in the routine examination of a patient in practice. The order in which they are done is unimportant and can be altered to suit the operator.

1.2   Neutral.

The easiest position of the patient for examination of the lumbar spine rotation in neutral is prone. For patients unable to lie prone it can be done sitting but this makes it less easy.

The examination is performed in exactly the same manner as that in forward bending; at L5 it is easier because the fascia is no longer tight. Note is made of any level where there is rotation of a lumbar or lower thoracic vertebra compared to the one below, paying particular attention to levels indicated by the scanning examination.

1.3   Extended.

For this examination also, the prone position is easiest, but with the difference that the patient props herself up on her elbows and holds up her chin in her hands as high as she can (i.e. with the elbows close together and almost directly below her chin, see Fig. 3.21). This has come to be known as the 'sphinx' position although the analogy is inaccurate. For this position to be effective it is necessary for the patient to relax her abdominal muscles. This examination can also be done with the patient sitting and arching her back as much as possible. The examination is done in the same manner as in the other two positions.

INTERPRETATION

If:

(a) in neutral the TPs of L2 are level or that on the left is rather more posterior and therefore easier to feel than that of L3,

(b) in flexion the left TP becomes more posterior and prominent,

(c) in extension the asymmetry disappears,

the inference is that the left facet joint at L2–3 will not open (flex). This means loss of right rotation and the associated sidebending with loss of flexion. Positionally the joint is extended, rotated and sidebent left, or *ERSlt at L2*.

If, on the other hand:

(a) in neutral the TPs of L2 are level or that on the left is rather more posterior than that of L3 (the same as above),

(b) in flexion the asymmetry disappears,

(c) in extension the left TP becomes more posterior,

the inference is that the right facet joint at L2–3 will not close (extend). This indicates that there will be loss of right rotation and sidebending but this time loss of extension at the L2–3 joint or it is flexed, rotated and sidebent to the left, *FRSlt at L2*. See Fig. 5.1.

Fig. 5.1 Diagram to show facet motion. In column 1 the spine is in neutral. In column 2 it is forward bent. In column 3 it is extended. In line A there is restriction of flexion at the left facet joint which automatically causes left sidebending and rotation at that segment when flexion is attempted. In line B the restriction is in extension and on the right side, also causing left sidebending and rotation but this time when the segment is extended.

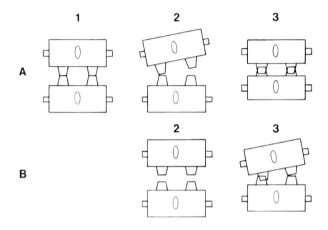

If:

(a) in neutral the TP of L2 is prominent on the right,

(b) the rotation may vary a little but is present in both flexion and extension,

(c) there is also rotation to the right at L1 and L3 but not at L4,

the inference is that there is a neutral group dysfunction centred at L2, sidebent left and rotated right or *NRrt* (Neutral, Rotated right).

If there is rotational asymmetry which does not change on flexion or extension but this does not appear to be a group of three or more vertebrae, there are three other possibilities;

(a) structural asymmetry,

(b) a congenital (or other) fusion,

(c) a bilateral dysfunction at the same joint with the facet joint on one side restricted in flexion and that on the other side in extension.

None of these can be regarded as rarities. Asymmetry is common and, in certain areas, the rule rather than the exception. The sacroiliac joint is an example; the auricular surface on one side is rarely, if ever, the same shape as that on the other side and this may in part account for the complexity of the dysfunctions found in the pelvis.

If a spinal joint has restricted flexion on one side (ERS) and restricted extension on the other side (FRS) there will be rotation and sidebending to the side of the ERS lesion but there may be no detectable flexion or extension movement and the rotation will not change when flexion or extension are introduced to that region of the spine.

Intervertebral fusion of any type will show on X-rays and, unless complicated by a neighbouring joint dysfunction, will not be accompanied by tissue texture changes.

Structural asymmetry can be distinguished by examining for flexion and extension at the interspinous interval. This motion will be normal in a joint where the asymmetry is structural but will be absent or much restricted if there is bilateral facet joint dysfunction, one flexed and the other extended.

2. Dynamic examination

This is most useful in the upper third of the thoracic spine but can be used lower if needed. It is normally done with the patient sitting on a stool or with her legs over the side of the examination table. It is important to see that the patient's feet are supported in case she is asked to bend forwards to the point where she might otherwise overbalance.

The examination can be performed actively by the patient initiating the movement, or passively when the operator does both the moving and the examination. The former is easier for the operator and is used unless the patient finds it difficult to understand or seems unable to follow the instructions. It is important that the flexion is performed as a segmental motion, curling down from the top, rather than a regional flexion.

When using the dynamic method it will sometimes be found easier to observe the upward motion of the TP and sometimes the forward motion (which makes the TP less prominent). These observations give the same information, if the TP on one side moves up, it is also moving forwards and vice versa. The starting posture is very important as any deviation from flexion/extension neutral will be reflected in the amount of movement available in the other planes. An easy way to get the patient to assume the neutral position when examining the thoracic spine is to ask her to 'sit up tall'. It is also important to make sure that the barrier has not already been passed in the starting position, that is, for a restriction of extension, the motion must be started from a point where the joint is free in flexion. In this region it is also helpful to make sure that the lower thoracic and lumbar joints are extended before assessing extension in the upper thoracic spine.

Active examination

The operator places his thumbs (fingers may be used if desired) over the TPs of the vertebra to be tested with the patient in neutral. The patient is then instructed to bend her head (or for lower down, head and shoulders) forwards and the relative motion of the TPs is observed. Abnormal motion is shown by the TP on one side rising and becoming less easy to feel while the other remains low and prominent (Fig. 5.2a–c).

The third observation is made by asking the patient to bend backwards. The relative motion is again noted; an abnormality this time would be a failure of one TP to descend and become prominent. Even in the upper thoracic spine it is often not enough for the patient simply to extend her

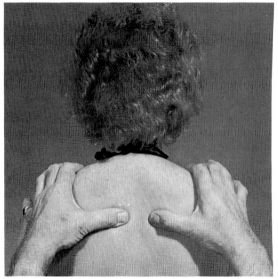

a

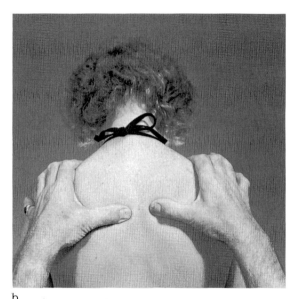

b

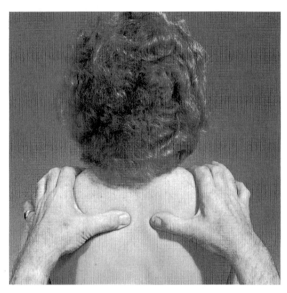

c

Fig. 5.2 Dynamic examination of upper thoracic spine asymmetry. (a) In neutral; (b) in flexion, the right thumb has moved up but the left has not, indicating restricted flexion on the left side; (c) in extension, the thumbs remain level. Either there is no restriction of extension or bilateral restriction.

neck. If extension from below is omitted the asymmetry may easily be missed. The necessary translation can be achieved by having her push her stomach forwards and bring her head back with her chin tucked in (extension of the neck on the thorax is required, not extension of the head on the neck). These observations are all made with reference to the next lower vertebra.

Passive examination

The operator uses the index and middle fingers of one hand to perform the examination while, with his other hand on her head, he controls the position of the upper spine. The finger tips should be one on the tip of each of the TPs of the vertebra being examined. Forward flexion from below can be produced by asking the patient to allow herself to slump. Extension from below is dependent on the patient's cooperation in pushing her stomach forwards when requested to do so. As in the active examination it is important to start from neutral. The active method is preferred because the operator can more easily concentrate on what he is feeling and thumbs are usually better than fingers for depth perception.

Interpretation

If the observation is of rotation of the vertebra, that is of which TP becomes the more anterior (or posterior), the argument is the same as in the static method of examination. If motion is being observed it is easy to see which is the restricted joint. If the restriction is of flexion (the joint is extended) the restriction of sidebending will be to the opposite (mobile) side because an extended joint causes sidebending to that side. For example, if it is the right facet joint that is extended, the segment will not sidebend to the left and it will be said to be ERSrt. If, on the other hand, the joint is flexed (with restriction of extension) the loss of sidebending is to restricted side. If it is the right facet joint that is flexed the segment cannot sidebend to the right and is said to be FRSlt.

Cervical

Static examination is difficult in the cervical spine and motion is used, chiefly by translation, because it introduces the movement from both above and below at the same time. *Translation to the left causes sidebending to the right and translation forwards causes extension etc.*

Although classed as a cervical joint, that between C7 and T1 is often more easily examined by the dynamic method described for the thoracic spine. Sometimes the joint between C6 and 7 is also more easily examined in this manner.

Typical cervical joints

The patient lies supine with her head close to the end of the table and the operator sits, kneels or stoops at her head. If the patient is unable to lie supine, the examination is done sitting. It is more difficult but can be done and it helps if the seat is low or if the operator stands on a stool. The examination is performed separately at each level indicated by alternately pushing on the lateral mass (articular pillar) of one vertebra, first in one direction (say left to right) then in the other (right to left). The indicated levels in the neck are most easily found by palpating for tissue texture change around the joints. For those whose fingers have not yet achieved the required sensitivity it is as well to examine each of the six joints in turn.

Examination

1. The patient is supine with the operator sitting at her head. If necessary the examination can be done kneeling; standing stooped over is not usually as satisfactory. The patient must be relaxed as is necessary for all motion testing.

2. The transverse process of C1 is easily felt on each side and the operator places his hand as in Fig. 5.3, with one finger in contact with the lateral mass of each vertebra from C2 to C5 inclusive. By light palpation around the lateral masses, it is usually possible to identify, by tissue texture changes, those levels that require detailed testing. If this is uncertain, it is better to test each level in turn.

Fig. 5.3 Four finger examination of cervical spine.

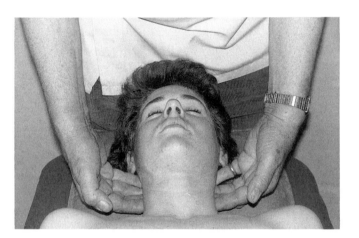

3. At one level at a time the vertebra is gently pushed sideways, into translation, first to one side then to the other. It is often easier to assess motion if the index fingers are used alone for that purpose (Fig. 5.4), moving them to the segment to be examined after the level has been identified with the four fingers as shown above. To make the diagnosis,

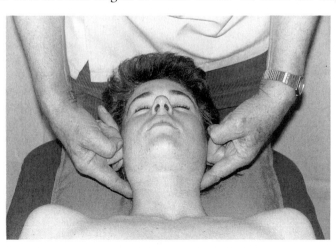

Fig. 5.4 Using index fingers for localisation in cervical spine.

the examination must be done in both flexion and extension although it is not necessary to go as far as the flexion or extension barrier. This is repeated at each indicated level. Some operators prefer to start in the mid position but there is no true neutral in the cervical joints.

Interpretation

If loss of translation to the RIGHT is found, there is restriction of LEFT sidebending at the joint between that vertebra and the one below.

If the restriction of sidebending is more marked in extension the segment has restricted extension and is said to be flexed; in the usual notation this would be FRS. If the restriction of translation is more marked in flexion, the joint is said to be extended or ERS.

Thus if a segment is found with restriction of translation to the left most marked in extension, it is said to be FRSlt because it is found in the flexed and left sidebent/rotated position. The restriction in this instance is at the right facet joint which will not close.

Similarly, if a segment is found with restriction of left translation more marked in flexion, it is extended, rotated and sidebent to the left (ERSlt), but this time the restriction is at the left facet joint which will not open.

Notes

1. The authors recognise that some operators are taught to use a notation that describes the lesion in terms of the joint that does not move. These different notations are very poor bedfellows. Any attempt to mix them, or to use both, leads to serious confusion and although both have been given so far, from this point on the FRS and ERS notation will be used almost exclusively for spinal joints.

2. Motion of the individual joints in this region can be tested sitting, the operator monitoring with the fingers of one hand while the other controls the patient's head (Fig. 5.5). This is easiest for flexion-extension

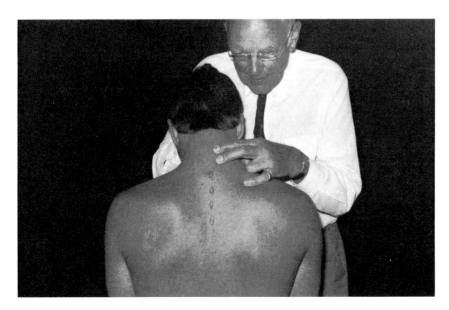

Fig. 5.5 Testing sagittal mobility in the cervical spine.

testing. For the typical cervical joints (C2–T1) most experienced operators prefer to have the patient supine and to test for sidebending by translation, rather than for rotation or flexion-extension. Testing for those
who are unable to lie supine can be done sitting with the operator standing behind supporting her back. Translation can be tested in this position
but it is less easy than in the supine position.

The occipitoatlantal (OA) and atlantoaxial (C1–2) joints

These two joints work as a complex with a wide range of flexion-extension at the OA and of rotation at C1–2. There are minor movements
also in both joints. In the OA there are a few degrees of sidebending
associated with a small range of rotation in the opposite direction. At the
C1–2 joint there is about 5° of sidebend[2] and the biconvex shape of the
facets causes a small range of superior to inferior (craniad to caudad) translation. The latter is of no importance in diagnosis or treatment but the
associated motions of the OA joint are used in both.

Examination of the atlantoaxial joint
  1. The patient is supine and the operator at her head, either sitting,
standing or kneeling.
  2. In order to localise the rotation as much as possible to the C1–2
level, in accordance with Fryette's third concept of spinal motion, the
operator flexes her neck as far as it easily goes. Forced flexion is not
required and it should be emphasised that the flexion is of the neck, not
of the head on the neck.
  3. With the patient relaxed the head is turned passively first to one
side, then to the other while monitoring with the index or middle
fingers at the C1–2 level on each side; the movement must be stopped
just before C2 begins to move. The normal range is more than 45° to
each side, of which probably only 30° to 35° takes place at the C1–2
joint itself[3]. The flexed position must be maintained during the rotation
or movement will occur at other joints and the examination will be
inaccurate. The range should be symmetrical. (Fig. 5.6a and b).

Examination of the occipitoatlantal joint
There are two different methods used; the first, which is easier to interpret and is usually the only one required, is by translation sideways in
flexion and in extension. The second, useful to confirm a doubtful
finding, is by anterior and posterior translation of the skull in 30° rotation
first to one side and then to the other.

  1. By side to side translation.
  1.1. The patient is supine and must be relaxed; the operator is at her
head, preferably sitting or kneeling.
  1.2. He cradles her head in his hands and lifts it a short distance off
the table. His index fingers are placed so that they can monitor motion
at the OA joint on each side but without pressing on the occipitoatlantal
membrane.

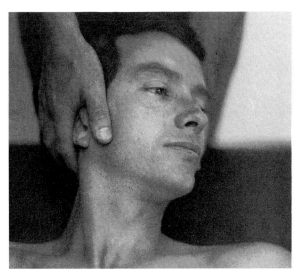

Fig. 5.6a and b Examination of motion at C1 by rotation.

a

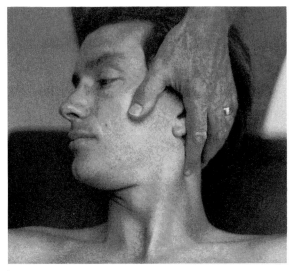

b

1.3. The operator introduces flexion at the OA joint by 'rolling the ball' around an imaginary axis through the external auditory meatus. This motion need not be taken to the barrier and extreme flexion is not required. With her head flexed, the operator translates it to one side, keeping the midline of the head parallel to that of the body. The distance between the midline of the head and that of the body is noted and the head then translated to the other side. The distance that the midline of the head moves should be symmetrical (Fig. 5.7a and b).

1.4. The 'ball' is then rolled into extension around the same axis and the examination repeated (Fig. 5.8a and b). Extreme extension is not needed, and it is as well to remember that the position of full extension

Fig. 5.7a and b Examination of motion at the occipitoatlantal joint by translation in flexion.

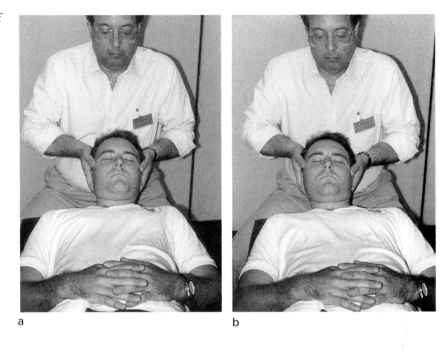

a   b

Fig. 5.8a and b Examination of motion at the occipitoatlantal joint by translation in extension.

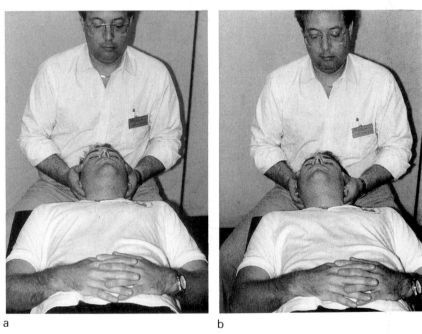

a   b

of the head on the neck is that which has been associated with development of stroke when combined with rotation. In some patients there will be restriction in both flexion and extension. The position with the greatest restriction is treated first and the joint reexamined; if restriction remains treatment is given in the other sagittal plane position.

Because restriction of sidebending in the typical joints can give a false positive when testing translation of the skull on C1, it is usual to examine and treat the lower joints first.

2. By anteroposterior translation.

2.1. The patient is supine and must be relaxed; the operator is at her head, either sitting or kneeling.

2.2. He cradles her head in his hands, lifts it off the table and turns it 30° to the right. This aligns the right facets of the occipitoatlantal joint so that they are nearly perpendicular to the table. The motion test is then performed by translating her head upwards (anteriorly) and downwards (posteriorly) thus sliding one facet on the other (Fig. 5.9a and b).

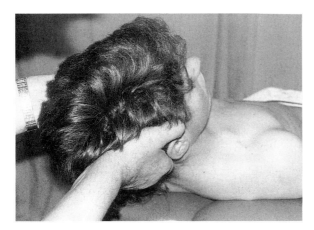

Fig. 5.9 A–P translation test for motion at the right facet of the OA joint. (a) Anterior translation; (b) posterior translation.

a

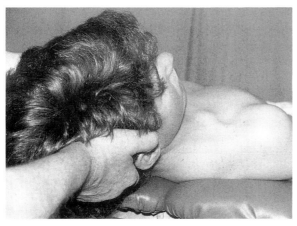

b

2.3. The head is then turned to 30° to the left of the mid position and the test repeated on that side. The amount of movement is normally symmetrical; the side with smaller range is the restricted side.

Interpretation

The interpretation of the standard method is similar to that of the translatory examination of the typical cervical joints.

(a) If there is restricted translation of the head to the right there is limitation of left sidebending at the OA joint, assuming that the lower cervical joints are mobile.

(b) If the restriction is more marked in the extended position, there is restriction of extension, written as *F*(flexed), *Rlt*(rotated left), *Srt*(sidebent right) or more simply *FSrt*.

(c) If the restriction is more in flexion of the head, there is restriction of flexion at the OA joint, written *E*(extended), *RltSrt* or *ESrt*.

(d) If on testing anteroposterior translation of the 30° rotated head there is restriction of anterior translation on the right, the indication is that the right facet of the occiput will not slide fully forward on the atlas; this signifies restriction of extension and of rotation to the left (NOT of flexion as in upward and forward sliding of intervertebral facets). Rotation and sidebending at the OA joint are to opposite sides and there is, therefore, restriction of right sidebending. This corresponds to restriction of left translation in the head extended position or *FRrtSlt* or *FSlt*.

(e) If there is restriction of posterior translation of the occiput on the atlas on the right, it means that the head will not fully flex or rotate to the right. This, in turn, means that there is restriction of left sidebending. This corresponds to restriction of translation to the right in the head flexed position, *ERltSrt* or *ESrt*.

(f) If the restriction is on the left side the inferences are the same with reversal of the side.

REFERENCES

1. Fryette, H.H. (1954). *The Principles of Osteopathic Technique*. Carmel: Academy of Applied Osteopathy.
2. Kapandji I.A. (1978). *The Physiology of the Joints*. Vol. 3, p. 184. London: Churchill Livingstone.
3. Penning L. (1968). *Functional Pathology of the Cervical Spine*. Amsterdam: Excerpta Medica.

Chapter 6

Manipulation

There is still disagreement as to the breadth of the meaning of the word manipulation. In Europe the term is used, in this context, almost solely for procedures involving a high velocity, low amplitude, thrusting movement. In North America it is used in a much wider sense, to include any active or passive movement initiated, assisted or resisted by the operator. This includes treatments sometimes listed as articulation, mobilisation, isometric and isotonic techniques, myofascial, functional or indirect and even craniosacral techniques.

In order to help resolve this difficulty the International Federation of Manual Medicine (FIMM) held a terminology workshop at Fischingen in 1983, following which the term 'mobilisation with impulse' was proposed for what is here called thrusting. 'Mobilisation without impulse' was proposed for the treatments that are here included under the heading 'manipulation' but which do not have a component of operator thrusting. These terms are somewhat cumbersome and in this edition the authors will use the term manipulation in the wide sense, as defined in the *Oxford English Dictionary*[1].

The phrase 'high velocity, low amplitude' is thought to have led some practitioners to emphasise the velocity too much and the simple word 'thrust' is becoming the preferred term. It is still important that the thrust is of high velocity, however small the amplitude because, if it is done slowly, the muscles will have time to tighten and prevent the movement. In this edition the term muscle energy will be used to cover those techniques which involve patient participation usually associated with operator resistance. It will include what in earlier editions had been called isometric, many of the techniques are indeed fully or in part isometric, but some use isotonic contraction in addition or instead. Some will also employ respiratory assistance from the patient and in some the operator may assist as well as resisting.

TYPES OF MANIPULATION

Many different techniques have been used to remove or alter the restrictive barrier and its associated tissue texture abnormalities. In the early editions of this book only high velocity techniques were described and of these some were quite non-specific. The non- and semi-specific techniques are omitted altogether from this edition. The semi-specific ones were retained in the fourth edition in the expectation that they would be a help to beginners. Further experience with teaching suggests that they are more confusing than helpful and are therefore better omitted.

Manipulative techniques may be direct or indirect. Direct techniques are those in which the barrier is located and directly addressed. High velocity and muscle energy treatments are both direct in type. The term indirect is used for techniques in which the joint is taken away from the barrier, usually localising at the point of maximum ease in the available range. The various functional techniques are all indirect. Combined techniques also exist in which some aspects are direct and some indirect.

A third class are known as exaggeration techniques. In these the joint is moved away from the dysfunctional barrier up to the opposite end of its normal range and a thrust is applied toward the normal end. Maigne[2] developed his own variety of this method in France and has many disciples, his belief is that the thrust should only be in the painless direction.

Mobilising forces

A variety of forces can be brought to bear on the joint to perform whatever treatment is needed. These are broadly classified as extrinsic or intrinsic. Extrinsic forces are those used when the operator does the work, as in thrusting, or when gravity or some mechanical apparatus is employed. Intrinsic forces are those generated by the patient whether by pushing or by breathing and also include the natural tendency of the body to correct itself when that is possible. Muscle energy treatment is regarded as using intrinsic force because the patient generates and is able to control the degree of force used, even if the operator must use an equal and opposite force to produce the desired effect.

Thrusting manipulation using extrinsic force was the standby of manual medicine practitioners for more than a century. It is probable that often these were only semi-specific techniques but they helped patients enough to justify research to improve and develop them. There are many reasons to look for other types of manipulation. In the first place thrusting is clearly unsuitable for certain classes of patient who still need help. Secondly thrusting is not always painless, although the more accurate the localisation and the less the force used the less unpleasant it is. Thirdly, thrusting is not entirely without disadvantage and occasional hazard, in particular to the vertebro-basilar circulation. In recent years a significant number of vascular accidents have occurred involving the upper neck. It was originally thought that these were due to obstruction of and injury to the vertebral arteries by high velocity manipulation and certainly some of them have happened at the moment of such a treatment. Recent evidence suggests that the problem is often one of intimal tear with development of a dissecting aneurysm, and it appears that this can happen even without any external force. Cases have been recorded in which the accident happened when the patient had merely held the neck in full extension with the head fully rotated to one side, without even being touched by another person.

The first sign of cerebral vascular insufficiency is anxiety. This symptom will appear before the onset of nystagmus and it is recommended that if a patient having examination or treatment to the neck becomes anxious, the manoeuvre should immediately be stopped and the situation reassessed before any similar position is again adopted. The problem is discussed in more detail in Chapter 12.

Types of technique

It was a wise man who said that 'If all you have in your tool box is a hammer, it is funny how many things look like nails.'

High velocity thrusting can be used to treat most dysfunctions if necessary. Until Dr Mitchell's work became known thrusting was all that was available to many practitioners in the field including one of the authors (JFB). Techniques which allow the patient to gauge the force applied have obvious advantages in those who have weakened bone from old age, osteoporosis or disease. An effective treatment other than thrust is highly desirable in the patient with a very acute condition in whom thrust could cause severe pain.

It has been shown that even such a simple injury as an ankle sprain materially increases energy expenditure and alleviation of skeletal dysfunctions may be of great value in those who are sick. Thrusting, on the other hand, would be out of place and even muscle energy techniques might require more effort than the sick person should do.

There are a variety of other methods. The oldest is probably what is now classed as soft tissue technique and can be regarded in part as an extension of physiotherapeutic massage and movement treatments. Before the Second World War physiotherapists were expert at massage but regrettably the advent of the electrical machine has changed that and many of the old techniques are either not taught or not practised.

Mobilisation is an extension of soft tissue technique and will be briefly described.

Muscle energy is now the most used method by many operators and is convenient and widely applicable but even the effort required for this treatment may be contraindicated in, for instance, those with congestive heart failure, even if they might stand to gain by reduction of unnecessary energy expenditure.

Functional or indirect techniques are relative newcomers with great promise. Myofascial techniques, which are even more recent, combine aspects of soft tissue, indirect and even craniosacral techniques and are applicable to situations where more orthodox treatment will sometimes fail. Neither of these puts any significant strain on the patient's cardiovascular system although the very gentle nature of the indirect techniques contrasts strongly with the physical handling of the patient by the operator in the myofascial variety.

Craniosacral techniques address primarily dysfunctions of the joints between the bones of the skull. It is surprising how widespread the changes can be if motion is restored to sutures which have lost their ability to move.

SOFT TISSUE TECHNIQUES

All somatic dysfunctions have a soft tissue component and in some it may be very important. In many patients correction of the skeletal component will allow the soft tissues to return to normal but, if they do not, the soft tissue abnormality may bring back a skeletal dysfunction that had been successfully treated. The local tissue texture alteration at the joint that helps with diagnosis is not usually the one that needs its own treatment, rather it is the secondary areas of change, often in peripheral or superficial muscle. Soft tissue techniques can be applied to skin and subcutaneous tissue and to deeper structures. They have a range of effects which include muscle and other tissue stretching, relief of oedema, toning of circulation etc. They may be used to 'tidy up' after a skeletal treatment or as preparation. To have the soft tissues relaxed certainly makes skeletal treatment easier.

One of the popular treatments for the superficial tissues is skin rolling. This can be used in both diagnosis and treatment because the palpable changes are maximal at the level of the causative joint dysfunction, allowing its level to be determined accurately. Used as a treatment, the area should first be rolled to find the abnormalities and those areas treated repeatedly until either they become normal or there is no further change. The technique for skin rolling was described under 'Scanning examination' in Chapter 3. After the skin rolling has been done it is wise always to check to see if there is a skeletal cause hiding under the area.

Muscles and their associated fascia can be treated by stretching either longitudinally or transversely or by deep pressure. These are perhaps the most commonly used techniques and, for instance, they can be very helpful when there is superficial muscle tightness associated with an intervertebral dysfunction. Stretching longitudinally can be direct, by traction or less direct by separating the origin and insertion of the muscle by sidebending, flexion etc. Techniques are described in Chapter 14. Traction can be localised to some extent in the neck with the patient supine. The operator can use his finger tips deeply in the muscles posterolaterally or on the articular pillars themselves to put the traction principally at one level. Elsewhere this is not so easy. Sidebending with or without sagittal plane positioning can also be used in the neck and may be combined with traction.

In the trunk lateral stretch is easier and can be done from either side. If the operator is on the side to be treated he pulls on the medial edge of the muscle mass with his finger tips. If from the opposite side he can push either with the heel of his hand or with the thumb and thenar eminence of one or both hands. The technique requires the application of steady pressure with the fingers or hand on the medial edge of the muscle and the hand must not be allowed to slip off the muscle mass so that only the skin is stretched. The stretch is continued until no further improvement is obtained or until the muscles are normally relaxed. Lateral stretch is also applicable to the cervical region where it can be done with the tips of the fingers of one hand while the other is used to steady the head and apply a counterforce.

Deep pressure can be used to persuade muscles to relax. The pressure may be quite painful, which does not help the patient to relax while it is being done, but the results can be good. This form of soft tissue treatment comes very close to some of the myofascial techniques described below, although the latter are more demanding in palpatory skill and are not usually worse than uncomfortable.

Deep pressure treatment can be done with the thumbs or, particularly in the occipital region, with the finger tips. Either tend to become quite uncomfortable for the operator especially if he has several patients needing the treatment in one session. For the long standing changes sometimes seen in the buttock muscles some practitioners even dig in deeply with the point of an elbow! This treatment was modified into her own system by Dr Ida Rolf.

Deep pressure is valuable in the suboccipital muscles and here is a part of the craniosacral treatment of occipital decompression. In many patients complaining of headache palpation of the suboccipital muscles with the patient supine will reveal areas which may be so tight that at first they feel almost like bone. The operator aligns the tips of his index and middle fingers of each hand so that they support the weight of the head in the area of the short posterior muscles, about 2.5 cm (1 inch) below the superior nuchal line. It is not difficult to feel which part of the muscle is most tense and the finger tip under that part should be advanced so that it is the principal support of the weight of the head. Within 30–90 seconds the muscles will begin to relax; it feels as if they were melting. As they relax it may be found that there is another area nearby that also needs attention but it is usual to be able to complete the treatment in about 90 seconds. It is always uncomfortable although often considered a 'good' hurt by the patient; reproduction of the usual headache is not uncommon. This should not be used alone except as emergency treatment, there will always be some other dysfunction needing to be addressed in the neck and often in the thoracic spine also. Similarly for a patient complaining of headache it is always wise to examine the suboccipital muscles in addition to whatever is done to the cervical and upper thoracic spine.

Muscle energy procedures can also be used as soft tissue treatment; isometric contraction of a tight muscle followed by stretching, which may be a simple taking up of the slack after the patient relaxes, will often relieve hypertonus and if the antagonists need strengthening that can be done by isometric or isotonic contractions. In this connection it is wise to stretch the tight tissues before attempting to strengthen the weak ones.

Spray and stretch is another method of treating hypertonic muscle. This was described originally by Travell for the true trigger point. The true trigger point is of great importance and should be looked for in any patient who is making less progress than expected. The cold spray and stretching will also help areas of muscle hypertonus that do not fit Travell's definition; it can be used for any such area and is particularly useful in patients in whom the area is so painful that other soft tissue treatments are difficult or impossible. Similarly, soft tissue treatments can be used for the true trigger points instead of the spray.

The techniques for the upper body are described in detail by Travell and Simons[3]. The cold spray is designed to chill, lightly, the skin over the hypertonic muscle; this results in relaxation, allowing the stretch. The muscle itself should NOT be chilled; cold muscle will tend to start shivering with recurrence of the hypertonus.

For the trigger points that do not respond well to spray and stretch, and those that are too acute to allow muscle energy treatment, injection of local anaesthetic is a valuable measure. The most important details are:

1. Use plain local anaesthetic, no adrenalin and no steroid.
2. ½ or 1% is strong enough.
3. Care is needed that the actual trigger point is not missed.
4. The muscle should be gently stretched after the injection.

Articulation or mobilisation

The articulatory techniques are direct in that they address the restrictive barrier. The techniques are based on the finding that if the joint is moved up to the barrier and the barrier is lightly 'teased', there will be a tendency for it to move away. The movement is repeated as long as there is gain. This procedure is painless; the operator must not push into the barrier. Not only is that painful but it can actually cause increased hypertonus. It should be remembered that the barrier is not a single point. It is more a curved plane and the object is to come up to part of that plane, move along it and then away again.

There are competent manipulators, well skilled in high velocity and muscle energy treatments who regularly start treating their patients with articulation and report that often that is all that they need to do in order to restore motion and relieve muscle spasm.

Detailed descriptions of articulatory technique can be found in a number of texts[4,5.]

Muscle energy techniques

The original concept of the bone setters was that a bone was out of place. It is remarkable how proficient some of them became at helping patients with their hands. The concept that muscle might be more important than actual position of bones in the production and maintenance of the symptoms seems only to have been seriously considered since the Second World War, although muscle had previously been treated incidentally by many practitioners.

The 'muscle energy' treatment, as we know it, was the brainchild of the late Dr Fred L. Mitchell Sr., DO and it is reported that his interest in this approach was partly based on work done by another osteopathic physician, Dr T.J. Ruddy, DO, who developed a contract–relax method of treating some of the conditions that he saw in his ophthalmological practice. Mitchell not only worked out the system of treatment but he also made a detailed study of anatomy, especially of the pelvis. His description of the mechanics of the pelvis has been developed by those who learned from him into the classification used in this book. Like so many innovators, when he first described his ideas they were not well received. Finally at about the time he was ready to give up trying, he taught a small group who became enthusiastic disciples, from three of whom the authors have had the privilege of learning.

Muscle energy treatments are classified as direct because the joint is taken up to the barrier. For the techniques to be effective the barrier must just be engaged and in all three planes. If the barrier has not been reached the effect is less and if the joint has been pushed into the barrier there may be no benefit at all. The techniques demand a fair degree of palpatory skill and beginners almost invariably fail to stop at the barrier but instead 'mash' into it with poor result. It is not uncommon in a basic class to see that, when treating the cervical spine supine, the trainee operator will think that he still has not reached the barrier when the amount of sidebending introduced has taken the localisation into the thoracic region!

The majority of muscle energy procedures are isometric but some are isotonic and other forces may be brought into play of which one of the most important is respiration. The physiological principles upon which muscle energy technique rests are post-isometric relaxation and reciprocal inhibition.

The direction of the patient effort is important. It must be away from the barrier. As has been said more than once, the barrier has to be found in all three planes; the patient may push away in any of these planes but, as the operator must prevent motion taking place, some directions are easier than others. As a general rule rotation is best avoided as being the most difficult for the operator to control. The effort may be sidebending, or whichever is appropriate of flexion or extension, or a resultant of the sagittal and coronal plane directions. Occasionally rotation is used and in some techniques the operator may use first one direction and then another. It is always worth trying a different direction if the first does not produce the desired result.

In order to make a contraction isometric, movement must be blocked. Many patients and physicians have tried to use these techniques on themselves but it is difficult both to attempt to move a joint and with some other part to prevent that movement. Prevention of movement in isometric contraction is done by the operator and he may have to warn the patient not to push too hard as otherwise he may be unable to prevent motion. Hard contraction is not only difficult for the operator, it is also less effective. The reason for this is that the muscles which are to be treated are small, many no thicker than a lead pencil, and they are only capable of generating a light force. If more force is used accessory muscles are recruited and the effect on the primary ones is diluted.

When treating isometrically the contraction should be maintained for a finite period; 3–5 seconds is the time usually advised. After the first period of contraction the patient is asked to relax and many will do no more than stop pushing. This is not the same thing. Before the second contraction effort by the patient the joint must be taken to the new barrier in all three planes and this cannot be found accurately if the patient is not relaxed. The instruction 'let go' is often effective or the patient may be asked a second time to relax fully. When relaxation has been secured, *and not before*, the joint is taken to the new barrier in all three planes and the contraction repeated. This is done three or more times in all; more is only useful if motion is still being gained. It is important at the end of a muscle energy treatment to re-examine the part to find if the treatment has been effective. It is not likely that there will be any audible sign of movement as often happens with high velocity treatment.

There are a number of muscle energy techniques in which the treatment is designed to cause movement of the joint. These, therefore, are not isometric and the majority are classed as isotonic. Occasionally a technique may be used in which a maximal effort by the patient is overcome by the operator; these have become known as 'isolytic' although purists would question the derivation of the word.

When used for treatment of the axial skeleton and pelvis, isotonic techniques are often combined with respiratory assistance, operator guiding and patient positioning to produce the desired effect. The method used is similar to the isometric techniques, with the difference that when the patient is positioned at the barrier it is so arranged that her attempt to push away against the operator's resistance causes motion at the dysfunctional joint. This is clearly seen in the treatment for inhalation restriction of ribs (Chapter 10). After the contraction has continued for 3–5 seconds, as in isometric methods, the patient is asked to relax. When relaxation is complete the operator takes up the slack to the new barrier in all three planes, and the procedure is repeated two or more times depending on response. Many of the techniques to be described utilise both isotonic and isometric principles.

High velocity thrusting

The term 'high velocity' in manual medicine is not complete unless followed by the rest of the description, which is 'low amplitude'. Mennell[6] in his description of joint play techniques describes the amplitude as 'less than an eighth of an inch at the joint', that restriction applies to almost any joint movement. The use of the lever principle to make this easier is discussed under the heading *Localisation of force* in this chapter. Once again it must be emphasised that we are not reducing a dislocation or subluxation, there is no 'little bone out of place' and the goal of the treatment is to restore, in the words of the workshop on terminology at Fischingen referred to above[7],

> . . . maximal pain-free movement of the musculoskeletal system in postural balance.

The feeling shared by some patients and some operators that if there is no noise nothing has happened is quite incorrect. The successful treatment of FRS dysfunctions, where the dysfunctional joint is being 'closed', is usually silent. Facet opening thrusts are more likely to be accompanied by a pop or other sound. The object is not simply to gap the joint, which could be noisy, it is to restore a normal range of gliding movement either by enabling the facets to open (flexion) or to close (extension). Dr Paul Kimberly, DO, FAAO used to say that ideally a (thrusting) manipulation should be noiseless and painless. It is important to remember that there is an anatomical barrier which, by definition, is the final limit of available motion in that joint. A thrust that forces the joint beyond the anatomical barrier will cause structural damage and the amplitude of the movement is as important as the amount of force. It is appropriate to compare the action of types of hammer. The steam hammer, with all its power but with its fine control, is a much easier tool than a hand hammer with which to break the glass of a watch without damaging the mechanism.

The present belief that the basic dysfunction being treated is of soft tissue rather than of joint or bone raises the question of what a high velocity treatment achieves. There is no doubt in the minds of the authors that such treatment can be very effective and sometimes seems to be the only really effective method. The concept that the basic need may be a reprogramming of the central computer (CNS) offers some help. It is believed that there is a short period of local proprioceptor silence following a high velocity treatment and this may bear some relation to the success of indirect treatment performed at the point of maximum ease (see the section on functional treatment).

High velocity treatment has been performed, often giving the patient relief, with scant attention paid to specificity; indeed there are at the present time operators using techniques that cannot even be described as semi-specific. Occasional accidents have occurred but, omitting the special case of the upper cervical spine, the majority appear to have been treated by manipulation incorrectly either because the diagnosis was in error or because the treatment was performed without accurate localisation. There is no total contraindication to treatment by thrusting manipulation other than hypermobility, provided that a proper diagnosis has been made and the force and amplitude used are suitable. If localisation is accurate, it will often be found that the joint moves on its own without any extra force. The better the localisation the less the force that will be needed.

Although the demands made on the operator's palpatory skill are greater, it is recommended that beginners should use muscle energy treatment until their ability to localise has developed.

Myofascial release techniques

Osteopathic physicians, especially in the United States, have found over the years that in addition to the orthopaedic and neuromuscular changes which can occur with manipulative therapy, in its widest sense, there are also more fundamental changes in the internal economy of the body. These are not limited to alterations in tone and function of structures segmentally related to the level treated. It has been found that when there are pre-existing pathological changes in the tissues, treatment by any form of manual intervention, in patients with apparently similar conditions, can be followed by changes which may be helpful or the reverse.

Physicians practising manual techniques find that, even when motion has been restored to the segment, there is often residual dysfunction which can be relieved by treating the soft tissues. Soft tissue treatments have been used for centuries by the physiotherapists and their predecessors who have found that release of soft tissue tensions will sometimes result in restoration of symmetry and motion to joints which at first appeared to need more direct mechanical treatment. Dr Robert C. Ward's[8] myofascial release approach is much more efficient than the classical physiotherapy treatments in this respect. The development of the various functional techniques has also given credence to the concept that the soft tissue changes are fundamental rather than secondary to the joint changes.

With this background and his observation of the work of many practitioners in the field, Dr Ward and others have developed techniques that address the soft tissues in ways that are based on their anatomical and physiological properties. Dr Ward is particularly interested in what he terms the 'tight–loose' phenomenon in soft tissues. This he ascribes to the complicated responses of an asymmetrical system to imposed asymmetrical loads. These are normal and self correcting unless the tissues are deformed beyond their innate ability to recover. Symptoms arise when the deformation persists and the tight–loose condition will be found if the soft tissues are carefully examined. To treat this with his myofascial techniques Dr Ward addresses the tissues with pressure applied with the hands in specific directions and continuously monitors the changes which take place, following 'releases' when they occur, or working against tight areas to produce release. A high degree of palpatory skill is required to make the necessary examination and monitor the tissue responses.

To those unfamiliar with this type of treatment the results may appear surprising. One of the authors (JFB) was present when Dr Ward was working in this manner on a fellow physician who, among other things, had a posterior subluxation of the third left rib. He did not at any time address the rib directly, treating only the trunk soft tissues and yet when the treatment was finished the rib position and function had returned to normal.

Once again the question is raised as to what the manual therapist is really doing. Is it in fact a means of addressing not just the musculoskeletal and neurological systems but rather a fundamental approach to the entire function of the body? If this is the case would it be better if the therapist approached primarily by functional, myofascial and cranial techniques rather than addressing the structure directly? Even if the answer to that question should prove to be affirmative, the necessity for the more mundane mechanical approach to the joints would be likely to remain because that does provide a means of developing palpatory skills while performing treatment helpful to the patient. It is appropriate at this point to say that while nearly anyone with adequate motivation can learn skill in palpation, it does come more easily to some than to others and it always requires patience and practice.

Functional techniques

The criterion that distinguishes functional techniques is that the segment being treated is taken away from the restrictive barrier towards the normal physiological barrier at the opposite end of the range of motion. In this they are different from thrusting or muscle energy techniques, or indeed articulation, all of which address the restrictive barrier directly.

Between the restrictive barrier and the opposite physiological barrier, there is a dynamic balance point (DBP) or point of maximum ease, which is the point reached when the joint is positioned so that the tensions in the soft tissues become balanced equally on either side. This must be done in all three planes in both translation and rotation, involving distraction or compression as well as the more usual movements. If motion in any plane is initiated away from the DBP, the soft tissue tension around the treated segment will rise and there will be an increased sense of palpatory bind.

Once the dynamic balance is reached, the operator has three treatment options:

1. *Position and hold.* In this method the segment being treated is maintained at the DBP for a period of usually 30–90 seconds.

2. *Operator active*, in which the operator initiates movement along the path of least resistance through the sequential releases of soft tissue tension which occur. An analogy would be that the segment is taken through a maze while the operator monitors the surrounding soft tissues to continue on the path of least resistance.

3. *Operator passive*, in which the operator passively follows the segmental unwinding through sequential releases of the segment being treated to the point of full soft tissue release, when the restrictive barrier is no longer detectable and normal motion is again possible.

With each of these three approaches, the end point should be normal motion of the segment being treated.

Another functional approach is the strain–counterstrain technique of Dr Larry Jones, DO, FAAO[9]. With this technique the operator monitors the Jones tender points while he positions the patient so that the tension at the monitor is at a minimum. The position is then held for 30–90 seconds, but the clinical end point is the same.

But how can techniques which are so gentle be so effective? It is postulated that, at the dynamic balance point, the afferent input from the proprioceptors (Golgi and Pacinian receptors, muscle spindles and mechanoreceptors) is 'shut down' and that this suppresses the local protective cord reflexes. This probably also changes reflex patterns of the cerebellar and cerebral cortices and thus changes and reprogrammes the software of the computer. At the dynamic balance point, fascial mechanical balance is also attained which would have a beneficial impact. On the other hand it has also been postulated that, with the operator active and operator passive techniques, the mechanoreceptors might be stimulated enough by the segmental movement to inhibit transmission of the pain impulses and by that means allow the paraspinal tissues to relax and the restrictive barrier to subside. Thus a multitude of possible mechanisms could be active with functional techniques. Some of these mechanisms previously have been labelled 'intrinsic' forces or factors.

Because of the time involved when utilising functional techniques, it is possible for dramatic physiological changes to occur, especially with chronic and complicated dysfunctional patterns. This probably occurs because the 'software' reflex patterns in the CNS can be altered as well by re-establishing normal physiological mechanical motion.

Thus functional techniques are indicated with acute traumatic injuries, chronic and complicated structural patterns, with acutely ill patients, with patients having osteoporosis, marked arthritic changes, spinal stenosis or disc pathology, and when it is necessary to rule out a mechanical component to the patient's pain pattern.

Functional techniques developed in the Osteopathic profession in the 1940s and 1950s under the guidance of Dr William G. Sutherland, DO, Drs Lippincott, Becker, Hoover, Johnston and Wales to name a few.

Dr Edward G. Stiles[10], while a student at the Kirksville College of Osteopathic Medicine in the early 1960s became interested in the unusual approach of Dr George Andrew Laughlin, DO, whose wife was a granddaughter of Dr A.T. Still. Although Dr Laughlin was not a member of the faculty, the success of his methods made him widely known and respected by patients from all over the mid west. He had some difficulty putting into words what he was doing but during three and a half years of observation, Dr Stiles became aware of the effectiveness of functional techniques which, in this case, were mainly operator passive and operator active techniques. Dr Stiles has recently started formal teaching of techniques of this type in the series of courses on Manual Medicine put on by the department of continuing medical education at Michigan State University College of Osteopathic Medicine.

The fact that the barrier is not directly addressed in these techniques might lead one to think that they are easier for those whose palpatory skills are not yet well developed. Unfortunately this is not so, indeed they require more palpatory skill than most. Finding and following the moving point of ease (DBP) is not simple even in one plane. In order to make the techniques work it must be followed in all degrees of freedom. Flexion or extension and sidebending are not enough. Rotation and translation in the antero-posterior (sagittal), coronal and transverse planes (long axis extension or compression), as well as the phase of respiration must be adjusted; in all there are seven degrees of freedom, all of which must be taken as their 'point of maximum ease' in order to reach the DBP.

One of the important uses of functional techniques is for the patient with a dysfunction so acute that no other treatment can be tolerated. As a concrete example, a former patient of one of the authors returned in great distress after a major upset with one of her superiors at work. She was totally rigid in her cervical spine and any attempt to position her for muscle energy treatment caused much too much pain. With her supine, the principal level was determined by the site of the maximum tissue tension and a simple attempt was made to hold that joint at the point of ease in all degrees of freedom. To the surprise of both patient and operator, within about 60 seconds she had relaxed, movement had returned to her neck and the pain had gone.

Craniosacral manipulation

That the skull was immobile has long been believed by the large majority of the orthodox medical profession. That there might be some reason for the maintenance of open suture lines into old age did not seem to influence that opinion. When Dr William G. Sutherland, DO started talking about his ideas in the osteopathic profession in 1932 he met with a similar response from his DO colleagues. In spite of his results with patients and the requests by individual physicians for instruction, it was not until about 1940 that he obtained academic recognition of any kind. Since then recognition has grown steadily and many different varieties of cranial treatment are now taught.

Sutherland's interest had been kindled in 1899 by studying the disarticulated skull when a student at the American School of Osteopathy as it was then called, now the Kirksville College of Osteopathic Medicine. He could not understand the suture anatomy in terms of immobility. After much studying and experimenting on himself and others he came up with concepts that have become the basis of this form of treatment[11].

The practical introduction experienced by one of the authors was convincing to a man who had only heard about it before. He was having his neck treated by the Dr Edward G. Stiles mentioned above when, in the course of the treatment, he put his hands lightly on the sides of the author's skull. The author felt apparent rhythmical motion and remarked on it. Dr Stiles suggested that it should be counted and it proved to be of the order of 10 oscillations a minute, quite different from pulse or respiration.

The motion, in the normal, is a rhythmical expansion and contraction of the transverse diameter of the skull, and an associated decrease and increase respectively in the vertical diameter. All the bones of the skull take part in the motion including those of the face and motion is also transmitted to the sacrum by the relatively rigid tube of dura mater. This is the reason for the name craniosacral. The normal rate of oscillation is 8–12 cycles per minute. In some states of disease, especially disease associated with coma, the rate may be either greater or less[12]. For descriptive purposes the movements are named starting at the sphenobasilar junction; this was regarded by Sutherland as the primary motion of the skull. In childhood the sphenobasilar junction is a synchondrosis but by age 25 is fused by bone[13]. As will be seen in the description of rib dysfunctions, living bone must be considered to be to some extent plastic and malleable, unlike the hard unyielding substance we see in the classroom. The mechanism is of flexion of the sphenoid on the occiput such that the angle formed inferior to the bones becomes less obtuse, the range of motion is small. There is also a torsional movement between the sphenoid and the occipital bone. Both movements involve the rest of the skull bones, even including the face.

When the sphenobasilar junction flexes, both sphenoid and ethmoid bones rotate about transverse axes, but in opposite senses. The anterior end of the sphenoid (and the posterior end of the ethmoid) become inferior and the anterior part of the ethmoid becomes superior. The occiput rotates so that the posterior part becomes more inferior, and the temporal bones are pushed into what is known as external rotation, with the tips of the mastoid processes becoming closer together and the squamous portions further apart. At the same time the temporals rotate about a transverse axis so that the tip of the mastoid process moves inferiorly and posteriorly. The resulting widening of the skull at the parietosquamous suture causes the inferior part of the parietal bones to separate and the skull to lose vertical diameter as the angle between the parietal bones at the sagittal suture becomes more obtuse. There are corresponding movements of the remaining skull bones and even the relationship of the mandible to the temporal surface at the temporomandibular joint is changed. These movements comprise what is called flexion and external rotation. The cycle is completed by the reverse movements known as extension and internal rotation.

When the occiput moves into flexion as defined here, the posterior rim of the foramen magnum becomes inferior with respect to the anterior rim. The tube of dura mater surrounding the spinal cord is attached to the margin of the foramen magnum, and when the occiput is flexed, the anterior aspect of the dura is raised and the posterior aspect allowed to drop. Although it has an attachment to C2 the dura is sufficiently rigid to transmit motion to its inferior attachment at the second sacral vertebra. Hence the confusion over 'flexion' of the sacrum; flexion of the occiput pulls the anterior aspect of the dura towards the skull and, for this reason, in craniosacral terminology flexion of the sacrum is what is termed posterior nutation in this volume. Among those unfamiliar with craniosacral work, the term sacral flexion is usually taken to mean what is here called anterior nutation.

If there is motion there must be a driving mechanism, and in the human there are few mechanisms that have no purpose. It is therefore pertinent to ask the nature of the driving mechanism and its purpose. The concept is that the known rhythmical motion of the cerebral hemispheres is the driving mechanism and put at its simplest the purpose is to pump fluid. There is no other known means by which the CSF is made to circulate and yet by analogy with the rest of the humoral mechanisms in the body, circulate it must. The hemisphere motion may be in response to the cyclical contraction and relaxation of the neuroglia which can be seen in cell culture.

To the mechanically minded it is difficult to understand how the relationship of bones like the skull can be accurately influenced from outside. We owe the development of these techniques to Dr Sutherland's persistence and experimentation.

No attempt will be made in this volume to describe specific techniques. Those wishing to study them can find descriptions in Magoun[14] and Upledger[12]. It is strongly recommended that no attempt be made to use these techniques without first taking a recognised course of instruction.

LOCALISATION OF FORCE

If a cabinet maker were to use a simple hammer to drive home his nails, the wood around the nail head would be marked by the face of the hammer. A nail punch is used as a means of localising the force accurately to the nail head. Similarly a manipulative force needs to be localised to one joint; the neighbouring joint may require treatment in a different direction or the bone nearby may be weakened and in danger of damage. For example, consider the osteoporotic spine. Osteoporosis is common in the elderly and more so in the female. Back pain is also common in the elderly; the two often are found together but the pain is frequently not due to the osteoporosis. Microfractures will cause pain and may not be visible even on good X-rays in the early stages. Even so, much of the back pain seen in osteoporotic patients is due to somatic dysfunction and can be relieved by suitable treatment. Muscle energy or functional treatment are preferred but one of the authors has extensive experience of using gentle thrusting treatment, with good results, on such patients in the days before Mitchell's work became widely known. It can sometimes be difficult to distinguish between pain from a microfracture and that from dysfunction. One observation that may help is the location of the tissue texture change. If it is solely unilateral a microfracture is unlikely. A gentle muscle energy treatment can be used as a diagnostic test and will do no harm as the patient doses the force; if thrust must be employed, the secret is good localisation and low amplitude. It is most important that the effect of the external force is accurately localised to the level of the dysfunction.

In this context, it is interesting to note the scant success of traction as a treatment for spinal joint dysfunction. It has been tried in hospital, in bed at home, in physiotherapy clinics, suspended from a beam and more recently upside down. Of course there will be an occasional patient who will benefit but, in spite of the claims of some of the manufacturers of traction apparatus, localisation is at best very imperfect. It is possible that an experienced operator could adjust the angle of the traction to localise correctly at the start but, as with functional balance and hold techniques, the barrier would move and the localisation would require to be changed as soon as it had started to help. If X-rays are taken of the neck of a patient while on traction, marked separation of some joints can be seen, but it appears to be the normal ones without muscle hypertonus rather than the ones it was hoped to treat.

Dr Fred Mitchell jr., DO uses the analogy of a garden hose to illustrate one of the principles of localisation. If a length of hose is twisted from one end the twist will travel along the hose and the more it is twisted, the further it will reach. If, for whatever reason, it is required that the twist go to a certain point and then stop, the control is very difficult. On the other hand if a kink is introduced at that point before the twist is started the hose can easily be twisted up to the desired point and no further.

Diagnostic localisation has been described in Chapter 5. The method of localisation of the manipulative force is an extension of the principles used in diagnosis. Both for muscle energy and for high velocity treatment it is by positioning the patient and, while there are minor differences, the position from which a high velocity treatment is performed is often the same as that required for muscle energy.

The precise position is determined by palpation; there is no 'rule of thumb' positioning that will do the job. Palpation can be for motion or for tension in the tissues or for both. Most experienced manipulators seem to use a combination; in some situations tension will be the easier to feel, in others motion. For the beginner the greatest difficulty is in feeling the 'feather edge' of the change and having missed that in going beyond and positioning the joint hard against the barrier when the muscles will tighten and make treatment much more difficult. It is sound advice to a beginner to stop slightly short of the barrier rather than to go too far.

When using thrust (high velocity, low amplitude treatment) it is an advantage to be able to control the dysfunctional joint through a long lever. Nature provides only short levers on the vertebrae, the transverse and spinous processes being the longest. Long and short lever and hybrid techniques will be described. The latter use a short lever on one side and a long lever on the other. Hybrid and short lever techniques have the advantage that, at least on the short lever side, the contact is on the actual vertebra to be treated. It might be thought that this would make overall localisation unnecessary; this is not so because if the tensions over neighbouring joints are adjusted, the treatment will be more successful. It is true that localisation through a long lever requires greater care but if the lever is long it requires less force to move the joint. Most of the supine thoracic techniques are hybrid with a long lever for the superior component and a short one for the inferior. The 'crossed pisiform' is an example of short lever technique for the thoracic spine and, as is pointed out in the description, it can easily be abused.

The principle of operation of a lever is that with a longer lever the distance travelled by the force is multiplied and the amount of the force divided by the ratio of the length of the long lever to that of the short one. In other words, if the tip of the transverse process is 2.5 cm (1 inch) distant from the facet joint and, by some means, a lever 15 cm (6 inches) long can be constructed, the force which has to be applied at the end of the lever is one sixth of that needed at the tip of the TP and the distance through which that force has to move is six times as much. This can be used to advantage because one of the difficulties is to apply a force of sufficient magnitude to overcome the resistance while stopping it before it has moved the bone more than the 'less than an eighth of an inch at the joint' which is the limit, as Dr John Mennell has so often reminded us.

Levers are constructed by a process known as 'locking' the spinal (and other) joints. The term locking is used to describe the process by which a joint is so positioned that no further movement is possible in the direction chosen. It should be pointed out that a locked joint is not the same as a joint with a restrictive barrier; the latter is what is found by examination, the former is what is done to a joint to prevent further motion in one direction. Locking can be produced by taking a joint as far as it will go in any direction, e.g. full flexion. The problem with that method is that spinal joints move a little like traffic lights in a busy street. In many places these are linked so that long before the first light has finished its green phase, the next and probably the third have turned green. In order to make a joint move it must be free and even the beginning of motion may spoil that freedom.

Fryette's third concept of spinal motion tells us that if motion in one plane is introduced in a spinal joint, motion in the other two planes is thereby restricted. By the same principle, locking can be produced by motion in more than one plane. If the dysfunction to be treated is FRS, so that part of the correction is the restoration of extension, the sagittal plane component of the locking, both from above and from below, should be extension. Similar considerations apply to the other planes of movement. If the dysfunction is a neutral group both flexion and extension should be avoided.

The object when introducing either flexion–extension or sidebending is to translate the vertebra being treated in such a way that it becomes the apex of a curve. This produces the required motion from below and from above giving more accurate localisation. Clearly the apices of the two curves should be at the same point. Translation in this manner has the advantage that the patient can remain balanced over her seat for most joints, instead of tending to fall and having to be supported. Ideally the tangent to the curve that is produced should be vertical.

The details of the localisation will be described under the various techniques but the principle is that the motion is continued only to the point when the tension in the tissues begins to increase at the next level above and the next level below the joint being treated. The same point will be reached if the motion itself is closely monitored. In localising from above the point is reached when the bone above the dysfunctional motor segment (i.e. L3 if the L4–5 joint is to be treated) can be felt to begin to move. The localisation from below also will be only as far as the next vertebra below; in the example above it would be the sacrum. Alternatively, the movement or the tension can be taken just to the point where it reaches the upper component of the motion segment (L4 in the example above) and the position then adjusted by a small reverse movement until that segment is relaxed. The locking from below can, of course, be done in the same manner. The final locked position will be at the barrier. The main difference between this and the positioning prior to muscle energy treatment is that it is done in such a way that a thrust can be applied as the treatment. That would not be possible in some of the techniques used to reach the barrier which are used for muscle energy treatments.

Reactions to treatment

Mild reactions to treatment are common, whether the treatment is thrusting or muscle energy or even of the indirect variety. They occur usually in the first 12 hours but may be delayed, although not commonly for more than 36 hours. The most common is soreness in the areas treated and is more likely in those whose state is more acute. More tiresome reactions sometimes occur, often in those with less stable autonomic nervous systems. These may include nausea, dizziness, tachycardia, sweating etc.

Reactions of any kind are only common at the initial treatment and are not necessarily a contraindication to follow up treatment. In those who are nervous it is wise to warn them that a reaction may happen. Reactions are likely to last for less than 24 hours but, in an old chronic case where extensive treatment has been performed at one session, exhibition of nonsteroidal anti-inflammatory drugs is often helpful and should be in anti-inflammatory rather than analgesic dosage.

SUBSEQUENT VISITS

When the patient returns for follow up, the examination must be repeated because with any successful manipulation the situation will have changed. There may be parts of the original examination which can be neglected at least on some occasions but any part that was treated should be re-examined. The concept that a structural diagnosis is once for all time is nonsense. It is common to find that the first treatment has 'peeled the outside skin off the onion' and under it are dysfunctions, many of which may not have been found at the first examination.

A special example of this is the patient who has had previous trouble in the same, or a neighbouring area, and who comes with symptoms following a fresh injury. Treatment of the recently injured level may make the him or her much better but, if the old dysfunctions are not looked for and dealt with, the recent dysfunction is likely to recur quickly. This is not unexpected because an old unresolved dysfunction will leave asymmetrical tension that will not only predispose to dysfunctions at other levels but will tend to make such dysfunctions recur precisely because of the asymmetry. It has been inferred but not explicitly stated that most patients will be found to have multiple dysfunctions. This is true and it will often be an old and no longer symptomatic joint that is the basic cause of recurrences. The manipulator's approach here differs sharply from that of the spine surgeon who at most may look at two or perhaps three levels. In this context it is important to recognise that much referred pain is 'paradoxical', that is to say that its site of origin is not what neuroanatomy would suggest. For example, pain in the buttock and leg is often found with dysfunction at the thoraco-lumbar junction. Similarly pain in the neck and arm seems to be associated with dysfunctions in the upper thoracic more than those in the neck itself.

Sometimes making a precise diagnosis is difficult even for those with experience and it would be unrealistic to deny that even they can occasionally take the wrong view of a problem. If the patient fails to improve with what appears to have been the right treatment, the first thing is to start from the beginning and check the diagnosis. If the diagnosis is confirmed as 'a manipulable lesion', the next thing is to start the structural examination again from the beginning. The findings in some patients are subtle enough for the state of wellbeing of the operator, as well as his state of health, to be important. It would be difficult to cancel one's appointments just because one was feeling 'off colour' but it is essential to check the findings carefully in such circumstances.

Re-examination

Almost, if not all, treatment techniques in this volume end with the instruction, 're-examine' or 'retest'. This is because there is no other way to find for certain if the object of the treatment has been achieved. With muscle energy, soft tissue, myofascial or indirect treatment there will not usually be a cavitation sound to indicate that motion has occurred. Sometimes during an isometric procedure a cavitation sound will be heard and the joint will be felt to move. For those who, like one of the authors formerly, think that muscle is the restrictor, that sound is proof that there is a mechanical factor as well.

Common dysfunctions

It is useful to know which dysfunctions are likely to prove to be more common than others. The list will vary with different patient populations; for instance inferior innominate shear is said to be much more common in areas where there is much horse riding, the mechanism of injury often being a fall with the foot trapped in the stirrup and the rider being dragged by the foot.

In general and from below up some of the most common findings are:

1. Left anterior nutation of the sacrum, often with a left posterior innominate.
2. Left on left anterior torsion.
3. Posterior torsion with right on left being rather the more frequent. This often is associated with FRSrt at L5.
4. Non-neutral dysfunction at L4–5; this may be ERS or FRS.
5. Non-neutral dysfunction at T11 or T12, ERS or FRS.
6. Non-neutral dysfunction, ERS or FRS at T8–9 or/and T4–5.
7. Neutral dysfunction of three joints in the upper thoracic spine often T2–3–4.
8. FRS dysfunction at C5–6 and C2–3.
9. ERS at T4–5 with external torsion of the 5th rib on the side to which T4 is rotated.

Recurrent dysfunctions

In those in whom the same dysfunction recurs after good treatment there are a number of different things to look for. The common ones, not necessarily in order of frequency, are:

1. Other dysfunctions, sometimes at a distance, that predispose to the abnormal tensions that are often the cause of the recurrence.
2. Abnormal anatomy; ERS dysfunctions are common on the side of

the coronal facing facet in cases of facet tropism and the more so if the under vertebra is asymmetrical in shape. Good X-rays are helpful.

3. Tilting of the sacral base due to a structurally short lower extremity or to asymmetry of size of the bones of the pelvis. This is particularly common in those who show recurrence of anterior sacral torsions.

4. Asymmetry of length or strength of the long hip and thigh muscles and abnormal firing patterns which are usually a sign of asymmetry in proprioception and may need special retraining programmes (see Chapter 14).

REFERENCES

1. *Oxford English Dictionary* (Compact Edition) (1980). Oxford: Oxford University Press.
2. Maigne Robert (1989). *Diagnostic et Traitment des Douleurs Communes D'origine Rachidienne*. Paris: Expansion Scientifique Francaise.
3. Travell J., Simons D.G. (1983). *Myofascial Pain and Dysfunction*. Baltimore: Williams and Wilkins.
4. Stoddard A. (1959). *Manual of Osteopathic Technique*. London: Hutchinson.
5. Maitland G.D. (1964). *Vertebral Manipulation*. London: Butterworth.
6. Mennell J.McM. (1964). *Joint Pain*. Boston: Little, Brown.
7. Dvorak J., Dvorak V., Schneider W. (1985). *Manual Medicine 1984*. Heidelberg: Springer-Verlag.
8. Ward Robert C. *Principles of Myofascial Release* in publication, East Lansing, Mi: Michigan State University.
9. Jones L.H. (1981). *Strain and Counterstrain*. Colorado Springs, Co.: American Academy of Osteopathy.
10. Stiles Dr E.G., of Norman, Oklahoma a member of faculty of other postgraduate courses at Michigan State University College of Osteopathic Medicine and recently teaching functional techniques also.
11. Magoun H.I. (1951). *Osteopathy in the Cranial Field*. Kirksville, Mo: Journal Printing Co.
12. Upledger J.E., Vredevoogd J.D. (1983). *Craniosacral Therapy*. Seattle: Eastland Press.
13. *Gray's Anatomy*. (1923) 22nd edn (English), p.206. London: Longmans, Green.
14. Magoun H.I. (1990). *Osteopathy in the Cranial Field*. Edn 3. Kirksville, Mo.: Journal Printing Co.

Chapter 7

Treatment of dysfunctions of the pelvis

It is of some importance that the treatment sequence should be observed, at least in the first steps. The recommended order is:

1. *Dysfunctions of the pubis.* Because the normal operation of the pelvic mechanism depends on free twisting at the symphysis, pubic dysfunctions will upset the diagnostic criteria and should be treated first.
2. *Innominate (iliac) shears* (upslip or downslip). These also upset the whole pelvic mechanism.
3. *Non-adaptive lumbar dysfunctions.* If they are not treated first treatment of the pelvis may prove difficult or even impossible. Many operators extend this recommendation to any non–neutral or even to all lumbar dysfunctions.
4. *Sacroiliac dysfunctions.* Anterior and posterior sacral torsions and sacral nutations which are also known as sacral shears (formerly as extended or flexed sacra).
5. *Iliosacral dysfunctions.* Anterior and posterior innominates and the uncommon in and out flares.
6. Any remaining lumbar dysfunctions.

The treatment techniques to be described will be arranged in the order in which the diagnoses were set out. Where available both muscle energy and thrusting (high velocity) treatments will be given. Only one side, usually the more common one, will be described; for the other it is only necessary to reverse the side descriptors. It is always good practice to test again after treatment to see if the desired result has been achieved; this is more important when using muscle energy because audible or palpable movement is the exception rather than the rule.

Whenever the patient lies prone her feet should be free over the end of the table. Forced plantar flexion affects the tensions even as high as the pelvis.

1   THE PUBIS

1.1   Superior pubis on the left

Diagnostic points. The standing forward flexion test is positive on the left. The left pubic tubercle is superior to the right and there may be tissue texture change at the insertion of the inguinal ligament.

1.1.1 Muscle energy.

1.1.1.1. The patient is supine, and her pelvis is moved to the edge of the table so that the left PSIS is only just on the table top. For stability her shoulders should remain in the centre of the table (Fig. 7.1a).

1.1.1.2. The operator stands beside her left leg and takes it off the table, supporting her ankle either between his lower legs or on the back of one ankle with the knee bent, while standing on his other leg. She should be asked to keep her knee straight (Fig. 7.1b and c).

Fig. 7.1 Treatment of the superior pubis. (a) Patient's position on the table; (b) supporting her leg between yours; (c) supporting her leg on your ankle.

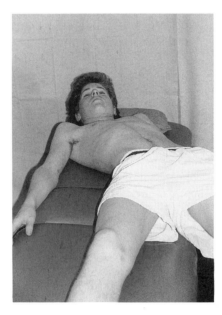

a

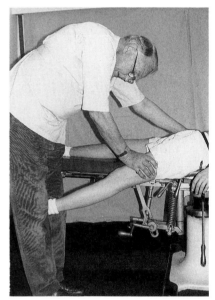

b

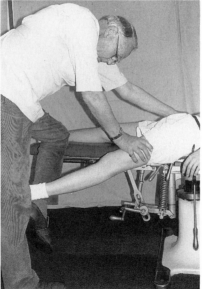

c

1.1.1.3. The operator uses his left hand to press down on the patient's right PSIS. This helps to prevent her feeling that she might fall off and is used to monitor the motion which should be stopped just before the ASIS begins to move.

1.1.1.4. The operator then places his right hand on the front of her left thigh to resist movement. The patello–femoral joint is sensitive and should be avoided.

1.1.1.5. The instruction is 'try to raise your left thigh against my hand'. The pressure should be no more than moderate and maintained for 3–5 seconds.

1.1.1.6. Have her relax and then wait for the second phase when relaxation is complete (if necessary asking again for full relaxation). When she has relaxed fully, allow her leg to slide down between your legs (or lower your ankle) until you reach the next barrier. There will be a sense of resistance and motion must not go so far that your hand on the opposite ASIS can feel movement. Her knee should not be allowed to hang bent.

1.1.1.7. Repeat steps 1.1.1.5 and 1.1.1.6 three or four times or until there is no further gain on relaxation.

1.1.1.8. Retest.

1.2 Inferior pubis on the right

Diagnostic points. The standing forward flexion test is positive on the right. The pubic tubercle is inferior on the right and there may be tissue texture change at the insertion of the inguinal ligament.

1.2.1 Muscle energy.

1.2.1.1. The patient is supine. For short operators it may be easier to stand on the side to be treated. The instructions for that will be shown in parentheses.

1.2.1.2. The operator stands on the left (right) side at the level of her pelvis and with his right (left) hand brings her right hip and knee into full flexion.

1.2.1.3. Rolling her pelvis towards (away from) him, the operator now inserts his left (right) hand under her right buttock so that the ischial tuberosity rests in the palm of his hand and his index and middle fingers can palpate either side of her right posterior superior iliac spine (Fig. 7.2a).

1.2.1.4. Having rolled the patient back to the supine position the operator leans over enough to be able to control her knee position with his trunk and, if on her left side, either presses down on her right PSIS with his right hand or grips the edge of the table to avoid being pushed away. He can then adjust the amount of hip flexion to that which just begins to move the ilium but does not move the sacrum, the fingers behind her pelvis being used as monitors (Fig. 7.2b). If standing on her right side he uses his left hand to help control the position of the patient's right thigh (Fig. 7.2c).

1.2.1.5. When the slack has been taken out, the instruction is '*gently push your right foot toward the foot of the table*'. This is resisted by an

Fig. 7.2 Treatment of the inferior pubis. (a) Placement of the under hand; (b) treatment position, contralateral; (c) treatment position, ipsilateral.

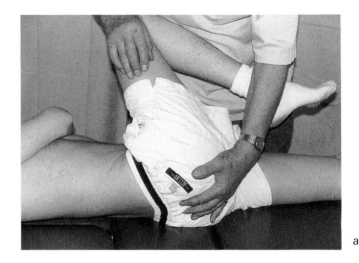

a

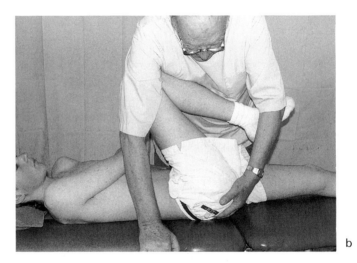

b

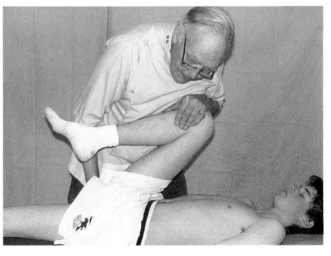

c

equal counterforce and, as the muscles concerned are powerful, the caution to be gentle is important.

1.2.1.6. After 3–5 seconds have her relax and, having waited for complete relaxation, take up the slack by lifting her ischial tuberosity with the palm of the left (right) hand in the direction of the pubic symphysis. At the same time the hip flexion should be increased slightly, but only to the point of the new barrier as found with the fingers as in step 1.2.1.4 above.

1.2.1.7. While maintaining tension with his left (right) hand, the operator has her repeat steps 1.2.1.5 and 1.2.1.6 three or four times or until there is no further gain.

1.2.1.8. Retest.

1.3 Pubis 'blunderbuss' technique for superior or inferior dysfunction

Diagnostic points. See under steps 1.1 and 1.2 above. In both technique 1.3.1 and 1.3.3 the patient will often feel a separation occur at the symphysis.

1.3.1 Muscle energy.

1.3.1.1. Distraction.

1.3.1.2. The patient is supine with both hips and knees flexed and feet flat on the table.

1.3.1.3. The operator stands to either side and separates her knees, inserting his forearm to prop them apart, the dorsiflexed palm of the hand being against the medial side of one knee and the back of the elbow against the medial side of the other knee (Fig. 7.3a).

1.3.1.4. The instruction is 'Try to pull your knees together' and the effort is maintained for not less than 3 seconds. If desired it may be

Fig. 7.3 Pubic symphysis dysfunction 'blunderbuss' technique. (a) Distraction phase; (b) compression phase.

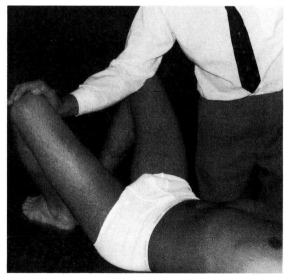

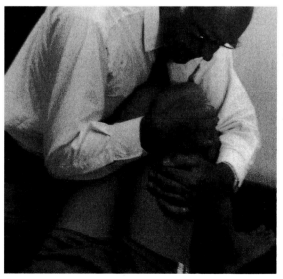

a   b

repeated and if this is done there is an advantage in sliding the 'prop' a short distance proximally to increase the abduction in the position of effort. There is no slack to be taken up in this technique.

1.3.1.5. Retest.

1.3.2. Compression.

1.3.2.1. The patient is in the same position as in step 1.3.1.1.

1.3.2.2. The operator stands to either side but this time puts both arms round the flexed knees and holds them tightly to his chest (Fig. 7.3b).

1.3.2.3. The instruction is 'try to separate your knees' which is prevented by the operator and usually repeated two or three times.

1.3.2.4. Retest.

1.3.3. Thrust.

1.3.3.1. The patient is in the same position as in step 1.3.2.1.

1.3.3.2. The operator places his hands on the medial side of her knees and has her attempt to bring them together.

1.3.3.3. While she is attempting to adduct, the operator separates his hands sharply, forcing her knees apart against resistance.

1.3.3.4. Retest.

2 INNOMINATE (ILIAC) SHEARS

2.1 Superior innominate (iliac) shear

This is inherently unstable and, in those with the joint configuration that permits this dysfunction, support of the pelvis after reduction is often necessary. A cinch type narrow sacroiliac belt is suitable and should be worn whenever out of bed for at least 6 weeks. The support may be used for longer if there is still a tendency for the dysfunction to recur. Because the belt should be worn even in a shower, at least two will be necessary. Suitable 'Hackett' belts with and without padding are available, for those in North America, from The Brooks Appliance Co[1]. These belts are about 5 cm (2 inches) wide and are made of a firm webbing with only a little 'give', they can be padded with felt.

Many patients have increased pain following correction of a superior shear dysfunction and this may last for several days while they adjust to the different mechanics. It is wise to warn each patient with such a dysfunction before the correction is performed.

Described for the left side
Diagnostic points. The standing forward flexion test is positive on the left. The left iliac crest is higher than the right, both prone and supine (but they are level when standing unless there is a structural leg length difference as well). The ischial tuberosity is higher on the left by at least a thumb's thickness. The left sacrotuberous ligament is lax and may be tender. Other landmarks on the left ilium are also higher than on the right.

2.1.1. Muscle energy.

2.1.1.1. The patient is shown supine but the same technique can be performed with her prone if preferred. Her feet should be just over the end of the table.

2.1.1.2. The operator stands at the foot of the table and lifts her left leg off the table, gripping just above the ankle with both hands. At the same time he should block downward movement of the right leg either by pressing against it with his left thigh, or with the help of an assistant.

2.1.1.3. The operator puts traction on her left leg, with enough abduction to loose-pack the sacroiliac joint and slight internal rotation to close pack her hip (Fig. 7.4).

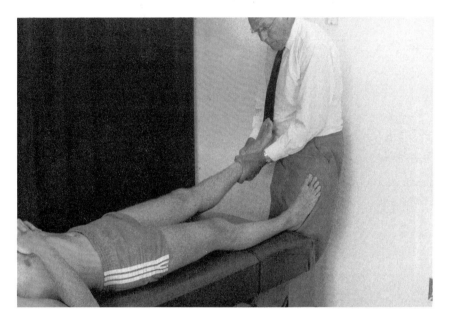

Fig. 7.4 Treatment of superior innominate shear (upslip).

2.1.1.4. The patient should be requested to inhale and exhale deeply to rock the sacrum between the ilia.

2.1.1.5. At the end of the third exhalation the patient is instructed to give a cough and at that moment the operator gives a moderately sharp tug on her left leg.

2.1.1.6. Retest.

2.1.2. Thrust.

This technique is NOT used if there are degenerative changes in either the hip or the knee of the same side.

2.1.2.1. The same as step 2.1.1.1.

2.1.2.2. The same as step 2.1.1.2.

2.1.2.3. The operator abducts her leg to the loose-packed position of the SI joint, but does not add internal rotation of the thigh which would close pack her hip.

2.1.2.4. The operator puts her hip and knee through a short series of flexions and extensions which end with a sharp tug in a caudad direction in the plane of the SI joint.

2.1.2.5. Retest.

2.2　Inferior innominate (iliac) shear

Unlike the superior shear, this is inherently stable when reduced and probably often is self-reduced by weightbearing. A supporting belt is not often required. When the patient is of the opposite sex, it is wise to explain carefully what is to be done as otherwise the procedure could be thought to be invasive.

Described for the right side
Diagnostic points. The standing forward flexion test is positive on the right. The left iliac crest is higher than the right, both prone and supine (or the right is lower). The ischial tuberosity is higher on the left by at least a thumb's thickness (or the right is lower). The right sacrotuberous ligament is tight and may be tender. Other landmarks on the right ilium are also lower than on the left.

2.2.1. Muscle energy or thrust

2.2.1.1. The patient lies on her left side.

2.2.1.2. The operator stands behind her hips and must raise her right lower limb either on his right arm or, and preferably, with the help of an assistant.

2.2.1.3. The operator contacts her right innominate bone with both hands. Both thumbs are medial to the ischial tuberosity. The index and middle fingers of his right hand pass forward to contact the body of her right pubic bone and his left index and middle fingers are on the medial side of her right PSIS (Fig. 7.5a and b).

M.2.2.1.4. The patient then breathes in and out deeply to rock the sacrum while the operator translates the innominate to the right and, with a rocking motion to help free the joint, translates it craniad.

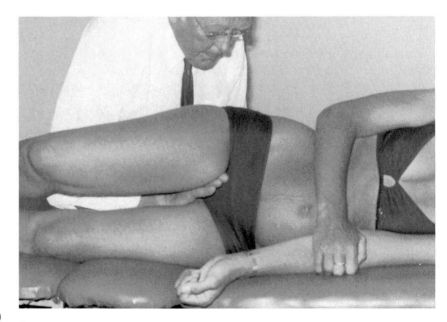

Fig. 7.5 Treatment of inferior innominate shear (downslip). (a) From anterior.

a

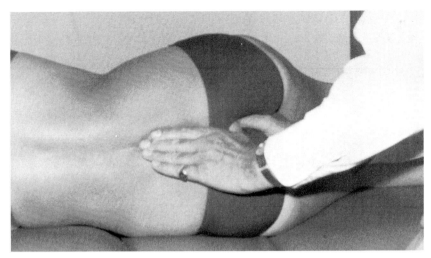

Fig. 7.5 (continued). (b) From posterior; (c) thrust, second technique.

b

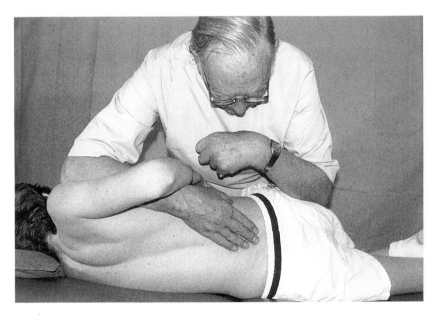

c

T.2.2.1.4. The patient is instructed to breathe deeply as for the muscle energy approach but the operator finishes with a specific craniad thrust. For this the help of an assistant to hold the leg up is essential.

2.2.1.5. Retest.

2.2.2. Thrust, second technique.

2.2.2.1. The patient lies on her left side and the operator stands in front of her. Her left leg should be extended as this will help to make the thrust come in the plane of the sacroiliac joint.

2.2.2.2. While monitoring at the sacrum with his right fingers, the operator pulls her left arm 'out from under' (anteriorly and caudad) to rotate her trunk to the right and introduce flexion to produce neutral locking down to and including the sacrum.

2.2.2.3. The thrust is given in a craniad direction with the upper part of his left forearm on her right ischial tuberosity with a high velocity movement (Fig. 7.5c)

2.2.2.4. Retest.

3   SACROILIAC DYSFUNCTIONS

3.1   Anterior sacral torsion

Described for anterior torsion to the left (left on left)
This is common, it is a restriction in part of the normal walking cycle of pelvic motion and may not be associated with severe symptoms. The major motion loss is of posterior nutation of the right sacral base. Because left rotation of the sacrum causes right sidebending the adaptive lumbar curve is convex right.

Diagnostic points. The sitting forward flexion test is probably positive on the right. The sacral base and the ILA are posterior on the left in flexion and probably when prone, but become level in extension. The lumbar spine is in lordosis and the spring test negative.

3.1.1. Muscle energy.

3.1.1.1. The patient lies prone with her right shoulder close to the side of the table and with her right arm hanging over the edge.

3.1.1.2. The operator lifts both her ankles with his left hand and her knees with his right hand and brings the knees up to her right side putting her in the left lateral 'Sims position'. The precise position is important; the hip flexion must be stopped at the point just before the sacrum begins to move and the movement is therefore monitored in its final stage by the fingers of his right hand on her right sacral base. Note that, in so far as she is on her side, that is the side of the axis of the torsion (Fig. 7.6a).

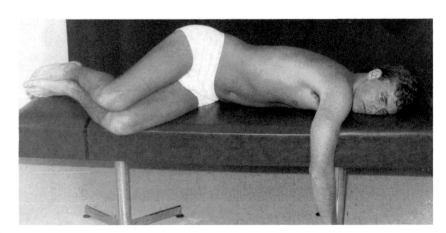

Fig. 7.6 Muscle energy treatment of left on left (anterior) sacral torsion. (a) Left lateral Sims position.

a

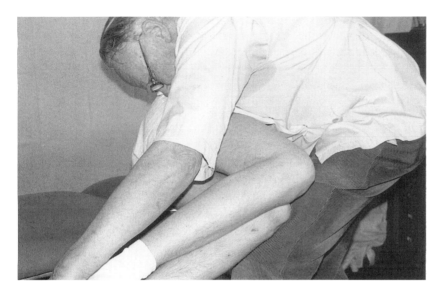

b

Fig. 7.6 (continued).
(b) Supporting her knees with
your knee; (c) the 'lazy man'
variant; (d) monitoring with the
right hand and resisting with
the left.

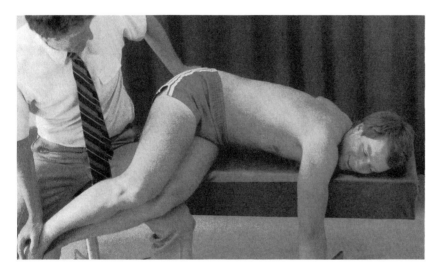

c

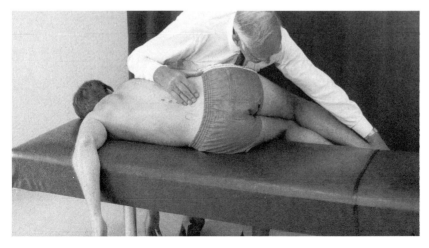

d

3.1.1.3. The patient should then breathe deeply and as she breathes out reach for the floor with her right hand. This movement also must be monitored and is stopped when L5 just begins to move. The operator uses his left hand to monitor at this stage because he may need to use his right hand to increase the patient's rotation by pressing down on her right shoulder as she breathes out. If necessary the exhalation and reaching for the floor is repeated until the point of tension is reached.

3.1.1.4. The necessary left sidebend is introduced by dropping the patient's feet over the edge of the table without losing the localisation from below. If this were done without protection, when the effort was made, the pressure of the table edge on the under thigh would be very uncomfortable. To avoid this one of four methods is commonly used.

3.1.1.4a. Place a small cushion under the thigh to protect it from the edge of the table.

3.1.1.4b. The operator stands so that he can support the patient's knees over his right knee (Fig. 7.6b).

3.1.1.4c. The operator sits on the foot of the table and, with legs apart, supports her knees on his left knee. This is sometimes known as the lazy man's technique; its disadvantage is that it is no longer possible for the operator to control the trunk with his right forearm. In order to monitor over the right sacral base he must change hands and his right hand now provides the resistance to the patient's effort in step 3.1.1.5. The patient should be told to maintain the twisted position. This technique is less easy if the operator is wearing a skirt as the abduction of the legs must be wide enough to allow the patient's feet to drop between them (Fig. 7.6c).

3.1.1.4d. The operator may balance the patient's legs over his thigh by placing it under her upper tibiae so that her thighs remain clear of the table top.

3.1.1.5. The instruction to the patient is 'raise your feet toward the ceiling' which the operator resists with an equal and opposite force with the left hand in variants 3.1.1.4a and 3.1.1.4b (Fig. 7.6d) but the right hand in variant 3.1.1.4c. The pressure is maintained for 3–5 seconds and the patient must then relax. It helps to tell her to 'drop her feet'. If the positioning is correct it should be possible to feel the right sacral base move back against the monitoring fingers during the patient's effort.

3.1.1.6. After full relaxation, the slack is taken up to the new point of tension as monitored by the fingers. This can usually be done by dropping the feet but sometimes an adjustment to the flexion of the hips may help.

3.1.1.7. Steps 3.1.1.5 and 3.1.1.6 are repeated two or more times.

3.1.1.8. Retest.

3.1.2. Thrust (sitting).

3.1.2.1. The patient sits astride the table, with her back close to the end, and holds her right shoulder with her left hand.

3.1.2.2. The operator stands to her right and contacts her left sacral base with his left pisiform bone.

3.1.2.3. With his right axilla over her right shoulder, the operator grasps her left humerus and bends her forward down to and including the sacrum, but not the innominates (Fig. 7.7a).

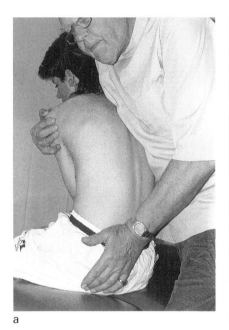
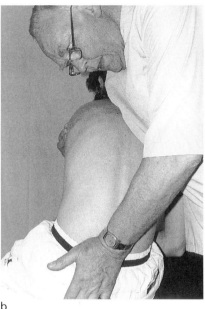

a   b

Fig. 7.7 Thrust treatment for L on L sacral torsion, sitting. (a) Starting position; (b) final position.

3.1.2.4. He then locks her spine by right sidebending and right rotation again including the sacrum but not the innominates (Fig. 7.7b). This will start the left sacral base moving forwards.

3.1.2.5. A low amplitude, high velocity thrust is now given by the operator's left pisiform against the left sacral base at the same time as the patient's trunk is taken into further sidebending and rotation; but in order to allow the sacrum to nutate anteriorly on the left and rotate right the flexion of the lumbosacral joint should be released at the same time.

3.1.2.6. Retest.

3.1.3. Thrust (sidelying).

3.1.3.1. The patient lies on her left side with shoulders perpendicular to the table and her trunk in slight flexion. The flexion must not take her spine out of the neutral range.

3.1.3.2. The operator stands in front of her and flexes her hips to a right angle (to help extend the right sacral base).

3.1.3.3. He then contacts the left inferior lateral angle of her sacrum with his left pisiform – with his elbow bent so that his forearm is nearly in line with the intended thrust.

3.1.3.4. With his right hand on her right shoulder, the operator introduces right sidebending by taking the shoulder caudad until all slack has been taken out, and, as the spine is in neutral, left rotation is produced (Fig. 7.8).

3.1.3.5. The operator then presses on her left inferior lateral angle with his left pisiform in the direction of her right shoulder until all the slack of that movement has been removed.

Fig. 7.8 Thrust treatment for L
on L sacral torsion, sidelying.

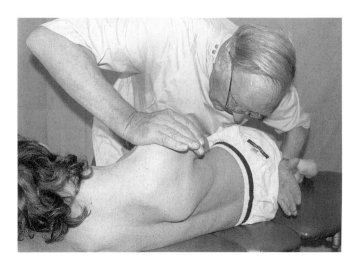

3.1.3.6. A low amplitude, high velocity thrust is given, by the pisiform, with a scooping motion, on the inferior lateral angle, directed towards her right shoulder, to bring the right side of her sacral base posterior.

3.1.3.7. Retest.

3.2   Posterior sacral torsion

Described for posterior torsion to the right (right on left)

This is not a position which occurs in normal walking. It can only occur when the lumbar spine is operating in non-neutral mechanics and is always associated with non-neutral dysfunction of the lumbar spine often with restriction of extension. Although a lot less common than anterior torsion, it is associated with marked symptoms and is very important. It is regarded as one of the most common causes of the 'failed back' syndrome. The major motion restriction is of forward nutation of the right sacral base.

The correction is thought to be produced by the combined action of the right piriformis pulling the sacrum (while acting as an abductor of the hip) and the gluteus medius with the tensor fasciae latae pulling on the ilium.

Diagnostic points. The sitting forward flexion test is positive on the right. The sacral base and the ILA are posterior on the right in extension and probably when prone but become level in flexion. The lumbar spine is flat and the spring test positive. There will often be a nonneutral dysfunction at L5–S1, most frequently FRSrt and, when such a nonadaptive dysfunction is present in the lumbar spine, it should be treated first.

3.2.1. Muscle energy. For illustrations of the earlier stages see Fig. 8.1a, b, c and d.

3.2.1.1. The patient lies on her left side, the side of the axis around which the torsion has taken place.

3.2.1.2. The operator stands in front of her and extends her spine by pulling her pelvis towards the front of the table while monitoring with his other hand to avoid locking the lumbosacral joint by too much extension. Localisation from above is to L5.

3.2.1.3. With his right hand monitoring at the sacral base, he extends the left hip by easing her left leg towards the back of the table leaving her right leg in front. This movement is part of the localisation and must be done by the operator with the patient relaxed. Any attempt by her to help must be stopped. The movement is taken to the point where the sacrum just begins to move but L5 does not.

3.2.1.4. Now monitoring with his left hand at L5 the operator takes the patient's right hand and, pulling it down enough to produce right sidebending, he rotates her right shoulder back introducing right rotation. This is taken to the point where the tension just reaches L5 as detected by the monitoring fingers. If that point is not reached more extension may be required in the spine. This can be obtained by lifting her shoulders and moving them back, a task that is difficult with a heavy patient when maintaining the monitoring contact. When that position is adjusted the patient should grip the back of the table to maintain it.

3.2.1.5. Monitoring again with his right hand over the right sacral base, the operator uses his right forearm against the front of her right shoulder to maintain rotation and uses his left hand to control movement of her right leg (Fig. 7.9).

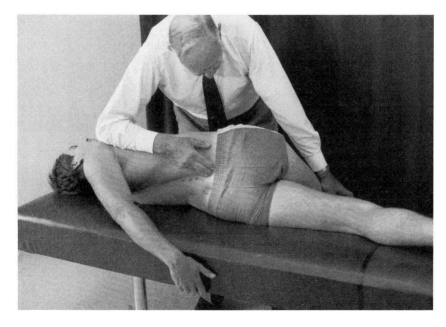

Fig. 7.9 Muscle energy treatment for right on left (posterior) sacral torsion

3.2.1.6. The instruction is 'try to raise your right leg against my hand'. The pressure should be maintained for 3–5 seconds and the patient must then relax. If the positioning is correct, it should be possible to feel the right sacral base move forwards away from the monitoring fingers during the patient's effort.

3.2.1.7. When relaxation is complete the slack is taken up to the new barrier and steps 3.2.1.5 and 3.2.1.6 are repeated three or more times.

3.2.1.8. Retest.

3.2.2. Thrust (sitting). This technique may also be used to correct a posterior nutation (superior sacral shear).

Described for right on left torsion.

3.2.2.1. The patient sits astride the table holding her right shoulder with her left hand.

3.2.2.2. The operator stands on her left side with the front of his left shoulder pressed against the side of her left shoulder and grasps her right shoulder with his left hand.

3.2.2.3. He contacts the right side of her sacral base with his right pisiform bone (or triquetrum or thumb) and then locks her spine down to and including the sacrum by sidebending to the right and rotating to the left to start the right sacral base moving forward (Fig. 7.10). Here the mechanics involve sacral rotation to start the movement and then extension of L5 to allow the sacral base to move forwards.

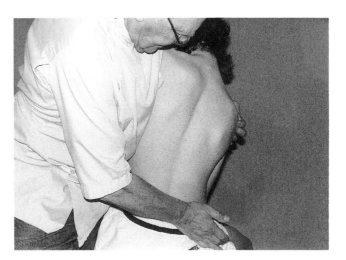

Fig. 7.10 Thrust treatment for R on L sacral torsion sitting.

3.2.2.4. The operator then extends her spine down to L5 and, when all slack has been taken out a low amplitude, high velocity thrust is given forwards on the right sacral base by his right pisiform. The triquetrum or thumb could be used but the smaller pisiform fits more easily into the narrow sulcus so that the sacral base itself is contacted.

3.2.2.5. Retest.

3.2.3. Thrust (supine). May also be used to correct a posterior nutation (superior sacral shear).

Described for right on left torsion.

3.2.3.1. The patient lies supine with her fingers laced together behind her neck and her elbows forward. Her pelvis should be close to the operator (at the left side of the table) and her feet and upper trunk are moved to the right side of the table producing a right sidebend of her trunk (Fig. 7.11a).

3.2.3.2. Leaning over, the operator threads his right forearm, from the lateral side, through the gap between her right arm and her chest and rests the back of his right hand on her sternum.

3.2.3.3. The operator then rotates her towards him, without losing her right sidebend, until her right ilium begins to lift.

3.2.3.4a. Either he holds the ilium down with his left hand and the correction is produced by a sharp increase in the rotation *without losing the sidebend*. Note that, in order to achieve this the spine must be locked down to and including the sacrum (Fig. 7.11b and c).

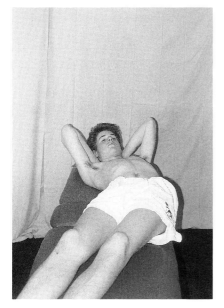

a

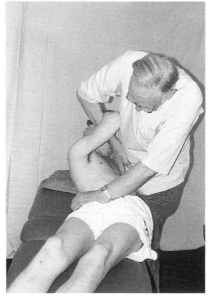

b

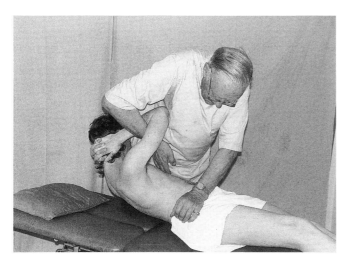

c

Fig. 7.11 Thrust treatment for R on L sacral torsion supine. (a) Starting position; (b) thrust position seen from patient's feet; (c) thrust position seen from right side of patient.

3.2.3.4b. Or the correction is made by a high velocity, low amplitude thrust posteriorly by the operator's left hand on her right ASIS while he holds her trunk flexed, rotated and sidebent.

3.2.3.5. Retest.

3.3   Anterior sacral nutation (inferior sacral shear or unilateral flexed sacrum)

Described for the left side

Diagnostic points. The sitting forward flexion test is positive on the left. The sacral base is anterior on the left in flexion and less so in neutral. In extension it becomes nearly, but not quite, symmetrical. The ILA is posterior on the left in flexion and nearly level in extension. The lumbar spine is in lordosis and the spring test is negative.

3.3.1. Muscle energy with thrust variant.

3.3.1.1. The patient lies prone and should have her feet free over the end of the table (not as in Fig. 7.12a).

3.3.1.2. The operator stands at her left side and monitors her left sacral sulcus with the index and middle fingers of his left hand.

3.3.1.3. With his right hand the operator lifts her left thigh and moves it to the point where the left sacroiliac joint is 'loose packed'. This is the point of maximum ease, as detected by the monitoring fingers, and is usually found in 10–15° of abduction. He then rotates her thigh internally to help to open the posterior aspect of the SI joint. The patient is then told to keep her leg in that position (Fig. 7.12a).

3.3.1.4. He then moves the heel of his right hand to the left inferior lateral angle of her sacrum so that he can apply a springing pressure. With his right elbow straight, he adjusts the direction of his right arm so that the springing pressure being applied with his right hand produces the maximum of movement in the sacral sulcus as detected by his monitoring fingers.

3.3.1.5. The patient is then instructed to breathe in as deeply as possible (which tends to bring the sacrum into posterior nutation) and then hold her breath. Many patients will stop before the limit of possible inhalation and it is often necessary to ask them to breathe more deeply and maybe even deeper still, to obtain the maximum. The operator then presses firmly in the direction discovered by the springing examination.

M.3.3.1.6. After about 5 seconds the patient should exhale slowly but the operator does not release the pressure (Fig. 7.12b).

M.3.3.1.7. Step 3.3.1.5 and 3.3.1.6 are then repeated two or three times and finally the operator slowly releases his pressure. Too rapid a release may allow the sacrum to spring back.

T.3.3.1.6. A thrust may be given at the end of one of the muscle energy efforts. It is given by a sudden but slight increase in the pressure with the hand on the ILA in the same direction.

3.3.1.8. Retest.

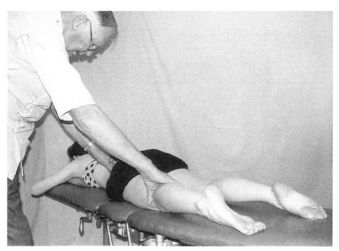

a

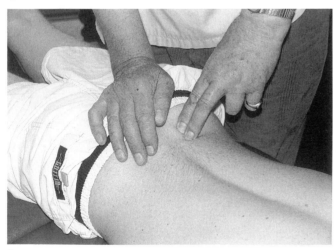

b

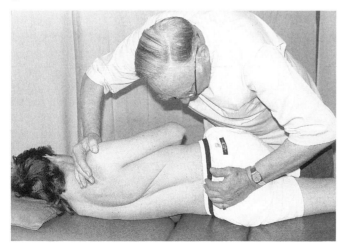

c

Fig. 7.12 Unilateral anterior sacral nutation on the left. (a) Muscle energy, positioning the leg; (b) muscle energy treatment; (c) thrust, sidelying.

3.3.2. Thrust, sidelying.

3.3.2.1. The patient lies on her left side.

3.3.2.2. The operator stands in front of her and flexes both her hips and knees to start posterior nutation of the sacrum but monitoring to ensure that the lumbo-sacral joint is not flexed.

3.3.2.3. He pulls her left shoulder forward and caudad to lock the spine by neutral mechanics down to L5.

3.3.2.4. He then flexes, a little further, her upper (right) knee and hip, being careful not to 'lock' the lumbo-sacral joint. This is to allow him to make contact with his left pisiform on the left inferior lateral angle of her sacrum.

3.3.2.5. With his left forearm parallel to the table he presses forward on her ILA to take out the slack from below.

3.3.2.6. With his right hand he takes out the slack down to L5 by pressure backwards on her right shoulder (Fig. 7.12c).

3.3.2.7. When all slack is taken out a high velocity, low amplitude thrust is given by the operator's left hand on her left ILA directed cranially.

3.3.2.8. Retest.

3.3.3. Alternative muscle energy.

The posterior innominate prone technique is described in step 4.1.3 below, with the modification that the counterforce is applied to the ipsilateral ILA (step 4.1.3.2). This will correct the very commonly associated posterior innominate at the same time.

3.4   Posterior sacral nutation (superior sacral shear or unilateral extended sacrum)

Described for the right side

Diagnostic points. The sitting forward flexion test is positive on the right. In flexion, and sometimes even in neutral, the sacral base and ILAs are almost symmetrical but in extension the right sacral base becomes posterior and the right ILA anterior. The lumbar spine is flat and the spring test positive.

3.4.1. Muscle energy.

3.4.1.1. The patient lies prone on the table and the operator stands at her left side and monitors with his left hand in her right sulcus. (The technique can be adapted to be done with the operator on the right side.)

3.4.1.2. The operator lifts her right thigh at or above the knee, avoiding the patellofemoral joint, and adjusts the ad- and abduction position until the SI joint is loose packed. He then externally rotates the thigh, to start to open the anterior aspect of her right sacroiliac joint, and puts the leg back on the table asking the patient to maintain that position.

3.4.1.3. He then places his left pisiform in contact with the right side of her sacral base and has her assume the sphinx position. (Extension of the lumbar spine tends to flex the sacrum.)

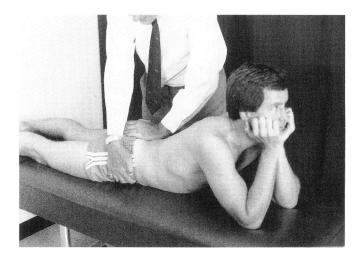

Fig. 7.13 Muscle energy treatment for posterior sacral nutation on the right.

3.4.1.4. The operator puts his right hand under her right ASIS to give counter-pressure (Fig. 7.13).

3.4.1.5. He then has her breathe out as far as possible and hold her breath, which tends to bring the sacrum into anterior nutation. At the same time he applies firm pressure on her right sacral base with his left pisiform while exerting a similar counterforce upwards on her right ASIS. It is wise to warn the patient that the sacral base contact will probably be quite uncomfortable. During the breath holding it may help if the patient pulls her ASIS down towards the table.

3.4.1.6. After 4 or 5 seconds he has the patient inhale slowly but does not let the pressure off.

3.4.1.7. Steps 3.4.1.4 and 3.4.1.5 are then repeated two or three times before the pressure is gradually released.

3.4.1.8. Retest.

3.4.2. Thrust. See the description of the thrust techniques for posterior sacral torsions (techniques 3.2.2 and 3.2.3) which will also correct this dysfunction (Figs 7.10 and 7.11a, b and c).

3.5 Bilateral anterior sacral nutation (bilateral inferior sacral shear or flexed sacrum)

Diagnostic points. Bilaterally positive sitting forward flexion test, both PSISs begin to move up at the start of forward flexion. This can be mistaken for a negative test; if there is doubt the stork test can be done and will be positive bilaterally. The standing test will also be positive. All landmarks are level but motion tests show stiffness and the lumbar spine is in lordosis with a negative spring test.

3.5.1. Muscle energy. Treat first one side and then the other as described in step technique 3.3.1 above.

3.5.2. Alternative muscle energy.

3.5.2.1. The patient sits on a stool, or on the front of a firm chair with her feet separated and toes turned in (to start opening the posterior aspect of both SI joints). She should be bent forward, as far as possible, with her arms between her legs.

3.5.2.2. The operator stands beside her and places the heel of his hand nearest to her back (the left hand if he is standing on her right), over the apex of her sacrum.

3.5.2.3. He contacts her upper trunk with his other hand and prepares to resist her extension effort.

3.5.2.4. The operator maintains pressure anteriorly on her sacral apex while the patient makes an effort to raise her shoulders towards the ceiling which he resists (Fig. 7.14).

Fig. 7.14 Muscle energy treatment for bilateral anterior sacral nutation.

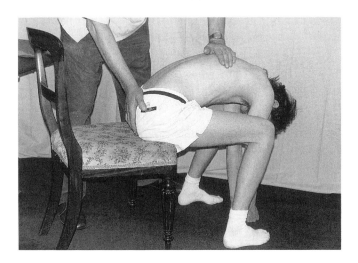

3.5.2.5. After 3–5 seconds she should relax. The operator keeps her position and takes up any slack with his hand on the sacrum.

3.5.2.6. Steps 3.5.2.4 and 3.5.2.5 are repeated two to four times.

3.5.2.7. Retest.

3.6 Bilateral posterior sacral nutation (bilateral superior sacral shear or extended sacrum)

Diagnostic points. All are the same as in 3.5 above except that the lumbar spine is flat and the spring test positive.

3.6.1. Muscle energy. Treat first one side and then the other as described in technique 3.4.1 above.

3.6.2. Alternative muscle energy.

3.6.2.1. The patient sits on a stool or on the end of a table with her feet together and her knees apart (to begin to open the anterior aspect of her SI joints). If on a table that is too high for her feet to reach the ground she should rest them on a stool. She should lean back and take hold of the edges of the stool or table behind her.

3.6.2.2. The operator prepares to resist her effort by standing beside her and placing his fist, or the heel of his hand, nearest her back against

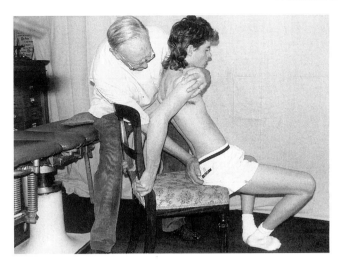

Fig. 7.15 Muscle energy treatment for bilateral posterior sacral nutation.

the base of her sacrum to press anteriorly. He places his other hand against her sternum to prevent her moving forwards (Fig. 7.15).

3.6.2.3. The patient makes an effort to bend forwards which the operator resists and after 3–5 seconds she should relax.

3.6.2.4. The operator takes up any slack by increasing her extension over his hand on the sacrum.

3.6.2.5. Steps 3.6.2.3 and 3.6.2.4 are repeated two to four times.

3.6.2.6. Retest.

4   ILIOSACRAL DYSFUNCTIONS

4.1   Posterior innominate on the left

Diagnostic points. After other pelvic dysfunctions, except flares, have been treated the standing forward flexion test remains positive on the left. The left ASIS is high, the PSIS a little low and the left sulcus deep. The left medial malleolus will be high supine if the legs are structurally equal.

Note that this dysfunction often accompanies anterior sacral nutation. *The effort required for treatment of the posterior innominate may cause recurrence of the nutation unless the sacral position is protected* (see step 4.1.3.2).

4.1.1. Muscle energy, sidelying.

4.1.1.1. The patient lies on her right side and the operator stands behind her at the level of her pelvis.

4.1.1.2. With his right hand the operator contacts the posterior part of her left iliac crest, preferably with the thumb placed so that he can monitor tension at her left sacroiliac joint.

4.1.1.3. With his left hand he picks up her flexed left knee and 'loose packs' the SI joint by abduction or adduction and/or external or internal rotation of the hip.

4.1.1.4. He then extends her left hip until the tension just reaches the sacroiliac joint and finally takes up the slack by pressing gently forwards on the iliac crest (Fig. 7.16a).

Fig. 7.16 Muscle energy treatment for left posterior innominate. (a) Sidelying, knee grip; (b) sidelying, ankle grip.

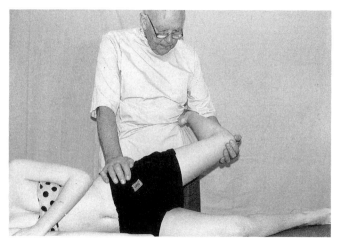

a

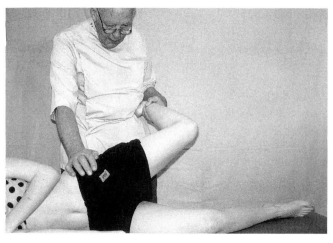

b

4.1.1.5. The instruction is 'pull your knee forward' and this the operator resists with an equal and opposite counterforce.

4.1.1.6 After 3–5 seconds she should be told to relax and, when full relaxation has occurred (and not before), the slack is taken up by further extension of the hip.

4.1.1.7. Steps 4.1.1.5 and 4.1.1.6 are repeated two or more times.

4.1.1.8. Retest.

Note. The operator may grip the ankle (Fig. 7.16b) instead of holding the knee. The advantage is that small operators do not have to reach so far. The disadvantage is that it is not as easy to position the limb properly in order to loose pack the SI joint.

4.1.2. Muscle energy, supine (compare superior pubis dysfunction technique 1.1; the difference allows the innominate to move anteriorly).

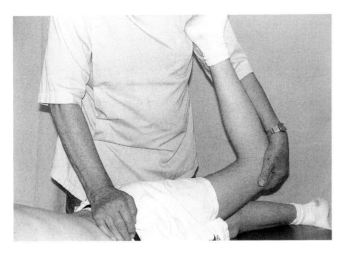

c

Fig. 7.16 (continued). (c) Prone; (d) prone, protecting anterior nutation correction.

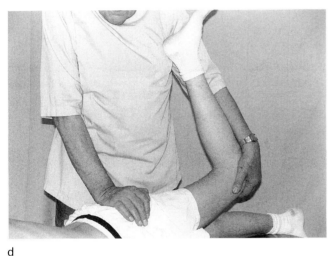

d

4.1.2.1. The patient is supine, and her pelvis is moved to the edge of the table so that the left PSIS is just *off* the table top. For stability her shoulders should remain in the centre of the table (see Fig. 7.1a.)

4.1.2.2. The operator stands beside her left leg and takes it off the table, supporting her ankle either between his lower legs or with his right ankle while standing on his left leg with his right knee bent (see Fig. 7.1b and c.)

4.1.2.3. The operator uses his left hand to press down on the patient's right ASIS. This helps to prevent her feeling that she would fall off and is used to monitor, the motion being stopped just before the ASIS begins to move.

4.1.2.4. The operator then places his right hand on the front of her left thigh to resist movement, being careful to avoid the patellofemoral joint.

4.1.2.5. The instruction is 'try to raise your left thigh against my hand'. The pressure should be no more than moderate and maintained for 3–5 seconds.

4.1.2.6. Have her relax and wait for the second phase when relaxation is complete, if necessary asking again for full relaxation. When she has relaxed fully, allow the leg to slide down between your legs (or lower your ankle) until you reach the next barrier. There will be a sense of resistance and motion must not go so far that your hand on the opposite ASIS can feel movement. Her knee should not be allowed to hang bent.

4.1.2.7. Repeat steps 4.1.2.5 and 4.1.2.6 three or four times or until there is no further gain on relaxation.

4.1.2.8. Retest.

4.1.3. Muscle energy, prone. (This is technique 4.1.1 turned through 90°.)

4.1.3.1. The patient is prone and the operator stands to either side. The left side may be easier for short operators but the right side is easier for many.

4.1.3.2. With his hand nearer her head the operator contacts the back of her left iliac crest to monitor and as counterforce (Fig. 7.16c). If an anterior nutation has been present and recently treated, the sacrum should be protected by the counterforce being applied to the left inferior lateral angle of the sacrum instead of the back of the crest (Fig. 7.16d). If this is not done the nutation may be brought back by the patient's effort.

4.1.3.3. With his caudad hand the operator lifts her left thigh, avoiding the patellofemoral joint. It is easier to lift if the knee is flexed to 90°.

4.1.3.4. With the SI joint loose packed and the slack taken up by lifting the thigh, the operator instructs the patient to pull the knee down toward the table. This he must resist and it is wise to caution the patient not to pull too hard.

4.1.3.5. After 3–5 seconds she should relax and, when relaxation is complete, the slack is taken up by further lifting of the thigh.

4.1.3.6. Steps 4.1.3.4 and 4.1.3.5 are repeated two or more times.

4.1.3.7. Retest.

4.1.4. Thrust. First technique.

4.1.4.1. The patient lies on her right side with her right leg moderately extended.

4.1.4.2. The operator stands in front of her pelvis and while monitoring over her sacral base with his right hand, he pulls her right shoulder forwards ('out from under'). In this way he induces right sidebending and left rotation of the spine down to and including the sacrum.

4.1.4.3. Changing to monitor with his left hand, the operator flexes her left leg to about 90°, leaving her left sacroiliac joint loose packed.

4.1.4.4. The operator now finds the ledge under her left PSIS and, leaning forward, contacts it with the heel of his right hand, usually with the pisiform bone. His forearm should be parallel to the table top and extend posteriorly and caudad at an angle of about 30° to the axis of her trunk (Fig. 7.17a).

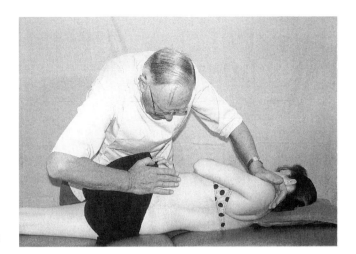

a

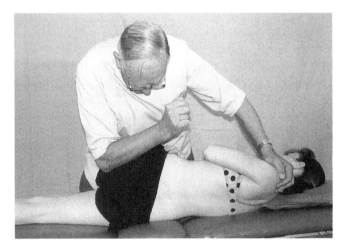

b

Fig. 7.17 Thrust treatment for left posterior innominate. (a) Using pisiform contact on PSIS; (b) using forearm contact on ischial tuberosity.

4.1.4.5. He now moves his left hand to the front of her left shoulder and takes up the slack by increasing slightly the left rotation of her trunk.

4.1.4.6. The thrust is given by a high velocity, low amplitude movement of his right hand in the direction in which his forearm is pointing and his pressure on her left shoulder is, at the same time, slightly increased to provide the counterforce.

4.1.4.7. Retest.

4.1.5. Thrust. Second technique.

Steps 4.1.5.1 to 4.1.5.3 are the same as steps 4.1.4.1 to 4.1.4.3.

4.1.5.4. The operator contacts the anterior part of her left ischial tuberosity with the upper part of his right forearm and takes up the slack in a craniad and posterior direction (Fig. 7.17b).

4.1.5.5. The thrust is given by the operator's forearm against her ischial tuberosity directed craniad and posteriorly while his left hand prevents loss of the position from above.

4.1.5.6. Retest.

4.2   Anterior innominate on the right

Diagnostic points. After other pelvic dysfunctions, except flares, have been treated the standing forward flexion test remains positive on the right. The right ASIS is low and anterior, the PSIS a little high and the right sulcus shallow. The right medial malleolus will be low in the supine position if the legs are structurally equal.

This dysfunction is common in association with a posterior sacral nutation on the same side. *If the patient has recently had such a nutation treated, the effort for treatment of the anterior innominate may cause recurrence of the nutation and the sacrum should be protected* as in step 4.2.2.4.

4.2.1. Muscle energy, supine. Compare technique 1.2 for inferior pubic dysfunction and note the difference in direction of the pull on the ischium.

4.2.1.1. The patient lies supine and the operator may stand to either side. For a small operator it may be easier to stand on the right side but, for a larger operator, it is easier to apply the force in the required direction if he is on the left side. The description will be for the operator standing on the left side and the differences will be noted in parentheses.

4.2.1.2. The patient's right knee and hip are flexed almost fully and the operator then rolls her so that he can insert his left (right) hand under her right buttock. His index and middle fingers should reach to be on either side of her right PSIS for monitoring (if they are long enough), while he holds her right ischial tuberosity in the palm of his hand.

4.2.1.3. With his axilla or shoulder (or other hand and trunk) the operator now blocks extension of her right hip and, while monitoring with his finger tips, takes up any slack by further hip flexion and by lifting her right ischial tuberosity in the direction of the right ASIS. If standing on her left the operator may increase his control by pressing posteriorly with his right hand on her right ASIS (see Figs 7.2a, b and c).

4.2.1.4. When the slack has been taken out, the instruction is '*gently push your right foot toward the foot of the table*'. This is resisted by an equal counterforce and, as the muscles concerned are powerful, the caution to be gentle is important.

4.2.1.5. After 3–5 seconds she should relax and, after full relaxation, the operator takes up the slack by pulling with the palm of his left hand *in the direction of her right ASIS.*

4.2.1.6. Steps 4.2.1.4 and 4.2.1.5 are repeated two or more times.

4.2.1.7. Retest.

4.2.2. Muscle energy, prone.

4.2.2.1. The patient lies prone with her right hip at the edge of the table.

4.2.2.2. The operator stands at her right side and takes her right leg off the table, allowing the knee to hang down in a position controlled by his right hand.

4.2.2.3. He so positions his legs that he can trap her right foot against his left leg and hold it there with his right leg (Fig. 7.18a).

4.2.2.4. While monitoring in the sacral sulcus with the tips of his left index and middle fingers, he moves her right knee to loose pack the sacroiliac joint by rotation, abduction/adduction and flexion/extension of

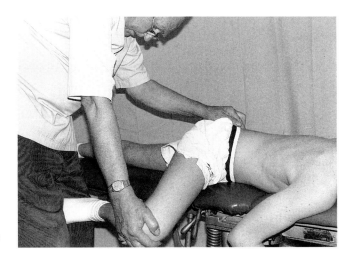

a

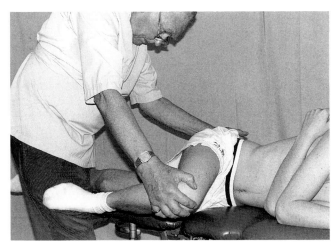

b

Fig. 7.18 Muscle energy treatment for right anterior innominate. (a) Prone; (b) sidelying.

the hip. If the patient has recently had a posterior sacral nutation on the right side the sacrum must be protected. This is conveniently done by the operator pressing anteriorly on the right sacral base with the heel of his left hand (or his left pisiform), the fingers of his left hand would otherwise simply be being used as monitors of the position and tension.

4.2.2.5. The instruction is 'gently push your right foot towards the foot of the table'. This movement is resisted by the operator's left leg and after 3–5 seconds the patient is told to relax.

4.2.2.6. Once again, when full relaxation has occurred, the slack is taken up, this time by the operator easing his left leg craniad until the monitoring fingers indicate that the new barrier has been reached.

4.2.2.7. Steps 4.2.2.5 and 4.2.2.6 are repeated two or more times.

4.2.2.8. Retest.

4.2.3. Muscle energy, sidelying.

4.2.3.1. The patient lies on her left side and the operator stands in front of her pelvis.

4.2.3.2. With his right hand the operator picks up her right knee and flexes knee and hip until he feels tension just begin to increase with the fingers of his left hand monitoring in her right sacral sulcus, between the PSIS and the sacral base (Fig. 7.18b).

4.2.3.3. The operator either stands in front and uses his trunk or thigh to block motion of her knee, or stands level with her left knee and resists her motion by placing her right foot against his right hip (or left thigh).

4.2.3.4. When all slack has been taken out by further controlled hip flexion the patient is instructed to try gently to push her right foot towards the foot of the table.

4.2.3.5. The pressure is maintained for 3–5 seconds and then relaxed.

4.2.3.6. After full relaxation the slack is taken, by further hip flexion, up to the new barrier and steps 4.2.3.4 and 4.2.3.5 are repeated two or more times.

4.2.3.7. Retest.

4.2.4. Thrust. First technique.

4.2.4.1. The patient lies on her left side and the operator stands in front of her pelvis.

4.2.4.2. He pulls her left shoulder out to lock her spine by neutral mechanics down to and including the sacrum.

4.2.4.3. With his left hand the operator picks up her right knee and flexes knee and hip until he feels tension just begin to increase with the fingers of his right hand monitoring in her right sacral sulcus, between the PSIS and the sacral base. Her foot may remain on the table top.

4.2.4.4. He now allows her right thigh to rest on the edge of the table and grasps her right ischial tuberosity with his left hand while with his right hand he contacts the front of her iliac crest (Fig. 7.19a).

4.2.4.5. Slack is taken out by a rotatory motion of her right innominate, his right hand pressing posteriorly on the anterior part of her right iliac crest, or the ASIS, and his left hand pulling anteriorly on her ischial tuberosity.

4.2.4.6. When the slack has been taken out (and this requires judgment as there is no monitor in the sulcus) a high velocity, low amplitude thrust is given by his left hand pulling her right ischial tuberosity forwards. The pressure of his right hand is increased slightly at the same time.

4.2.4.7. Retest.

4.2.5. Thrust. Second technique.

Steps 4.2.5.1 and 4.2.5.2 are as steps 4.2.4.1 and 4.2.4.2.

4.2.5.3. Her right thigh is allowed to hang over the edge of the table and he contacts the posterior part of her right ischial tuberosity with his left upper forearm taking up the slack with pressure anteriorly and craniad.

4.2.5.4. The operator controls the position of her right ASIS with his right hand and the thrust is given by his left forearm on her ischial tuberosity anteriorly and craniad (Fig. 7.19b).

4.2.5.5. Retest.

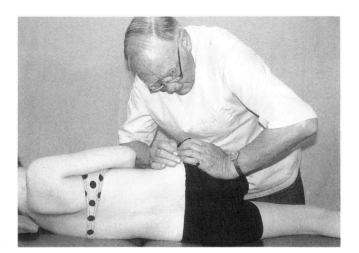

Fig. 7.19 Thrust treatment for right anterior innominate. (a) Using heel of hand on ischial tuberosity; (b) using forearm on ischial tuberosity.

a

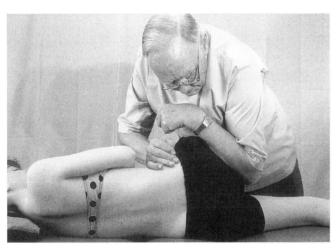

b

4.3   Iliac outflare

Diagnostic points. These are described for the left side. After all other pelvic dysfunctions have been treated the standing forward flexion test remains positive on the left, and the ASIS is further from the midline on the left side than on the right.

4.3.1. Muscle energy.

4.3.1.1. The patient lies supine and the operator stands to either side of her pelvis.

4.3.1.2. The patient's left hip and knee are fully flexed and, if standing to her left, the operator leans forward so that he can control abduction movement with his trunk. If on her right he controls her thigh with his left hand.

4.3.1.3. With his right hand the operator reaches his finger tips under her to monitor and to grip her left PSIS and pull it laterally.

4.3.1.4. With his left hand he controls the position of her left thigh

Fig. 7.20 Muscle energy
treatment of left iliac outflare.

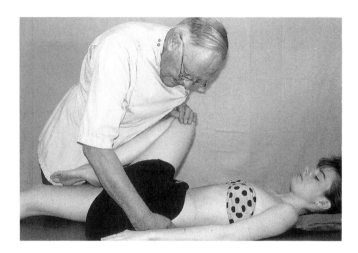

(Fig. 7.20) but if is standing on her left side he may use it to apply
counterforce to her right ASIS.

4.3.1.5. The slack is taken out by further adduction of her left thigh,
to the point of tension (before the sacrum begins to move) and the
instruction is then 'try to push your left knee to the left'.

4.3.1.6. After 3–5 seconds she should relax.

4.3.1.7. When relaxation is complete steps 4.3.1.5 and 4.3.1.6 are
repeated two or more times.

4.3.1.8. Retest.

4.4   Iliac inflare

Diagnostic points. These are described for the right side. After all other
pelvic dysfunctions have been treated the standing forward flexion test

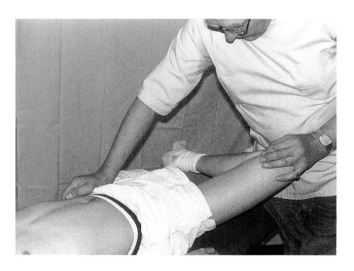

Fig. 7.21 Muscle energy
treatment of right iliac inflare.

remains positive on the right, and the ASIS is nearer the midline on the right side than on the left.

4.4.1. Muscle energy,

4.4.1.1. The patient lies supine and the operator stands to the right of her lower thighs.

4.4.1.2. The patient's right hip is fully flexed and abducted and her knee flexed enough to allow her right foot to rest on the table, lateral to her left knee.

4.4.1.3. The operator holds her right knee with his left hand to keep her hip abducted and places his right hand against the medial side of her left ASIS for counterforce (Fig. 7.21).

4.4.1.4. When any slack has been taken out by abduction of her right thigh as far as it easily goes (and without moving her left ilium), the instruction is 'try to press your right knee forward (into adduction) against my hand'.

4.4.1.5. After 3–5 seconds she should relax.

4.4.1.6. When relaxation is complete steps 4.4.1.3 and 4.4.1.4 are repeated two or more times.

4.4.1.7. Retest.

REFERENCE

1. Brooks Appliance Co., 310 E. Michigan Avenue, Marshall, Michigan 49068, USA.

Chapter 8

Treatment of the lumbar spine

Both muscle energy and thrusting techniques will be described. All the thrust techniques for the lumbar spine can be modified to become muscle energy procedures but the reverse is not true. The modification is at the point when localisation is complete. Instead of an external force being used to break through the barrier, the patient is asked to attempt to push away from it. This movement is blocked by the operator and the treatment relies on post–isometric muscle relaxation to make the barrier recede. As has been pointed out earlier, muscle energy treatment will only work well if localisation is accurate. Accurate localisation is also needed for good thrust treatment; much less force is then required.

1   SIDELYING, SIDEBENDING ACTIVATION TECHNIQUES

These make use of sidebending for the correction and, to allow the required rotation, the patient will be on the side of the posterior transverse process for the FRS and on the side of the anterior TP for ERS and neutral dysfunctions. Contrast the rotatory force techniques for which the posterior TP is always down on the table.

Muscle energy only
1.1. For non-neutral dysfunction with restriction of extension and of sidebending and rotation to the same side. Described for L3 rotated to the left, FRSlt. Compare the similar treatment for posterior sacral torsion described in Chapter 7, technique 3.2.1.

Diagnostic points. There is tissue texture change at the segment. The left transverse process of L3 is posterior to that on the right in extension (sphinx) but they are level in flexion. There may be some prominence on the left in neutral.

   1.1.1. The patient lies on her left side and the operator stands facing her. He moves her pelvis near to the front of the table, while monitoring at the segment in order to avoid moving too far. This starts extension of the spine and is best done by lifting with one hand under her waist while using the other as monitor (Fig. 8.1a).

   1.1.2. Monitoring at L4 with his right hand, the operator extends her under (left) hip, by moving her leg back, until L4 is about to move (Fig. 8.1b).

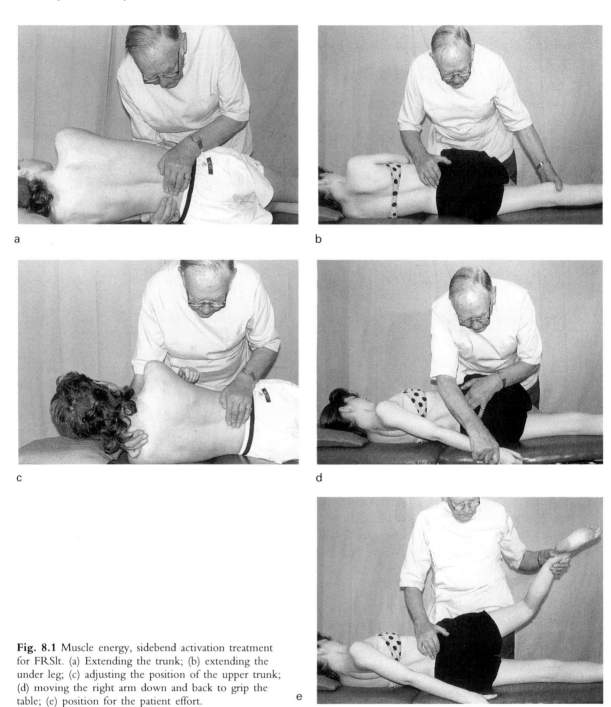

Fig. 8.1 Muscle energy, sidebend activation treatment for FRSlt. (a) Extending the trunk; (b) extending the under leg; (c) adjusting the position of the upper trunk; (d) moving the right arm down and back to grip the table; (e) position for the patient effort.

1.1.3. The operator now changes to monitor at L3 with his left hand while he localises from above. If step 1.1.1 has been carried out, it may be found that only rotation is needed to bring the tension to the right place. If this does not happen the position of the upper spine should be adjusted by lifting under her neck and sliding her left shoulder backwards (or forwards because it is possible to extend too far in the initial movement) until the tension reaches the monitoring finger at L3. The shoulder is not pulled out from under her; that would reverse the sidebend (Fig. 8.1c).

1.1.4. Rotation is introduced and sidebending increased in extension by the operator picking up her right hand and pulling her arm down and back until the tension is just felt at L3, that is up to but not beyond the barrier. She is then asked to hold on to the table edge to maintain the position (Fig. 8.1d).

1.1.5. The operator then changes back to monitor with his right hand while with his left hand he lifts her right ankle directly above her left knee by abduction and internal rotation until he begins to feel the tension with his right fingers (Fig. 8.1e).

1.1.6. The instruction is 'pull your right foot down towards your left knee'. When she does this he should feel the muscles tighten at L3 with his monitor if the position is correct.

1.1.7. After 3–5 seconds both relax but the position must be maintained.

1.1.8. After full relaxation the slack is taken up to the new barrier by lifting her right leg and if necessary asking her to move her grip further down the table which increases both extension and sidebending. Steps 1.1.6 and 1.1.7 are repeated two or more times.

1.1.9. Retest.

1.2. For non-neutral dysfunction with restriction of flexion and of sidebending and rotation to the same side. Described for L3 rotated to the right, ERSrt. Compare the treatment for anterior sacral torsion Chapter 7, technique 3.1.1.

> *Diagnostic points.* There is tissue texture change at the segment. The right transverse process of L3 is more posterior than the left in flexion and they are level in extension. There may be some prominence on the right in neutral.

1.2.1. The patient lies prone with her right shoulder close to the side of the table and with her right arm hanging over the edge.

1.2.2. The operator lifts both her ankles with his left hand and her knees with his right hand and brings the knees up to her right side putting her in the left lateral 'Sims position'. The precise position is important; the hip flexion must be stopped at the point just before L4 begins to move and the movement is therefore monitored in its final stage by the fingers of his right hand at the L4 level. Note that, in so far as she is on her side, it is the side of the anterior transverse process (Fig. 8.2a).

1.2.3. The patient should then breathe deeply and as she breathes out reach for the floor with her right hand. This movement also must be monitored and is stopped just before L3 begins to move. The operator uses his left hand to monitor at this stage because he may need to use his right hand to increase the patient's rotation by pressing down on her right shoulder as she breathes out. If necessary the exhalation and reaching for the floor is repeated until the point of tension is reached.

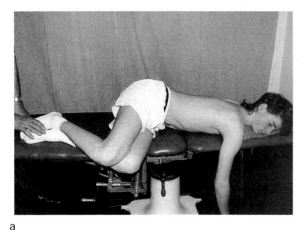

a

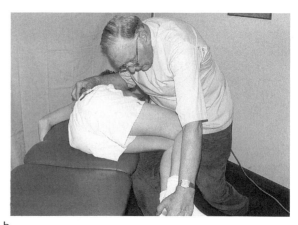

b

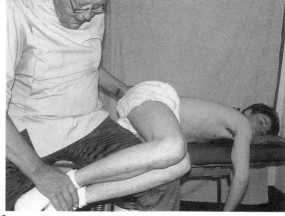

c

Fig. 8.2 Muscle energy, sidebend activation treatment for ERSrt. (a) Left lateral Sims position; (b) position for effort, supporting her knees on yours; (c) position for effort, operator seated.

1.2.4. The necessary left sidebend is introduced by dropping the patient's feet over the edge of the table without losing the localisation from below. If this were done without protection, when the effort is made the pressure of the table edge on the under thigh would be uncomfortable. To avoid this one of three methods is commonly used.

1.2.4a. Place a small cushion under the thigh to protect it from the edge of the table.

1.2.4b. The operator stands so that he can support the patient's knees over his right knee (Fig. 8.2b).

1.2.4c. The operator sits on the foot of the table and, with legs apart, supports her knees on his left knee. This is sometimes known as the lazy man's technique; its disadvantage is that it is no longer possible for the operator to control the trunk with his right arm. In order to monitor at L3–4 he must change hands and his right hand now provides the resistance to the patient's effort.

1.2.4d. The patient's lower limbs may be supported under the upper tibiae as described in Chapter 7, technique 3.1.1.

1.2.5. The patient should be told to maintain the twisted position. While easier for the small operator, the 'lazy man' technique is difficult for those operators wearing skirts because of the abduction required to allow the patient's feet to drop (Fig. 8.2c).

1.2.6. The instruction to the patient is 'raise your feet toward the ceiling' which the operator resists with an equal and opposite force with the left hand in variants 1.2.4a and 1.2.4b but the right hand in variant 1.2.4c. The pressure is maintained for 3–5 seconds and the patient must then relax. It helps to tell her to 'drop her feet'.

1.2.7. After full relaxation, the slack is taken up to the new point of tension as monitored by the fingers. This can usually be done by dropping the feet but sometimes an adjustment to the flexion of the hips may help.

1.2.8. Steps 1.2.6 and 1.2.7 are repeated two or more times.

1.2.9. Retest.

1.3. For neutral (type I, or group) dysfunction with restriction of right rotation and left sidebending at L2, 3 and 4, NRlt (rotated to the left and sidebent right).

Diagnostic points. There is tissue texture change at the group. The left transverse processes of L2, 3 and 4 are more posterior than those on the right. This is most marked in neutral flexion–extension but in no position do they become level.

1.3.1. The patient lies on her right side and the operator stands in front of her.

1.3.2. The operator flexes her hips and thighs with his right hand while monitoring with his left at L3. This time, because neutral is required in the sagittal plane, the end point is not tension but *maximum ease* at the apex of the group (L3).

1.3.3. The operator then introduces left sidebending by lifting her feet until he feels motion at L4, *but not at L3*, remembering that the most common fault is to go too far (Fig. 8.3).

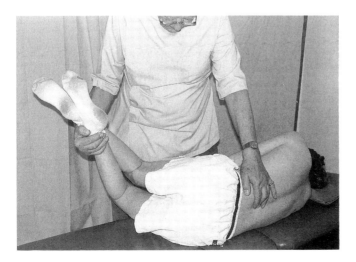

Fig. 8.3 Muscle energy sidebend activation treatment for NRlt.

1.3.4. The instruction is 'try to pull your feet down to the table' which the operator resists. The effort is maintained for 3–5 seconds and then she should relax.

1.3.5. After relaxation is complete the feet are lifted to the new barrier and steps 1.3.4 and 1.3.5 are repeated two or more times.

1.3.6. Retest.

2   SIDELYING, ROTATORY TECHNIQUES

These three are easy to remember because in each the patient lies with the most posterior transverse process down on the table. When thrust is used it is important to remember the 'low amplitude' part of the description because the lumbar joints are designed not to rotate and each joint has only about 3° of rotation before reaching its anatomical barrier.

2.1. For non-neutral dysfunction with restriction of extension and of sidebending and rotation to the same side. Described for L3 rotated to the right, FRSrt.

Thrust or muscle energy

Diagnostic points. There is tissue texture change at the segment. The right transverse process of L3 is posterior to that on the left in extension (sphinx) but they are level in flexion. There may be some prominence on the right in neutral.

2.1.1. The patient lies on her right side and the operator stands in front of her. He moves her pelvis near to the front of the table which starts extension of the spine while monitoring at the segment in order to avoid moving too far. (Compare technique 1.1 but note that the opposite side is being described.)

2.1.2. Monitoring at L4 with his left hand, the operator extends her under (right) hip until L4 is about to move. Her left leg lies on the table with the knee bent and, if the foot is placed in front of her right knee, the tendency of the patient to flex the right leg (and spoil the localisation) can be reduced. See Fig. 8.1b (but note that the opposite side is involved).

2.1.3. The operator now monitors at L3 with his right hand while he localises from above. If step 2.1.1 has been carried out, it may be found that only rotation is needed to bring the tension to the right place. If this does not happen the position of the upper spine should be adjusted by lifting under her neck and sliding her right shoulder backwards (or forwards) until the tension reaches the monitoring finger at L3. In order to preserve the left sidebend the right (under) shoulder is not 'pulled out' (Fig. 8.4a).

2.1.4. The operator slides his left forearm through her left axilla and places his fingers as an additional monitor at L3 while his upper forearm rests against the front of her left shoulder. Alternatively his left hand can press on the front of her shoulder but the additional monitor is not then available.

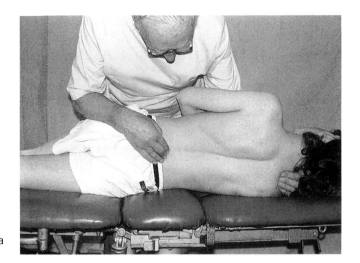

a

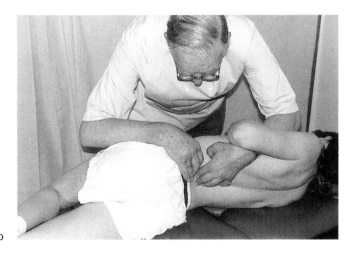

b

Fig. 8.4 Rotatory activation treatment for FRSrt. ME or thrust. (a) Localisation from above; (b) position for patient effort.

2.1.5. With his right fingers monitoring at L4 the operator places his right forearm over the upper part of her left buttock between the iliac crest and the trochanter (Fig. 8.4b).

2.1.6. The position is 'fine tuned' by rotation backwards of her shoulder and forwards of her left buttock until all slack is taken out and the tension is localised at the L3–4 joint, that is when the tension just reaches L4 from below and L3 from above.

T.2.1.7. Thrust variant. The high velocity, low amplitude thrust is given by the right forearm on the buttock placed so that while rotating the ilium forwards it will help to sidebend the L3–4 segment to the left. The pressure with the left forearm must be increased enough to stabilise the patient's upper trunk. In order to increase the force available for the thrust, which makes it easier to be accurate, the operator should try to 'lock' his forearm against his trunk and use a trunk/forearm movement for the thrust. The thrust may be given against the ischial tuberosity, directed craniad to produce sidebending but the fingers of the right hand can no longer monitor accurately.

M.2.1.7a. Muscle energy variant. Instead of a thrust the patient is asked to try to change her position against resistance. This can be done by the operator maintaining the position at the barrier while she is instructed 'try to untwist yourself', or 'push your left shoulder forwards', or, if the operator moves his right hand to the lateral aspect of her left knee, 'try to lift your left knee against my hand'. Some patients will push too hard and need to be cautioned to be gentle because, for it to be isometric the operator must be able to prevent motion.

M.2.1.7b. After 3–5 seconds the patient should be told to relax and, when relaxation is complete, the operator adjusts her position to reach the new barrier. This can usually be reached by increasing the rotation but further extension may be added if required.

M.2.1.7c. The last two steps are repeated twice, or sometimes more depending on the response. The final adjustment of the position ('taking up the slack') is important as it is then that the gain in range of motion is completed.

2.1.8. Retest.

2.2. For non–neutral dysfunction with restriction of flexion and of sidebending and rotation to the same side. Described for L3 rotated to the right, ERSrt.

Thrust or muscle energy

Diagnostic points. There is tissue texture change at the segment. The right transverse process of L3 is more posterior than the left in flexion and they are level in extension. There may be some prominence on the right in neutral.

2.2.1. The patient lies on her right side and the operator stands in front. She should be positioned towards the back of the treatment table.

2.2.2. While monitoring at L4 with his left hand, the operator flexes her right leg until L4 is about to move. The left foot may be hooked into the back of the right knee or the legs may be moved together.

2.2.3. The operator must now monitor at L3 with his right hand while he localises from above. The flexion of the upper spine is increased by lifting under her neck and sliding her right shoulder forwards until the tension just reaches L3. In order to preserve the left sidebend the right (under) shoulder is not 'pulled out' (Fig. 8.5a).

2.2.4. The operator slides his left forearm through her left axilla and places his fingers as an additional monitor at L3 while his upper forearm rests against the front of her left shoulder. Alternatively his left hand can press on the front of her shoulder but the additional monitor is not then available.

2.2.5. With his right fingers monitoring at L4 the operator places his right forearm over her left buttock roughly half way from the ischial tuberosity to the ASIS, behind the greater trochanter.

2.2.6. The position is 'fine tuned' by rotation backwards of her shoulder and forwards of her left buttock until all slack has been taken out

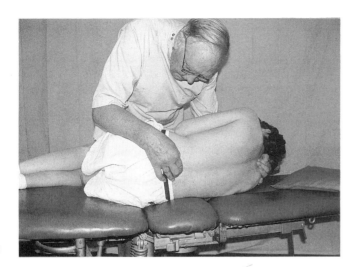

a

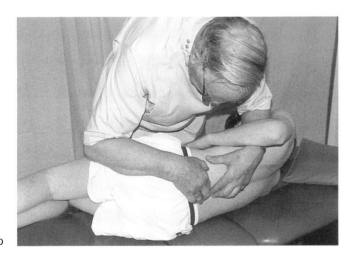

b

Fig. 8.5 Rotatory activation treatment for ERSrt. ME or thrust. (a) Localisation from above; (b) position for patient effort.

and the tension is localised at the L3–4 joint, that is when the tension just reaches L4 from below and L3 from above (Fig. 8.5b).

T.2.2.7. Thrust variant. The high velocity, low amplitude thrust is given on the buttock to produce left sidebending and left rotation and slight flexion of the pelvis by having the forearm contact posterior and caudal to the greater trochanter. The pressure with the left forearm must be increased enough to stabilise the patient's upper trunk. In order to increase the force available for the thrust, which makes it easier to be accurate, the operator should try to 'lock' his forearm against his trunk and use a trunk/forearm movement for the thrust.

M.2.2.7a. Muscle energy variant. Instead of a thrust the patient is asked to try to change her position against resistance. This can be done by the operator maintaining the position at the barrier while she is instructed 'try to untwist yourself', or 'push your left shoulder forwards', or, if the operator moves his right hand to the lateral aspect of her left knee, 'try to lift your left knee against my hand'. Some patients will push too hard and need to be cautioned to be gentle because, for it to be isometric, the operator must be able to prevent motion.

M.2.2.7b. After 3–5 seconds the patient should be told to relax and, when relaxation is complete, the operator adjusts her position by rotation, with added flexion if needed, to reach the new barrier.

M.2.2.7c. The last two steps are repeated twice, or sometimes more depending on the response. The final adjustment of the position ('taking up the slack') is important as it is then that the gain in range of motion is completed.

2.2.8. Retest.

2.3. For neutral (type I, or group) dysfunction with restriction of left rotation and right sidebending at L2, 3 and 4, NRrt (rotated to the right and sidebent left). The most posterior TP will be that of L3 on the right.

Thrust or muscle energy

Diagnostic points. There is tissue texture change at the group. The right transverse processes of L2, 3 and 4 are more posterior than those on the left. This is most marked in neutral flexion–extension but in no position do they become level.

2.3.1. The patient lies on her right side and the operator stands in front.

2.3.2. Her left foot should be hooked behind her right knee and the flexion–extension position of her legs is then adjusted so that the centre vertebra of the group is at the point of maximum ease with respect to the ones above and below.

2.3.3. The rotation required is the same as in techniques 2.1. and 2.2, but the sidebend has to be reversed. To achieve this the operator monitors with his left hand while he pulls her right shoulder out from under her. The movement is continued caudad until the barrier is reached in rotation and flexion (when the tension just reaches the L3 level from above) (Fig. 8.6).

2.3.4. With his arms positioned as for techniques 2.2.4 and 2.2.5, the operator fine tunes the position by rotation. The point of localisation should be just below the apex of the group (on and just below the TP of L3).

T.2.3.5. Thrust variant. The high velocity, low amplitude thrust is given by the right forearm on the buttock by rotation anteriorly without a flexion or extension component. In order to increase the force available for the thrust, which makes it easier to be accurate, the operator should try to 'lock' his forearm against his trunk and use a trunk/forearm movement for the thrust.

M.2.3.5a. Muscle energy variant. Instead of a thrust the patient is asked to try to change her position against resistance. This can be done by the operator maintaining the position at the barrier while she is instructed 'try to untwist yourself', or 'push your left shoulder forwards', or, if the operator moves his right hand to the lateral aspect of her left knee, 'try to lift your left knee against my hand'. Some patients will push too hard

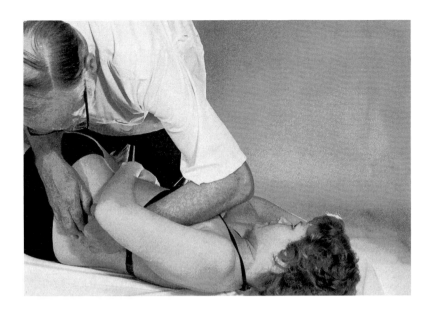

Fig. 8.6 Rotatory activation treatment for NRrt. ME or thrust.

and need to be cautioned to be gentle because, for it to be isometric, the operator must be able to prevent motion.

M.2.3.5b. After 3–5 seconds the patient should be told to relax and, when relaxation is complete, the operator adjusts her position by rotation to reach the new barrier.

M.2.3.5c. The last two steps are repeated twice, or sometimes more depending on the response. The final adjustment of the position ('taking up the slack') is important as it is then that the gain in range of motion is completed.

2.3.5. Retest.

3 SITTING

These can also be used for thoracic dysfunction up to about T5. Except for the first technique, they are described with the patient sitting astride the table because that improves stability; they can be done with the patient on a stool or sitting across the table if necessary. Alternative grips for the operator can be used especially for the muscle energy variants and some of these will be described at the end of this chapter.

3.1. For non-neutral dysfunction with restriction of extension and of sidebending and rotation to the same side. Technique using neutral mechanics to restore left rotation before addressing the sidebending and extension components. Described for L3 rotated to the right, FRSrt.

Muscle energy
Diagnostic points. There is tissue texture change at the segment. The right transverse process of L3 is posterior to that on the left in extension (sphinx) but they are level in flexion. There may be some prominence in neutral.

3.1.1a. The patient sits on a stool with her right buttock near the left edge of the stool and her left buttock resting on the knee of the operator who sits on a stool or chair behind her. The patient's stool should be of such a height that the operator can support her left buttock either above or below the right one by raising and lowering his knee. By reversing the knee movements the operator may have the patient sit with her right buttock on his right knee and her left buttock on a stool.

3.1.1b. Alternatively the patient may sit on a table or stool and the sidebending is then introduced from above by the standing operator as in technique 3.2. The remainder of the technique is the same.

3.1.2. The patient should sit in 'erect neutral', that is erect or as nearly erect as still preserves flexion–extension ease. The operator monitors with his right hand at the L3 level and holds the patient's left shoulder with his left hand.

3.1.3. The first part of the technique is designed to restore the lost left rotation and for this 'neutral mechanics' are used. The operator lowers his left knee and drops the left side of the patient's pelvis enough to produce right sidebending from below up to the L4 level. At the same time he sidebends her to the right from above down to the top of L3, as always monitoring the tension and motion until the level is reached. This results in translation of L3 to the left (Fig. 8.7a).

3.1.4. The operator then asks the patient to rotate her left shoulder back as far as it easily goes which should bring the tissue tension to the L3 level. (Left rotation with right sidebending.)

3.1.5. He then holds her left shoulder with his left hand and she is asked to attempt to rotate it forwards which he resists. The effort is maintained for 3–5 seconds and when she relaxes the slack is taken up by further left rotation and steps 3.1.4 and 3.1.5 are repeated until there is no more gain of rotation (Fig. 8.7b).

3.1.6. The patient is then returned to non-neutral mechanics by the operator raising his left knee and gently depressing her left shoulder *while maintaining the left rotation that has been achieved*. This produces the required left sidebending with translation of L3 to the right (Fig. 8.7c).

3.1.7. Extension to the barrier is now needed and can be introduced by asking the patient to push her stomach out in front. The movement must be monitored by the operator's right hand and if she has moved too far the position must be adjusted by asking her to slump a little or some similar instruction.

3.1.8. The corrective effort can either be further pulling forward or elevation of the left shoulder which must be resisted by the operator.

3.1.9. After 3–5 seconds the patient should relax and the operator takes up the slack by asking the patient to push her stomach a little further out and fine tuning by backward rotation of the left shoulder with or without more sidebending at the same time.

3.1.10. Steps 3.1.8 and 3.1.9 are repeated two or more times or until there is no further gain of motion.

3.1.11 A further extension effort may be made if the patient is returned to the sagittal plane without losing the existing extension. The operator then puts his left arm across the front of her chest and

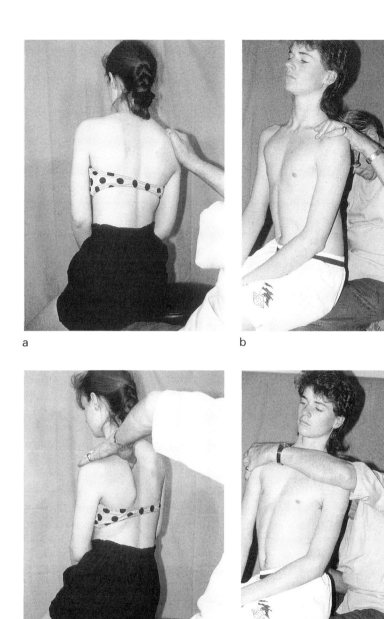

a

b

c

d

Fig. 8.7 Muscle energy sitting treatment for FRSrt with preliminary correction of rotation. (a) Starting position, sidebent right by translation left; (b) rotation left in neutral; (c) changing to left sidebend and starting extension; (d) position for patient's flexion effort.

grips her right humerus. At the same time he transfers his right hand to the segment below (L4) and, by pressure anteriorly, blocks backward translation of that vertebra. Her effort should be to attempt to bend forward which is resisted and the effort repeated two or three times (Fig. 8.7d).

3.1.12. Retest.

3.2. For non-neutral dysfunction with restriction of extension and of sidebending and rotation to the same side. Simpler technique not using preliminary correction of rotation. Described for L3 rotated to the right, FRSrt.

Thrust or muscle energy

Diagnostic points. There is tissue texture change at the segment. The right transverse process of L3 is posterior to that on the left in extension (sphinx) but they are level in flexion. There may be some prominence in neutral.

3.2.1. The patient sits astride the table with her back close to the end and puts her right hand on her left shoulder. The patient may sit on a stool with her feet on the floor or she may sit across a table but in the latter example the pelvis is less well controlled.

3.2.2. The operator stands behind and to her left and with his left hand grasps her right shoulder with his arm in front of her and his left axilla resting on her left shoulder or see note below for alternative (Fig. 8.8a).

3.2.3. With his right thumb (or the heel of the hand) the operator contacts the right transverse process, or the left side of the spinous process, of L3. This serves both as monitor and thrusting contact.

3.2.4. Extension is introduced by having the patient push her stomach out to obtain anterior translation bringing the tension just down to L3 and just up to L4. Translation to the right by downward pressure on her left shoulder is then used to sidebend from above and below with the same monitor. Rotation to the left will 'fine tune' so that the tension just reaches L3 from above (Fig. 8.8b which shows the alternative grip described in the note below).

T.3.2.5. Thrust variant. When all the slack is taken out, the operator brings his right hip close behind his elbow and the high velocity, low amplitude thrust is given through the thumb or the heel of the hand, against the right transverse process or on the left side of the spinous process of L3, while the trunk position is slightly exaggerated. Control is improved by the thrust coming mainly from movement of the operator's right hip (Fig. 8.8c).

M.3.2.5a. Muscle energy variant. The patient is asked to try to raise her left shoulder or pull it forwards, or to bend to the right. This is resisted by the operator and to keep the contraction isometric it may be necessary to tell the patient to be gentle in her effort.

M.3.2.5b. After 3–5 seconds she is asked to relax and, when relaxation is complete, the operator adjusts her position to reach the new barrier in all three planes.

M.3.2.5c. The last two steps are repeated twice or more and the slack is finally taken up.

M.3.2.5d. If necessary an isometric flexion effort may be used as well, or instead. For this the operator reaches across the front of the patient's chest and grips her opposite arm. The patient is asked to bend forwards while the operator resists and after 3–5 seconds the contraction is stopped to be repeated after positioning at the new barrier (Fig. 8.8d).

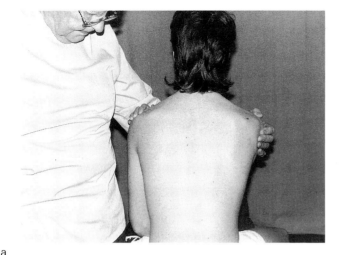

a

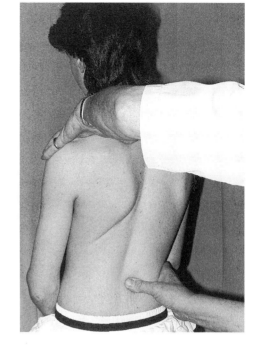

b

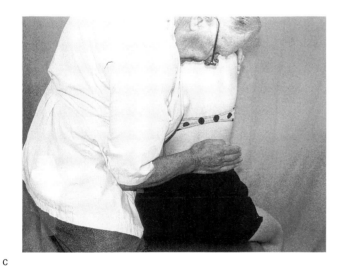

c

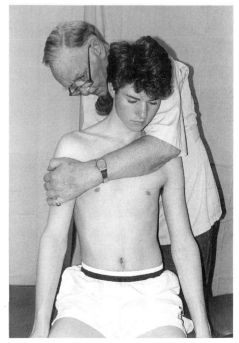

d

Fig. 8.8 Treatment for FRSrt without preliminary correction of
rotation. ME or thrust. (a) Starting position; (b) position for patient
effort, showing alternative grip; (c) thrust position using hip to
reinforce elbow movement; (d) position for final flexion effort.

3.2.6. Retest.

Note: the operator can use his hand on the top of the patient's left shoulder instead of his axilla. If that position is used the patient's effort is to attempt to lift her left shoulder and for short operators it is helpful if the table is low or the patient is sitting on a low stool.

3.3. For non-neutral dysfunction with restriction of flexion and of sidebending and rotation to the same side. Described for L3 rotated to the right, ERSrt.

Thrust or muscle energy

Diagnostic points. There is tissue texture change at the segment. The right transverse process of L3 is more posterior than the left in flexion and they are level in extension. There may be some prominence on the right in neutral.

3.3.1. The patient sits astride the table with her back close to the end and puts her right hand on her left shoulder. She may sit on a stool with her feet on the floor or she may sit across a table but in the latter example the pelvis is less well controlled.

3.3.2. The operator stands behind and to her left and with his left hand grasps her right shoulder with his arm in front of her and his left axilla resting on her left shoulder.

3.3.3. With his right thumb, or the heel of the hand, the operator contacts the right transverse process or the left side of the spinous process of L3. This serves both as monitor and thrusting contact.

3.3.4. The operator introduces flexion by translation of her trunk from before backwards ('allow yourself to slump') and sidebending by translation

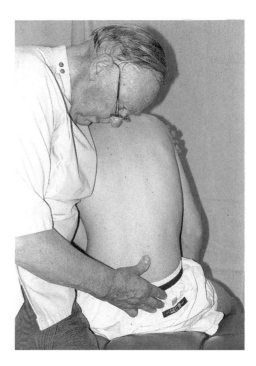

Fig. 8.9 Sitting treatment for ERSrt. ME or thrust.

from left to right, both being adjusted to bring the tension from above just to L3 and from below just to L4. Rotation to the left will 'fine tune' the position so that the tension just reaches L3 from above and all slack is taken out (Fig. 8.9).

T.3.3.5. Thrust variant. A high velocity, low amplitude thrust is given against the right TP, or the left side of the spinous process, of L3 by the right thumb, or the heel of the hand, supported by the hip which is brought up behind the elbow for the purpose as in Fig. 8.8c, while the trunk position is slightly exaggerated.

M.3.3.5a. Muscle energy variant. The patient is asked to try to raise her left shoulder or to bend to the right. This is resisted by the operator and to keep the contraction isometric it may be necessary to tell the patient to be gentle in her effort.

M.3.3.5b. After 3–5 seconds she is asked to relax and, when relaxation is complete, the operator adjusts her position to reach the new barrier in flexion, sidebending and rotation.

M.3.3.5c. The last two steps are repeated twice, or more if desired, and the slack is finally taken up.

M.3.3.5d. If necessary an isometric extension effort may be used as well, or instead. The patient is asked to bend backwards while the operator resists and after 3–5 seconds the contraction is stopped to be repeated after positioning at the new barrier.

3.3.6. Retest.

3.4. For neutral (group) of at least three vertebrae with restriction of left rotation and right sidebending, NRrt. Described for L2–3–4 rotated right and sidebent left. The most posterior TP will be that of L3 on the right.

Thrust or muscle energy
Diagnostic points. There is tissue texture change at the group. The right transverse processes of L2, 3 and 4 are more posterior than those on the left. This is most marked in neutral flexion and extension but in no position do they become level.

3.4.1. The patient sits astride the table with her back close to the end and puts one hand on the other shoulder. She may sit on a stool with her feet on the floor or she may sit across a table but in the latter example the pelvis is less well controlled.

3.4.2. The operator stands behind her and to her left and threads his left forearm through her left axilla to grip her right shoulder from in front (Fig. 8.10a and b).

3.4.3. With his right thumb, or the heel of the hand, the operator contacts the right side of L3 at and a little below the right transverse process, *not on the left side of the spinous process* because that would tend to prevent the necessary right sidebending.

3.4.4. With his left arm he then introduces right sidebending and left rotation of her trunk down to L3. Her lumbar spine should remain in neutral flexion–extension (Fig. 8.10c).

T.3.4.5. Thrust variant. The high velocity, low amplitude thrust against and a little below the right TP of L3 is given by the thumb, or the heel

Fig. 8.10 Sitting treatment for NRrt. ME or thrust. (a) Operator's grip with left forearm through axilla; (b) the same grip seen from behind; (c) position for patient effort; (d) thrust variant.

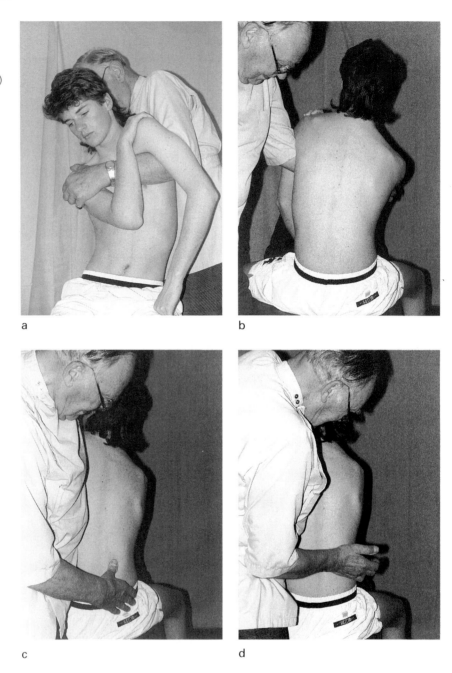

a

b

c

d

of the hand, supported by bringing his right hip behind his elbow and using body movement (Fig. 8.10d).

M.3.4.5a. Muscle energy variant. The patient is asked to attempt to sidebend to her left and the operator resists the movement.

M.3.4.5b. After 3–5 seconds she is asked to relax and, when relaxation is complete, the operator adjusts her position to reach the new barrier in sidebending and rotation.

M.3.4.5c. The last two steps are repeated twice, or more if desired, and the slack is finally taken up.

3.4.6. Retest.

3.5. Sitting technique for bilaterally restricted backward bending. Described for L3–4 level.

Thrust or muscle energy

Diagnostic points. The TPs are level in neutral, in forward bending and in backward bending but there is tissue texture change at the segment. The spinous process interval is wide at L3–4 and on motion testing the joint does not move.

3.5.1. The patient sits astride the table with her back close to the end with each hand holding the other shoulder.

3.5.2. The operator stands behind and to one side (either). He places the heel of one hand (right if he stands on the patient's left) across the spinous and both transverse processes of L4 (Fig. 8.11a).

3.5.3. The operator then grasps the patient's elbows with his free hand and extends her spine taking out all slack until the tension reaches L3 (Fig. 8.11b).

T.3.5.4. Thrust variant. The thrust is given by a high velocity, low amplitude, forward translation of L4 with his lower hand and further extension of the trunk with his upper hand.

M.3.5.4a. Muscle energy variant. The patient is asked to attempt to bend forwards against the operator's resistance.

M.3.5.4b. After 3–5 seconds she is asked to relax and, when relaxation is complete, the operator adjusts her position to reach the new barrier by extension alone.

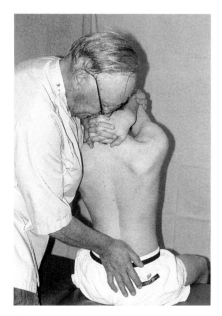
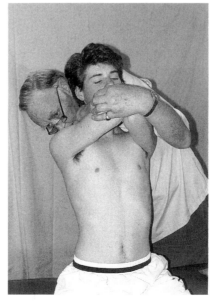

a   b

Fig. 8.11 Treatment for bilaterally restricted extension. ME or thrust. (a) From behind; (b) from in front.

M.3.5.4c. The last two steps are repeated twice, or more if desired, and the slack is finally taken up.

3.5.5. Retest.

There are several positions for the patient's arms by which the operator can control her upper trunk in the manner that is needed before a treatment can be given with accuracy. They are not all as applicable as each other in any given situation. For instance, if the operator wishes to sidebend the patient away from him, the under axilla grip has certain advantages. With the under axilla grip, however, it is not easy to control the patient in flexion. Control of extension is simple. If, on the other hand, sidebending towards the operator is required, the over-the-shoulder position gives better control but, in this instance, flexion is easier and extension more difficult to control. In both grips the operator stands behind and to one side of the patient. For the under axilla grip the operator threads his left arm through the patient's left axilla (or his right arm through her right axilla) and grips her opposite shoulder from in front. For the over-the-shoulder grip he grasps her far shoulder from in front with his hand (of the opposite side) and brings his axilla down on top of her near shoulder (Figs. 8.10a and 8.8d).

When muscle energy treatment is planned, the operator can stand on either side and the decision as to the grip used will depend on convenience and the above considerations. However, for thrust treatment with the patient sitting, the operator will want to stand on the side away from which the thrust is to be applied. It follows that in those cases where thrust may be needed, even if the primary corrective attempt will use

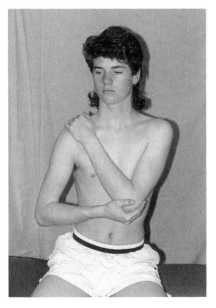 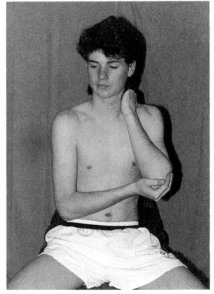

Fig. 8.12 a and b Alternative placement of arms to enhance control.

a   b

muscle energy, it may be that the operator will want to use a position from which either can be done without him having to move.

There are also several variations of grips by which the patient can stabilise her shoulder–trunk connection so that motion introduced by the operator holding her shoulders is transmitted accurately to her trunk joints. The most simple is for the patient to hold one shoulder with the other hand. This can be on either side and gives reasonable stability. If more is needed she can use her other hand to hold the elbow of the arm with which she is holding the shoulder (Fig. 8.12a). This also can apply to either side, the object being to enhance the patient's stability rather than the operator's contact. Some operators prefer to have the patient use one of her hands to hold her neck on the same side and then, with her other hand to hold her fully flexed elbow (Fig. 8.12b). This gives excellent stability but some patients find it very uncomfortable. For certain thrusting techniques the patient's hands are laced tightly together behind her neck and this grip could be used for muscle energy techniques if circumstances made it necessary (see Fig. 3.25).

The position with the patient astride the table is useful for certain techniques because it increases the stability of the innominates. The model in Fig. 8.12b also illustrates this position. It can only be used on tables that are not so wide that it becomes too uncomfortable for the patient to separate her knees that far.

Chapter 9

Treatment of the thoracic spine

Treatment for the thoracic spine can be done by thrusting in a variety of positions; some lend themselves to muscle energy variants but this is not true of all. Only in this region are there more thrusting than muscle energy techniques available.

At the lower end of the region both the rotary and the sidebending activation lumbar techniques can be used but accurate localisation becomes more difficult as one gets higher up. As in the lumbar spine, only the rotary activation techniques are available for thrusting. For descriptions see under the lumbar spine, Chapter 8, techniques 1.1, 1.2, 1.3, 2.1, 2.2 and 2.3.

The sitting techniques described for the lumbar spine (3.1, 3.2, 3.3 and 3.4) are applicable to the thoracic spine below T5, both in their muscle energy and thrust variants. Sitting techniques which are similar in many respects (1.2.1, 1.2.2 and 1.2.3) are the great standbys for the upper thoracic joints and these can be used with either activation. There are also the 'knee-in-back' techniques which can only be used with thrust activation.

The prone position can be used for thrust treatment of restrictions of extension and, in the upper joints, for neutral dysfunctions but care is required as rib subluxations can be produced by incorrect technique.

Supine techniques are available for thrust treatment of FRS, ERS and neutral dysfunctions.

When positioning the patient for ERS and FRS techniques the apex of the anteroposterior (sagittal plane) curve, introduced by the translation, should coincide with that of the lateral (coronal plane) curve.

Occasionally it may be found that there is an ERS dysfunction of a joint, usually between T4 and T10, with which there is also an external rib torsion. This combination will sometimes prove difficult to resolve unless both are treated at the same time and a combined technique is described in Chapter 10 as technique 5.9.

Bilateral restrictions of flexion or extension are not uncommon in the lower thoracic spine.

1 SITTING TECHNIQUES

It is important that the joint being treated should be in neutral at the start. It is easy to assume that the joint will be in neutral in the middle of the normal range of motion but this is not always so; the restriction may be severe enough for the barrier to be engaged already in that position. Examination will show when the joint has a free range in the restricted direction and the positioning should start from within that free range.

1.1 For the lower thoracic spine, T6 down (sometimes a little higher)

The techniques described for the lumbar spine in Chapter 8 as 3.1, 3.2 and 3.3 may be used for either thrusting or muscle energy treatment, or the 'knee-in-back' method may be used if thrusting is the treatment of choice (see 1.3, below).

1.2. For the upper thoracic spine, C7 to T5

Thrust or muscle energy
When treating FRS dysfunctions in the upper half of the thoracic spine the neck position is important for both thrust and muscle energy treatment. In order to bring the dysfunctional segment to the extension barrier the spine must be extended, but in many patients with these dysfunctions the neck is stiff and painful and may be very uncomfortable if the extension is not introduced correctly. The requirement is for the lower cervical segments to be extended down to the required point of tension in the thoracic spine. The upper neck joints should not be extended, nor should the head be extended on the neck. Extension of the upper neck may actually worsen the condition of the cervical spine and protecting the neck by the operator supporting it with his forearm is not always enough. It seems that the problem only arises when FRS dysfunctions are being treated.

The difficulty can be resolved by having the patient extend the low neck only. This can be achieved by having her pull her chin back while leaving the head upright. Some patients have difficulty understanding what is being asked of them but the request 'let me bring your chin back' is usually successful. There may then be some difficulty in persuading the patient to relax in that position. The use of the operator's forearm to protect the neck is an additional help (Fig. 9.1a, b and c).

There is another variant applicable to muscle energy treatment for FRS dysfunctions. To treat FRSrt at T3 the operator can have the patient hold her right shoulder with her left hand. He then lifts her left elbow in front of her face while monitoring with his other hand and at the same time introduces left sidebending and left rotation until the barrier is reached. The right arm may be used if preferred. Both movements are by translation rather than simple extension or sidebending and it may help to ask the patient to push her stomach forwards as the elbow is raised. The patient's effort is then to try to push her elbow down and forwards, which the operator resists in the usual way (Fig. 9.1d). This variant may be used down to the mid thoracic region and is particularly useful in the upper joints in those patients who have dysfunctions in the cervical region that make it undesirable to use the neck as a lever.

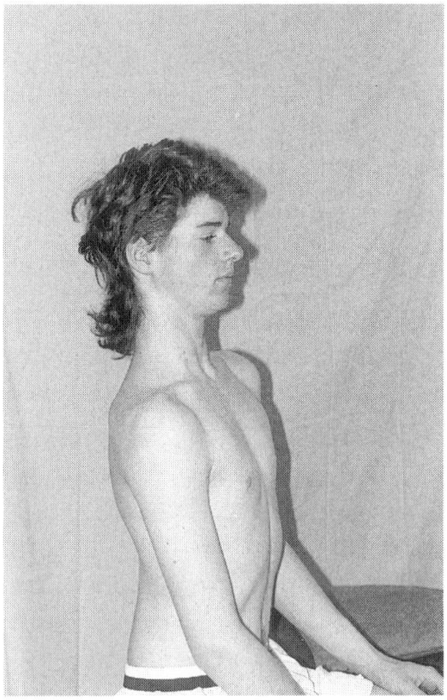

a

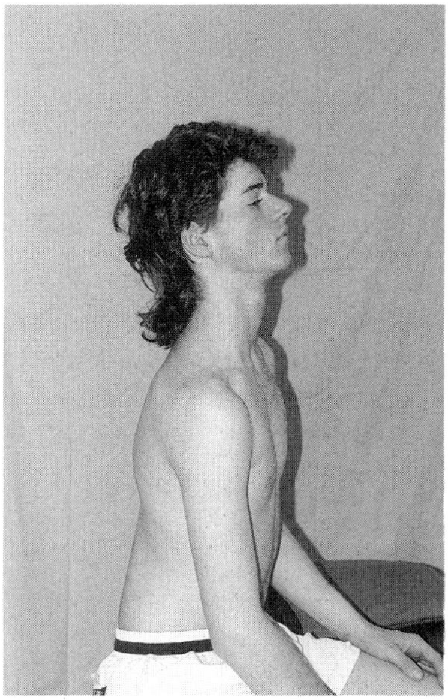

b

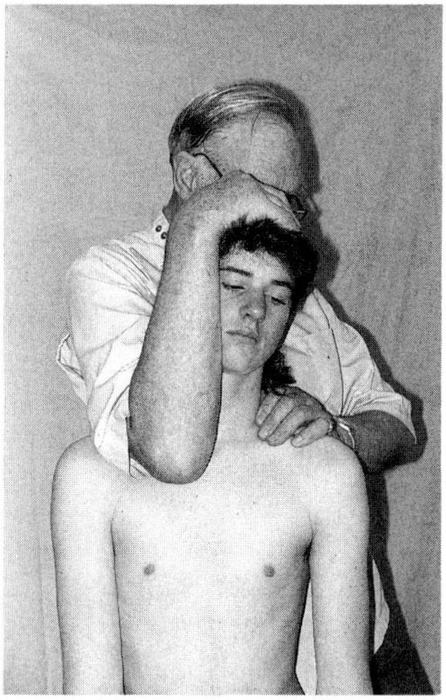

c

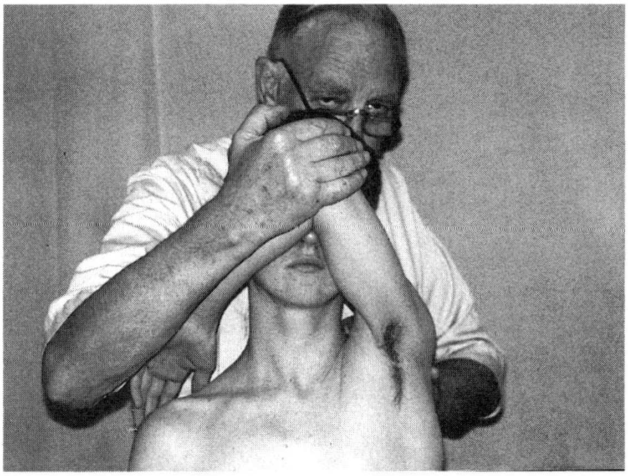

d

Fig. 9.1 Methods of protecting the cervical spine when treating FRS dysfunctions in the upper thoracic region. (a) 'Chin in', extension of the neck with the face vertical; (b) head extension which is to be avoided; (c) protecting the neck with the operator's forearm; (d) variant using the patient's elbow.

When there is difficulty in lateral translation of the upper thoracic region the technique described in Chapter 10 for first rib sitting treatment may be useful. The operator puts his foot, on the table top with his thigh beside the patient's chest, on the side towards which the patient is to be translated. If the patient then drapes her arm over the operator's thigh he has an extra means of controlling her lateral movement by moving his thigh to one side or the other as required (see Fig. 10.15).

1.2.1 For extension restriction

Described for restriction of rotation and sidebending to the left at T3, FRSrt.

Diagnostic points. There is tissue texture change at the segment. In the neutral position the right TP of T3 may be a little more prominent (posterior) than the left. On forward flexion the TPs become even but on backward bending the right TP becomes more inferior and posterior while the left stays superior and anterior.

1.2.1.1. The patient sits on a table or stool and the operator stands behind her.

1.2.1.2. The operator places his left hand over the shawl area of her left shoulder with his thumb (as monitor) on the posterior aspect of the transverse process of T3 close to the side of the spinous process (Fig. 9.2a). With his right hand and forearm he controls her head.

1.2.1.3. By forward pressure of his left thumb and asking the patient to push her abdomen forward and bring her chin back T3 is translated forward to reach the barrier in extension from above and below. It is wise to protect the cervical joints by the operator bringing his right forearm against the right side of her neck. The forearm length can be made to match the neck by sliding the elbow more or less forward (Fig. 9.2b and cf. Fig. 9.1c). For the alternative patient position that does not put so much force through the neck see Fig. 9.1d and the description to which it refers.

Fig. 9.2 Treatment of FRSrt in upper thoracic spine. ME or thrust. (a) Placement of thumb monitor and sidebend by translation; (b) position for patient effort, for thrust the operator's forearm would be in line with his thumb.

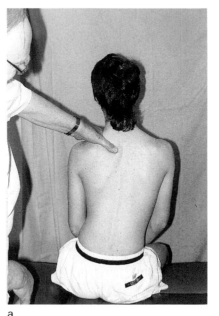
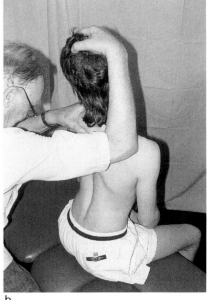

a   b

1.2.1.4. By pressure of his left hand caudad and to the right and sidebending of her head to the left (by his right hand) the operator introduces translation of T3 to the right to give left sidebending from above and below. Both these movements must be monitored by his left thumb and stopped as soon as the tension begins to reach the area.

1.2.1.5. Left rotation is introduced by the operator turning her head to the left and this can be used as the 'fine tuning' of the position to take up all the slack.

T.1.2.1.6. Thrust variant. The thrust is given by a high velocity, low amplitude movement of the operator's left hand caudad and to the right, mainly over the shawl area with the web of the hand, but also with his thumb to the right at the base of the spinous process or as near as he can reach. In order to have enough power for the movement to be easy to control, the operator's forearm should be in line with the direction of the thrust.

M.1.2.1.6a. Muscle energy variant. The patient is asked to attempt to push her head to the right gently and the operator resists with an equal and opposite force. A flexion effort could be used instead and may be valuable if the response to sidebending is inadequate. Rotation is best avoided as being more difficult to control.

M.1.2.1.6b. After maintaining the effort for 3–5 seconds she is asked to relax. When relaxation is complete, the operator takes her position to the new barrier in all three planes, and steps M.1.2.1.6a and b are repeated two or more times.

1.2.1.7. Retest.

1.2.2 For flexion restriction
Described for restriction of left rotation and sidebending at T3, ERSrt.

Diagnostic points. There is tissue texture change at the segment. In the neutral position the right TP of T3 may be a little more prominent (posterior) than the left. On forward flexion the right TP stays inferior and posterior while the left moves superior and anterior, but on backward bending the TPs become even.

1.2.2.1. The patient sits on a table or stool and the operator stands behind her.

1.2.2.2. The operator places his left hand over the shawl area of her left shoulder with his thumb on the posterior aspect of the transverse process of T3 close to the side of the spinous process. With his right hand he controls her head (as in Fig. 9.2a).

1.2.2.3. The forward flexed position is obtained by having the patient slump into backward translation of T3 and by forward bending of her neck until the tension just reaches the upper border of T3 from above and the lower border of T4 from below.

1.2.2.4. By pressure of his left hand caudad and to the right and sidebending of her head to the left (by his right hand) the operator introduces translation of T3 to the right to give left sidebending from above and below, monitored by his left thumb and stopped as soon as the tension begins to reach the area.

1.2.2.5. Left rotation is introduced by the operator turning her head to the left and this can be used as the 'fine tuning' of the position to remove all the slack (Fig. 9.3).

T.1.2.2.6. Thrust variant. The thrust is given by a high velocity, low amplitude movement of his left hand on the shawl area increasing both the left sidebend and the flexion. In order to have enough power for the

Fig. 9.3 Treatment of ERSrt in upper thoracic spine. ME or thrust. See caption for Fig. 9.2b.

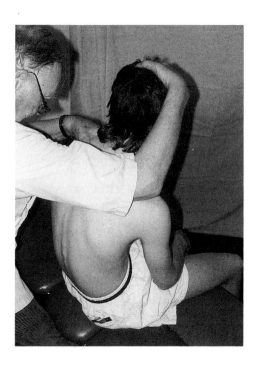

movement to be easy to control, the operator's forearm should be in line with the direction of the thrust.

M.1.2.2.6a. Muscle energy variant. She is asked to attempt to push her head to the right gently and the operator resists with an equal and opposite force. An extension effort could be used instead and may be valuable if the response to sidebending is inadequate. Rotation is best avoided as being more difficult to control.

M.1.2.2.6b. After maintaining the effort for 3–5 seconds she is asked to relax. When relaxation is complete, the operator takes her position to the new barrier in all three planes and steps M.1.2.1.6a and b are repeated two or more times.

1.2.2.7. Retest.

1.2.3   For a neutral group
For neutral (type I, or group) dysfunction.

Described for T2–3–4 convex left, that is sidebent right and rotated left, NRlt.

Diagnostic points. There is tissue texture change at the group. In neutral the TPs of T2, 3 and 4 are all rotated to the left. In both flexion and extension the rotation remains although it may change in amount.

1.2.3.1. The patient sits on a table or stool and the operator stands behind her.

1.2.3.2. The operator places his left hand over the shawl area of her left shoulder with his thumb between the transverse processes of T3 and T4 with pressure anteriorly *not* against the spinous process. With his right hand he controls her head and neck.

1.2.3.3. Because this is a neutral dysfunction the upper thoracic spine is maintained in neutral flexion–extension although minor adjustment of the sagittal plane position may help with localisation.

1.2.3.4. By pressure of his left hand caudad and to the right with sidebending of her head to the left (by his right hand) the operator introduces translation of T3 to the right to give left sidebending from above and below, monitored by his left thumb and stopped as soon as the tension begins to reach the apex of the curve.

1.2.3.5. Right rotation is introduced by the operator turning her head to the right and this can be used as the 'fine tuning' of the position to remove all the slack. As in the non-neutral techniques, the neck may be protected by the operator's forearm (Fig. 9.4).

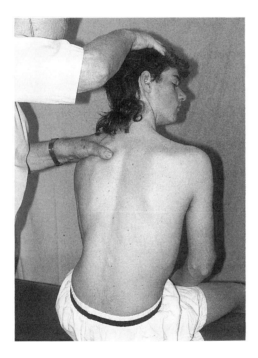

Fig. 9.4 Patient position for treatment of NRlt. ME or thrust.

T.1.2.3.6. Thrust variant. The thrust is given by a high velocity, low amplitude movement with the web of the hand caudad and to the right, and anteriorly by the operator's left thumb, increasing the left sidebend while the right rotation is increased slightly by his right hand. The operator's left forearm should be in line with the thrust.

M.1.2.3.6a. Muscle energy variant. She is asked to attempt to push her head to the right gently and the operator resists with an equal and opposite force. Extension or flexion efforts are not appropriate for this dysfunction. Rotation is best avoided as being more difficult to control.

M.1.2.3.6b. After maintaining the effort for 3–5 seconds she is asked to relax. When relaxation is complete, the operator takes her position to the new barrier by sidebending and rotation and steps M.1.2.1.6a and b are repeated two or more times.

1.2.3.6. Retest.

Note: when treating neutral dysfunctions the point at which to monitor and at which to apply any external force is a little below the centre of the group. This is because the upper vertebra is less rotated than the middle one and does not usually require individual attention.

1.3. Knee-in-back techniques

These are applicable to the lower two-thirds of the thoracic spine. Except for the neutral dysfunction, the techniques to be described have the knee supporting and stabilising the lower member of the motion segment being treated. There are variants in which the upper vertebra is contacted by the knee, which then becomes the thrusting agent, but when this is done the lower vertebra is not as well stabilised.

The position of the knee requires careful adjustment. The 'ladder' stool (Fig. 9.5a and b) is useful for this purpose, having bars at various heights. Without such a stool the required position can often be obtained by using

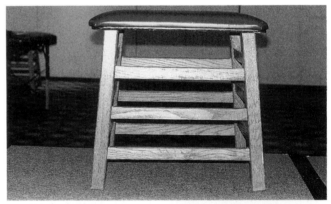

a

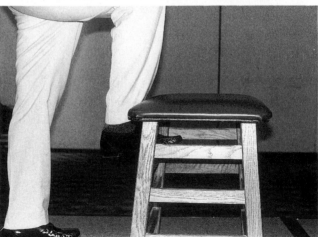

b

Fig. 9.5 a and b Ladder stool showing possible foot placement.

whatever support is available and, if necessary, having the leg tilted to one side to adjust the height of the knee.

Thrust only.

1.3.1 *For restriction of extension*

Described for restriction of right rotation and sidebending at T6, FRSlt.

Diagnostic points. There is tissue texture change at the segment. In the neutral position the left TP of T6 may be a little more prominent (posterior) than the right. On forward flexion the TPs become even but on backward bending the left TP becomes more inferior and posterior while the right stays superior and anterior.

1.3.1.1. The patient sits on a table or stool with her hands clasped behind her neck.

1.3.1.2. The operator stands behind her and with his foot on the table top, or a support of suitable height, he places his knee against the right transverse process of T7 (the lower vertebra).

1.3.1.3. He threads one hand through her axilla of the same side and grasps her wrist (Fig. 9.6a).

1.3.1.4. Monitoring at T6 with his other hand he introduces forward translation controlled by his knee, then translation from right to left and finally right rotation to localise the forces to T6 from above and T7 from below.

1.3.1.5. He then grips her other wrist, threading his free hand through her other axilla. Any remaining slack is taken out by adjustment of rotation and the thrust is given by a high velocity, low amplitude movement translating her upper trunk backward and slightly craniad while maintaining the sidebend and the rotation (Fig. 9.6b).

1.3.1.6. Retest.

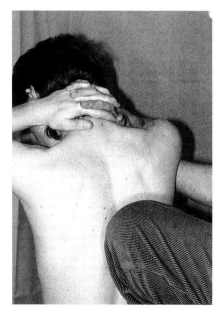 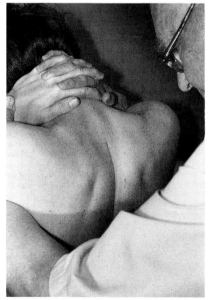

a   b

Fig. 9.6 'Knee in back' (KIB) treatment of FRSlt. Thrust only. (a) Knee in position and first hand gripping wrist; (b) Position at barrier, note extension at T6 although the upper joints are flexed.

1.3.2   For restriction of flexion

Described for restriction of right rotation and sidebending at T6, ERSlt

Diagnostic points. There is tissue texture change at the segment. In the neutral position the left TP of T6 may be a little more prominent (posterior) than the right. On forward flexion the left TP stays inferior and posterior while the right moves superior and anterior, but on backward bending the TPs become even.

1.3.2.1. The patient sits on a table or stool with her hands clasped behind her neck.

1.3.2.2. The operator stands behind her and with his foot on the table top, or a support of suitable height, he places his knee against the right transverse process of T7 (the lower vertebra).

1.3.2.3. He threads one hand through her axilla of the same side and grasps her wrist.

1.3.2.4. Monitoring at T6 with his other hand, he introduces backward translation, controlled by his knee, then translation from right to left and finally right rotation to localise the forces to T6 from above and T7 from below.

1.3.2.5. He then grips her other wrist by threading his free hand through her other axilla. Any remaining slack is taken out by adjustment of rotation and the thrust is given by a high velocity, low amplitude movement translating her upper trunk craniad and backward so as to produce flexion at T6–7, while maintaining the sidebend and the rotation (Fig. 9.7).

1.3.2.6. Retest.

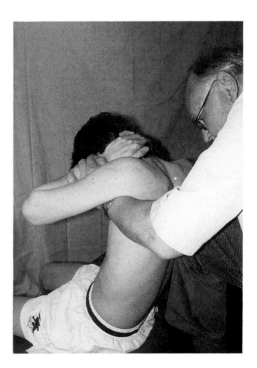

Fig. 9.7 KIB treatment for ERSlt.

1.3.3   *For neutral group restriction*

Described for T6, 7, 8 with restriction of left rotation and right sidebending, NRrt (rotated to the right).

Diagnostic points. There is tissue texture change at the group. In neutral the TPs of T6, 7 and 8 are all rotated to the right. In both flexion and extension the rotation remains although it may change in amount.

1.3.3.1. The patient sits on a table or stool with her hands clasped behind her neck.

1.3.3.2. The operator stands behind her and with his foot on the table top, or a support of suitable height, he places his right knee just below the right transverse process of T7 (or just below the apex of the curve). See note after technique 1.2.3.

1.3.3.3. He threads his right hand through her right axilla and grasps her right wrist. At this point he must see that her spine is in neutral in the sagittal plane.

1.3.3.4. Monitoring at T7 with his left hand, he introduces right sidebending by translation from right to left, and left rotation to localise the tension to T7 (Fig. 9.8).

1.3.3.5. He then threads his left hand through her left axilla and grips her left wrist. Any remaining slack is taken out by rotation and the thrust is given by a high velocity, low amplitude movement translating her upper trunk backward and slightly craniad, to rotate the group to the left, while maintaining the sidebend.

1.3.3.6. Retest.

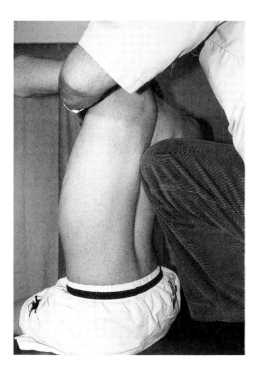

Fig. 9.8 KIB treatment for NRrt.

1.3.4 For bilateral restriction of flexion (extended)

This dysfunction is found mostly in the lower thoracic joints. Described for T9–10.

   Diagnostic points. The TPs of T9 are level in neutral, in flexion and in extension but there is tissue texture change at that segment. Motion testing reveals no movement at the T9–10 joint and the interspinous interval is unusually narrow.

   1.3.4.1. The patient sits on a table or stool with her hands clasped behind her neck.

   1.3.4.2. The operator stands behind her and with his foot on the table top, or a support of suitable height, he places his knee against the spinous process of T10 (the lower vertebra).

   1.3.4.3. He threads one hand through her axilla of the same side and grasps her wrist.

   1.3.4.4. Monitoring at T9 with his other hand, he introduces flexion by backward translation controlled by his knee.

   1.3.4.5. He then threads his other hand through her other axilla and when all slack is taken out by flexion the thrust is given by a high velocity, low amplitude movement of his arms directed posteriorly and slightly craniad (Fig. 9.9).

   1.3.4.6. Retest.

Fig. 9.9 KIB treatment for bilateral restriction of flexion.

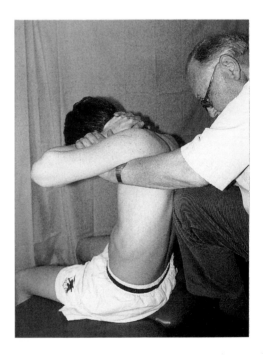

1.3.5 For bilateral restriction of extension (flexed)

This dysfunction is found mostly in the lower thoracic joints. Described for T9–10.

Diagnostic points. The TPs of T6 are level in neutral, in flexion and in extension but there is tissue texture change at that segment. Motion testing reveals no movement at the T9–10 joint and the interspinous interval is wide.

1.3.5.1. The patient sits on a table or stool with her hands clasped behind her neck.

1.3.5.2. The operator stands behind her and with his foot on the table top, or a support of suitable height, he places his knee against the spinous process of T10 (the lower vertebra).

1.3.5.3. He threads one hand through her axilla of the same side and grasps her wrist.

1.3.5.4. Monitoring at T9 with his other hand, he introduces extension by forward translation (controlled by his knee) (Fig. 9.6b).

1.3.5.5. He then threads his other hand through her other axilla and when all slack is taken out the thrust is given by a high velocity, low amplitude movement lifting and translating backward her upper trunk over the fulcrum of his knee.

1.3.5.6. Retest.

2   THORACIC SUPINE TECHNIQUES

Used for T5–T12 (and in some patients down to L2 or 3). These are all thrust techniques and, although primarily for the lower thoracic vertebrae, in some patients they can be used even as high as T3; above that level localisation becomes very difficult.

2.1   For restriction of extension

Described for T7 with restriction of rotation and sidebending to the left, FRSrt.

Diagnostic points. There is tissue texture change at the segment. In the neutral position the right TP of T7 may be a little more prominent (posterior) than the left. On forward flexion the TPs become even but on backward bending the right TP becomes more inferior and posterior while the left stays superior and anterior.

2.1.1. The patient is supine and the operator stands to her right (the side of the most posterior transverse process). She should cross her arms over her chest so that her left elbow is directly in front of her right with her hands in the opposite axillae.

2.1.2. The operator reaches across and lifts her left shoulder with his left hand so that he can insert his right hand under her with the base of the thenar eminence in contact with the left transverse process of T8, the thumb pointing craniad and her spinous processes in the hollow of his hand. His fingers support the right side of her spine (Fig. 9.10a). For those operators whose knuckle joints will flex fully without pain, the fingers can be flexed as in Fig. 9.10b which gives more support to the right side of the spine. If it is necessary to use the fingers fully flexed but that is painful, as it is for one of the authors, a small fold of material held

Fig. 9.10 Supine thrust treatment for FRSrt at T7. (a) Position adopted by under hand with fingers extended; (b) position adopted by under hand with fingers flexed; (c) placing the hand under the supine patient; (d) thrust position, using lower chest on elbows.

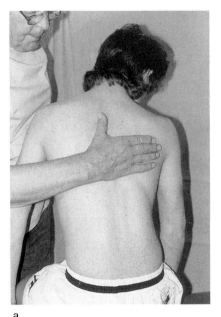

a

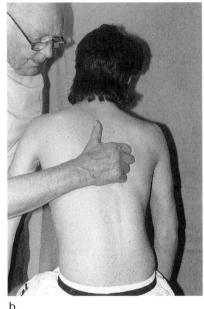

b

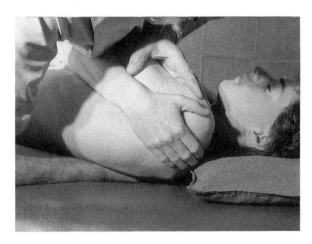

c

d

in the bent knuckles will stabilise the position but prevent maximum flexion and can be helpful.

2.1.3. The operator then returns her to the supine position with his hand underneath (Fig. 9.10c).

2.1.4. With his left hand on her elbows, the operator introduces flexion until movement is felt at T7 and then allows her to extend just so that the T7–8 joint is no longer flexed.

2.1.5. He then takes her into left rotation and left sidebending monitored by his right hand so that the tension only just reaches T7.

2.1.6. Bringing his chest or upper abdomen over his left hand, the operator then gives a high velocity, low amplitude thrust by dropping his weight on to the patient's arms in the direction of T6 (i.e. just above the level of the dysfunction) to extend T7 on T8 (Fig. 9.10d).

2.1.7. Retest.

2.2   For restriction of flexion

Described for T7 with restriction of rotation and sidebending to the right, ERSlt.

Diagnostic points. There is tissue texture change at the segment. In neutral the left TP of T7 may be a little more posterior than the right. In extension the TPs will become level but in flexion the left TP will remain posterior and prominent while that on the right will become superior and anterior.

2.2.1. The patient is supine and the operator stands to her right (opposite the most posterior transverse process). She should cross her arms over her chest so that her left elbow is directly in front of her right with her hands in the opposite axillae.

2.2.2. The operator reaches across and lifts her left shoulder with his left hand so that he can insert his right hand under her with the base of the thenar eminence in contact with the transverse process of T8, his thumb pointing craniad and her spinous processes in the hollow of his hand. His fingers are used to support the right side of her spine. For alternative finger position see technique 2.1.2 above.

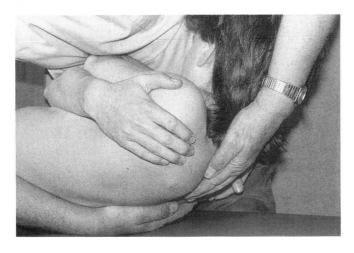

Fig. 9.11 Supine thrust for ERSlt. Note position of hand giving flexion.

2.2.3. After returning her to the supine position the operator reaches down to the upper thoracic vertebrae with his left hand to support her head and neck and flexes, rotates and sidebends her to the right until movement just begins at T7 (Fig. 9.11).

2.2.4. Bringing his chest or upper abdomen over the patient's elbows, the operator then gives a high velocity, low amplitude thrust by dropping his weight on to her elbows in the direction of T8, i.e. in the direction of his right hand, which produces flexion of T7 on T8 and the required rotation and sidebending.

2.2.5. Retest.

2.3 For a neutral group dysfunction

Described for T6–7–8 with restriction of right rotation and left sidebending, NRlt (rotated left).

Diagnostic points. There is tissue texture change at the group. In neutral the TPs of T6, 7 and 8 are all rotated to the left. In both flexion and extension the left rotation remains although it may vary in amount.

2.3.1. The patient is supine and the operator stands to the side away from which the group is rotated; in this example he stands on her right side. She should cross her arms over her chest with her left elbow anterior to her right and her hands in the opposite axillae.

2.3.2. The operator lifts her left shoulder with his left hand so that he can insert his right hand under her with the base of the thenar eminence just below the left transverse process of T7, his thumb pointing craniad and her spinous processes in the hollow of his hand. His fingers are used to support the right side of her spine. For alternative finger position see technique 2.1.2, above. See note after technique 1.2.3.

2.3.3. After she is returned to the supine position the operator leans over her with his chest or upper abdomen to bring the tension to his right thumb. With his left hand he lifts her head, but not beyond the neutral range, and rotates her neck and upper trunk to the right and sidebends her to the left down to T7.

2.3.4. The thrust is given by dropping his body weight on to her elbows in the direction of his right thenar eminence.

2.3.5. Retest.

2.4 For bilateral restriction of flexion

This dysfunction is found mostly in the lower thoracic joints. Described for T9–10.

Diagnostic points. There is tissue texture change at the segment. The TPs of T9 are level in neutral, in flexion and in extension. On motion testing the T9–10 joint does not move and the spinous processes are very close together.

2.4.1. The patient is supine with her fingers laced together behind the base of her neck and with her elbows together in front (Fig. 9.12a).

2.4.2. The operator stands at either side. If he stands on her right side he lifts her left shoulder with his left hand so that he can insert his right hand under her with the base of the thenar eminence in contact with the left transverse process of T9. His fingers support the right transverse process and his thumb points craniad. For alternative finger position, see technique 2.1.2 above.

2.4.3. She is then returned to the supine position with the operator's hand under her.

2.4.4. The operator then uses his left hand to flex her trunk by pressing posteriorly and caudad on her elbows until the tension is brought down to just above T9.

2.4.5. When all slack is taken out the high velocity, low amplitude thrust is given by the operator leaning his chest (or upper abdomen) over his left hand on her elbows and dropping his weight on her in the direction of his right thenar eminence (Fig. 9.12b).

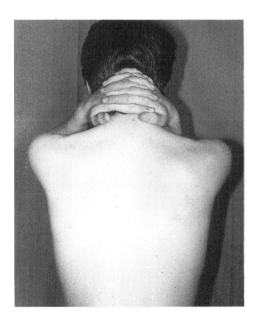

a

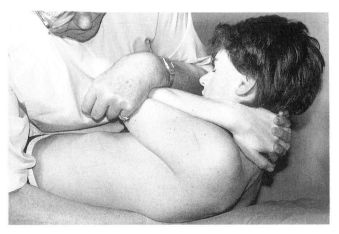

b

Fig. 9.12 Supine thrust for bilateral restriction of flexion. (a) Position of hands behind base of neck; (b) thrust position, hand as in fig. 9.10a, b and c.

2.4.6. For the upper thoracic joints the arm position described in techniques 2.1.1, 2.2.1 and 2.3.1 may be easier. In that event the operator's left hand lifts her head and upper trunk to reach the barrier. The thrust is then given by the operator's chest directly against her elbows and a folded towel or small cushion may be inserted for the operator's comfort.

2.4.7. Retest.

2.5 For bilateral restriction of extension

This dysfunction is found mostly in the lower thoracic joints. Described for T9–10.

Diagnostic points. There is tissue texture change at the segment. The TPs of T9 are level in neutral, in flexion and in extension. On motion testing the T9–10 joint does not move and the spinous processes are wide apart.

2.5.1. The patient is supine with her fingers laced together behind the base of her neck and with her elbows together in front.

2.5.2. The operator stands at either side. If he stands on her right side he lifts her left shoulder with his left hand so that he can insert his right hand under her with the base of the thenar eminence in contact with the left transverse process of T10. His fingers support the right transverse process and his thumb points craniad. For alternative finger position see technique 2.1.2 above.

2.5.3. She is then returned to the supine position.

2.5.4. The operator then uses his left hand to flex her down to T9 by pressing posteriorly on her elbows. She is then allowed to extend just so that T9 is extended on T10 (Fig. 9.13).

Fig. 9.13 Supine thrust for bilateral restriction of extension.

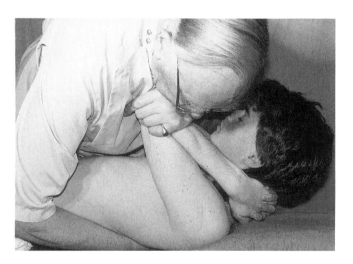

2.5.5. When all slack is taken out the high velocity, low amplitude thrust is given by the operator leaning his chest (or upper abdomen) over his left hand on her elbows and dropping his weight on her in the direction of T8.

2.5.6. For the upper thoracic joints the arm position described in techniques 2.1.1, 2.2.1 and 2.3.1 may be easier. In that event flexion is introduced by pressure of the operator's chest on the patient's elbows until the tension reaches the vertebra to be moved. She is then allowed to extend by a slight reverse movement until that vertebra is extended on the one below. The thrust is given by the operator's chest against her elbows in the direction of the upper vertebra or even the next vertebra higher.

2.5.7. Retest.

3   THORACIC PRONE TECHNIQUES

These are used for FRS lesions and in the upper joints there is a technique for neutral dysfunctions. All use thrusting force only.

3.1   'Crossed pisiform'

This technique is powerful but is only useful for restrictions of extension (FRS) primarily between T4 and T10. It must be done correctly as, if repeated force is applied to the posterior aspect of the ribs, anterior subluxation of the rib can result. There are several variants of this technique but this is one presented as if performed as indicated with transverse process and *not* rib contact, it is a safe method. Regrettably the technique has often been used incorrectly and the patient thereby harmed.

Described for restriction of extension and of left rotation and sidebending at T7, FRSrt.

Diagnostic points. There is tissue texture change at the segment. In the neutral position the right TP of T7 may be a little more prominent (posterior) than the left. On forward flexion the TPs become even but on backward bending the right TP becomes more inferior and posterior while the left stays superior and anterior.

3.1.1. The patient is prone with her head turned to the left.

3.1.2. The operator stands at her left side and puts his left pisiform in contact with the superior aspect of the left transverse process of T7 (Fig. 9.14a). It is important that the contact is on the TP and not on the rib.

3.1.3. With his right pisiform he contacts the posterior aspect of the right TP of T7 (Fig. 9.14b). Again, the rib must be avoided.

3.1.4. The slack is taken out by a combination of caudad pressure with the left pisiform on her left TP and anterior pressure by the right on the right TP. The high velocity, low amplitude thrust is given, at the end of exhalation, in those directions, introducing left rotation and left sidebending. As this is a short lever technique with contact on the transverse process on either side the distance to be travelled by the force is very small and the 'low amplitude' part of the instruction is correspondingly important.

3.1.5. Retest.

Fig. 9.14 Prone 'crossed pisiform' thrust. (a) Left pisiform contacts upper surface of left TP of T7; (b) right pisiform on posterior aspect of right TP of T7.

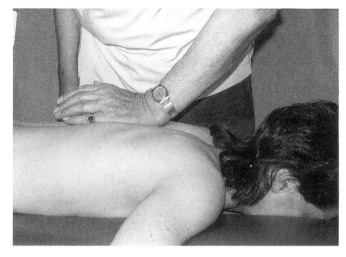

a

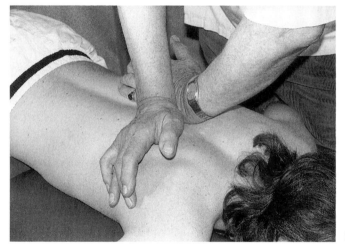

b

3.2 For extension restrictions T1 to T5

Described for T3 rotated and sidebent to the left, FRSlt.

Diagnostic points. There is tissue texture change at the segment. In the neutral position the left TP of T3 may be a little more prominent (posterior) than the right. On forward flexion the TPs become even but on backward bending the left TP becomes more inferior and posterior while the right stays superior and anterior.

3.2.1. The patient is prone and the operator stands a little to her right at the head of the table.

3.2.2. The operator lifts her head and moves her chin to her right and, at the same time, rotates her head to face right allowing it to rest on the left side of the chin (Fig. 9.15a).

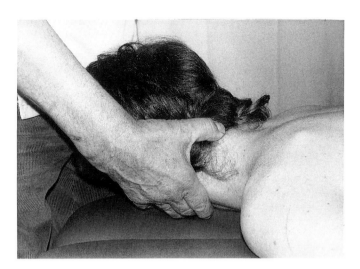

a

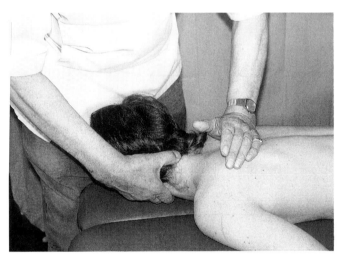

b

Fig. 9.15 Prone upper thoracic thrust for FRSlt at T3. (a) Chin and head position; (b) thrust position.

3.2.3. With the pisiform of his left hand, the operator contacts the posterior surface of the right transverse process of her T4 and takes up the slack by pressing anteriorly.

3.2.4. The operator's right hand maintains the right sidebending and rotation of her head.

3.2.5. The high velocity low amplitude thrust is given by the left hand in an anterior direction. This produces extension and left rotation of T4 under T3, thereby producing relative right rotation of T3 (Fig. 9.15b). It would be possible to use the left hand contact on the left TP of T3 to rotate it directly but there is then no block to rotation of T4.

3.2.6. Retest.

Fig. 9.16 Prone upper thoracic thrust for NRrt. (a) Chin and head position; (b) position if more sidebend required for localisation.

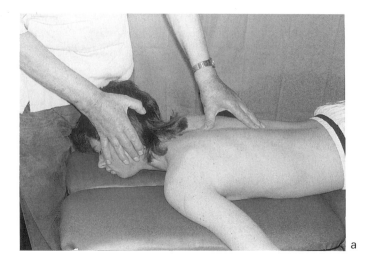

a

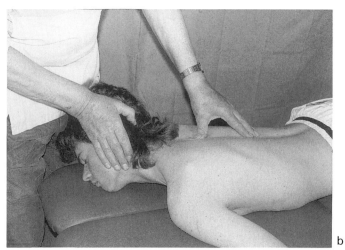

b

3.3　For neutral group restrictions T1 to T5

Described for T3–4–5 with restriction of left rotation and right sidebending, NRrt (rotated right and sidebent left).

　　Diagnostic points. There is tissue texture change at the group. In neutral the TPs of T3, 4 and 5 are all rotated to the right. In both flexion and extension the rotation remains although it may change in amount.

　　3.3.1. The patient is prone with her head resting on her chin in the midline and the operator stands at the head of the table controlling her head with his right hand (Fig. 9.16a).

　　3.3.2. The operator places his left thumb on the right of her spine just below the apex (T4) pressing in the direction of the facet joint between T4 and T5.

3.3.3. By rolling her head to her right on the chin, with his right hand, the operator introduces right sidebending and left rotation until the tension approaches his left thumb. If rolling the head does not bring the tension to the required level, the head should be lifted and sidebent a little to the right before putting the chin down and trying the rotation again (Fig. 9.16b).

3.3.4. When all slack has been taken out the high velocity, low amplitude thrust is given by the operator's left thumb on the right transverse processes ventrally and to the left while the position of the head is slightly exaggerated to help both the rotation and the sidebending.

3.3.5. Retest.

Chapter 10

Diagnosis and treatment of dysfunctions of the rib cage

Excerpts from this chapter have previously been published as three articles in *The Journal of Orthopaedic Medicine* and permission from the Society for them to be included with minor modifications is gratefully acknowledged.

DESCRIPTION AND DIAGNOSIS

There are several different dysfunctions to which ribs are subject. Many of them are associated with spinal joint problems, often at the joint at which the head of the rib articulates with the demifacet above and below. That is, the 5th rib will often be influenced by dysfunction of T4, at the T4–5 joint.

The simpler dysfunctions consist of restriction of excursion in either inhalation or exhalation and are commonly known as 'respiratory rib dysfunctions' or simply 'respiratory ribs'. These are associated with hypertonus in the intercostal muscles above or below and, although they may not cause much pain, the restriction of motion may predispose to recurrence of the spinal joint problem if it is not treated. For this reason it is important to add to one's armamentarium techniques for treatment of these respiratory ribs.

There is another group of rib dysfunctions which also may be associated with, and some probably caused by, disturbances of spinal joint function. These also are accompanied by hypertonus in the intercostal muscles. They are known as 'structural ribs' or 'structural rib dysfunctions' and comprise a diverse group. They are important in that they are often the cause of chest pain which may be severe and may be mistaken for pain of cardiac origin. It is of interest, and can be confusing, that this type of rib pain will apparently often be relieved by nitroglycerine.

In both types treatment of the associated spinal joint may allow the rib function to return to normal, and, if it does, treatment of the rib itself is unnecessary. For this reason it is usual to treat thoracic joint dysfunctions before those of the ribs, but see the remarks under technique 5.9 at the end of the chapter.

RESPIRATORY RIBS

Rib motion may be restricted in inhalation or in exhalation. As the treatment is different, it is important to distinguish between them. Inhalation restriction is common in the upper ribs on the right, exhalation restriction is common in the lower ribs on the left.

The diagnosis of respiratory rib dysfunction is made by observing the excursion of the ribs on forced inhalation and exhalation. For this observation to be accurate precautions must be taken because the difference between one side and the other may be quite small.

1. The first precaution is that the operator must stand with his dominant eye over the midline of the patient. It is surprising how inaccurate are observations made from even a short distance away from the point of symmetry. Determination of the dominant eye is described in Chapter 3. For those who have so little eye dominance that they are unable to be certain with which eye they are looking, it is wise to close one eye and look with the open eye over the patient's midline.

2. The observations are made both with the eye and the hands. The eye should focus on the midline of the patient so that, with his peripheral vision, the operator observes the rib movement on both sides at the same time. The hands should be placed symmetrically on the chest and it is possible to use either the flat hand or the tips of the fingers. The latter is sometimes more suitable for a male operator examining a female patient (Fig. 10.1).

It is most important that the hands should make very light contact with the ribs. This is partly because firm contact will tend to modify the rib movement and partly because the operator's proprioceptors will be more sensitive if they are not overloaded by too much pressure. The point of palpation can be either the rib itself or the intercostal space. It is important that the same point be used on both sides and the fingers should be on symmetrical parts of the rib or space on the two sides.

3. The question to be answered is on which side does the movement stop first. This is a much easier observation than that sometimes taught in medical schools, namely to estimate which side moves furthest. It is important to remember the possibility of acapnia from overbreathing, and

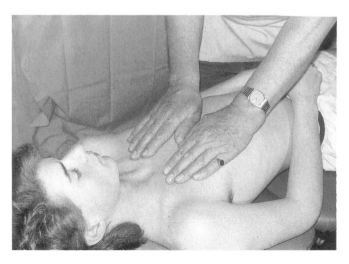

Fig. 10.1 Examination for restriction of respiratory motion. (a) Upper ribs, using flat hand.

a

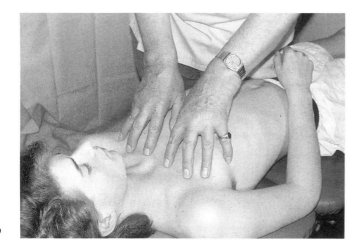

b

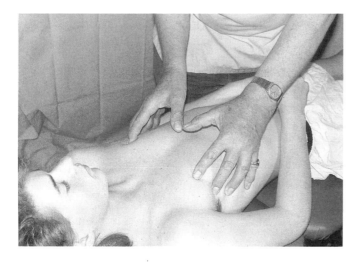

c

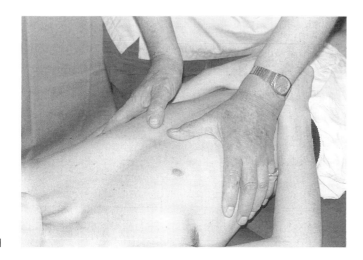

d

Fig. 10.1 (continued) (b)
Upper ribs, using finger tips; (c)
middle ribs; (d) lower typical
ribs.

the discomfort caused by it. This can be avoided if, after finding out at which end of the respiratory range there appears to be a restriction, repeated examinations are limited to that end of the range. For example, if an inhalation restriction is suspected, the instruction should be 'breathe out a little and then breathe in as far as you can' rather than 'breathe in and out deeply'.

For descriptive purposes, normal rib motion can be divided into two types. These are commonly referred to as 'pump handle' and 'bucket handle' although as will be mentioned later the terms are not without their difficulties. The terms refer to the rise and fall of the anterior end of the rib (pump handle) and the rise and fall of the lateral part of the rib (bucket handle). All ribs have some component of each in their motion; the relative proportion varies from above down, and is determined by the angle formed between the line joining the costovertebral and costotransverse joints with the coronal plane (see Fig. 2.10). The upper ribs have very little bucket handle component while the lower ribs have mainly that motion.

Although the proportion of sagittal plane to coronal plane motion is fixed for each rib by the orientation of the line joining the costovertebral to costotransverse joint, the direction of the restriction is more dependent on which tissue is tight. Bucket handle restrictions may be found at the first rib and pump handle restrictions sometimes in the lower ribs. It is of less importance to distinguish between pump and bucket handle motion than to distinguish inhalation from exhalation restriction.

Diagnosis of respiratory dysfunctions of ribs 1–10

To assess restriction of pump handle motion, the hands need to be near the anterior end of the ribs and to assess bucket handle motion they should be further lateral on the rib shaft. The first rib presents some difficulty because much of it is covered by the clavicle or by the brachial plexus and its associated vessels. The costal cartilage can be felt immediately distal to the medial end of the clavicle but, to assess bucket handle motion, palpation must be in the anterior triangle of the neck, posterolateral to the neurovascular bundle.

The rib cage is first examined to find if there is a group of restricted ribs. This is started in the front for the upper ribs and the upper three or four can be assessed together. Moving more laterally, because of the increasing bucket handle component of the motion, the next group down is tested. Then with the hands in the axilla the lower rib motion is estimated. The rib cage down to R10 can normally be tested using just three positions.

Respiratory rib restrictions tend to occur in groups and when a restriction of inhalation or exhalation is found it is important to discover the 'key' rib. The key rib is the uppermost restricted rib in a group with inhalation restriction and the lowest restricted one in a group with exhalation restriction. The importance of the key rib is that, partly for mechanical reasons, the neighbouring ribs (those above if the restriction is of exhalation and those below when there is restriction of inhalation) will not move fully if the key rib remains restricted. There is sometimes more than one key rib in a group and, partly for this reason, it is always wise to re-examine the area after treatment.

The key rib is found by testing the movement of individual ribs starting at the top for an inhalation restriction and at the lower end of the group if it is exhalation that is restricted. This is done using one finger on the corresponding rib on each side and both the anterior ends and the lateral aspects of the ribs may need to be examined to discern between pump and bucket handle restrictions. Structural rib dysfunctions will often cause respiratory restriction and may act as key ribs.

Diagnosis of respiratory dysfunctions of ribs 11 and 12

Examination of the motion of the 11th and 12th ribs is performed with the patient prone. Their movement characteristics are different because they have no anterior attachment and it is usually described as a 'calliper' type of movement. The examination is made by placing the two thumbs symmetrically over the medial ends of the rib on each side and the index finger of the same hand on the shaft as far laterally as the ribs can be felt. If the rib on one side is short, the finger on the other side should not be further from the midline than that on the short rib side (Fig. 10.2a and b).

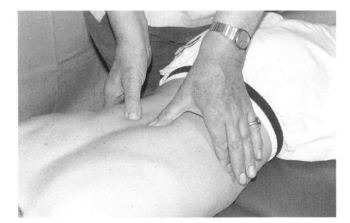

a

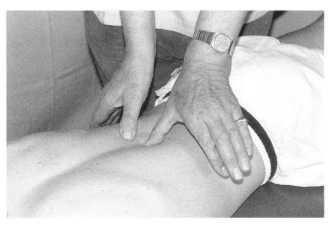

b

Fig. 10.2 For restriction of respiratory motion of ribs 11 and 12. (a) Position in exhalation; (b) position in inhalation.

The purpose of the examination is to assess the relative opening and closing of the calliper formed by the rib on either side at the same level. Failure of one side to close properly indicates an exhalation restriction; failure to open an inhalation problem.

STRUCTURAL RIBS

There are several types of structural rib dysfunction, as follows.

(a) Subluxation, anterior, posterior or superior.
(b) Torsion, external or internal.
(c) Lateral flexion.
(d) Anteroposterior compression.
(e) Lateral compression.

Structural rib dysfunctions are mostly found after injury or in patients who have been subjected to major chest surgery. In post surgical patients the dysfunctions are often multiple and may be difficult to treat. Structural rib dysfunctions are the cause of the pain in most cases of so-called costochondritis and treatment will often remove the symptoms immediately. Structural dysfunctions in the upper three ribs are a frequent cause of shoulder pain.

In those who have chest wall pain, if there is no structural rib dysfunction, there is likely to be some truly pathological cause. Of the possibilities one of the most common is herpes zoster.

Diagnosis will depend on finding asymmetry of position and tissue texture change but there will often be tenderness as well. A rib with a structural dysfunction will often act as a key rib for a group of ribs with respiratory restriction.

The important landmark for most of the structural rib dysfunctions is the rib angle. This is the most posterior part of the rib and, being the point of insertion of the iliocostalis muscle, is the place where tissue texture change may be palpable. In the upper ribs (2 to 5 particularly) the rib angle is usually concealed by the scapula and in order to find it the shoulder must be protracted. It is usually enough to instruct the patient to cross her hands in her lap.

The line of the rib angles normally forms a smooth curve from before backwards and from medial to lateral. Any deviation from either curve should be a cause for further examination. The curve formed by the anterior ends of the ribs should also be smooth. When the alteration is in the same direction in both front and back an anterior or a posterior subluxation is probable but if the anterior end is anterior (prominent) and the posterior end of the same rib is posterior (also prominent) a lateral compression is likely. Similarly if both front and back of the same rib are depressed suspect antero-posterior compression.

Subluxations

These are true subluxations of the costovertebral joint with the whole rib moving slightly anteriorly or posteriorly, or, in the first rib only, with the posterior end moving superiorly. Anterior subluxations are somewhat more common than posterior ones.

Anterior

Anterior subluxations are fairly common and may be seen in those patients who have had repeated treatment for thoracic joint problems by the 'crossed pisiform' technique. When performed well, that technique is excellent for joints with restriction of extension; regrettably it is often applied incorrectly and if the ribs are repeatedly thrust forward subluxation may result.

It is as well to remember that subluxated joints are hypermobile and should not be treated with a high velocity thrust.

Diagnosis

The head of the rib slides forward on the vertebrae with which it articulates and, because of the direction of the line joining the costovertebral and costotransverse joints the rib angle not only becomes less prominent posteriorly (out of line in the A–P curve) but it also becomes more medial and out of the line of the lateral curve. The rib angle will usually be tender and be the site of tissue texture changes.

When examined in front the anterior end of the same rib is prominent and usually tender. The examination is best performed with the patient sitting. If supine the other ribs may be pushed forward by contact with the table and make the asymmetry less easy to see. Similarly, if prone, the anterior rib may be pushed back enough to make it difficult to find.

Posterior

This again is a true subluxation; the joint is hypermobile and thrusting manipulation is contraindicated. Posterior subluxations are common; they may be caused by a blow on the front of the chest, as in road traffic accidents, and are often found in those who have had sternal splitting surgery.

In the posterior subluxation the rib has moved laterally and posteriorly in relation to the vertebrae with which it articulates. The rib angle will be more prominent than that of the neighbouring ribs and there will usually be tissue texture change at the insertion of iliocostalis associated with tenderness. Anteriorly the costochondral junction will be posterior to that of the neighbouring ribs, but, if the patient is supine, the rib may be pushed forward enough to make the position appear normal. As for the anterior rib, the examination is best performed with the patient sitting. Here also tenderness at the anterior end of the rib is common.

Diagnosis

The anterior end and the angle of the rib are posterior to the smooth curve made by the corresponding parts of the neighbouring ribs. The rib angle will also be lateral to the expected position in the lateral curve. There will be tissue texture change at the insertion of iliocostalis at the rib angle.

Superior

In the first rib only, the costotransverse joint may be subluxated superiorly by the pull of the scalene muscles. This is not uncommon and will often be associated with dysfunction of either C7–T1 or T1–2. These joints should always be checked and treated first if they are dysfunctional. When the first rib is pulled up its angle will tend to become 'hitched' on the superior aspect of the transverse process of T1 and the rib will then need to be eased forward (anteriorly) before the subluxation can be reduced.

Symptoms are often severe and may be long lasting. There is usually pain all up the neck to the base of the skull on the side of the subluxation and it will often involve the shoulder and the arm down to the hand. There will be associated cervical joint dysfunctions which will need to be treated in order to avoid recurrence from tightness in the scalene muscles. There may be an associated bucket handle restriction of respiratory motion when the subluxation has been treated.

In patients in whom it proves difficult to reduce a superior subluxation of the 1st rib, a laterally flexed 2nd rib should be considered and treated, if present, before proceeding.

Diagnosis

The first rib position can be felt by the operator standing behind the seated patient. With one index finger on either side he pulls the trapezius posteriorly to find the superior aspect of the rib in front of the main part of the muscle (Fig. 10.3). In a first rib subluxation the difference in height of the rib on the two sides will be not less than 6 mm ($\frac{1}{4}$ inch). Examination for this must be gentle; even in the normal the posterior

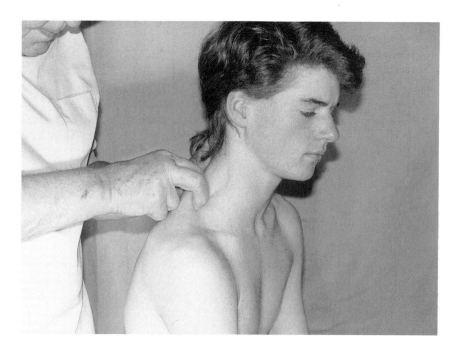

Fig. 10.3 To find the superior aspect of the head of rib 1.

end of the first rib is tender, and when subluxation is present the tenderness may be severe. There will be marked restriction of respiratory excursion and if the patient is asked to flex her neck the rib can often be felt to move forward on the subluxated side.

Rib torsions

When one thoracic vertebra is rotated on the one below, the two demifacets that make up the vertebral component of the costovertebral joint are not correctly aligned. This change in shape tends to twist the rib head, the more so if the upper vertebra is extended on the lower because this leaves less room for the rib head. If the upper vertebra is rotated to the right on the lower, the rib head on the right side will be twisted so that the upper border of the rib becomes more prominent at the posterior end; this is known as external torsion of the rib. At the same time the rib head on the left side will be twisted so that the lower border of the rib will become relatively more prominent; this is internal rib torsion. This happens in normal movement; it is only likely to be found if there is intervertebral dysfunction and the rib torsion will usually be corrected when the intervertebral joint has been successfully treated.

Rib torsions only need treatment when the rib position has been present for long enough for it to become self perpetuating. The restriction in rib torsions is within the normal range of motion at the costovertebral joints and, in the absence of hypermobility, thrusting treatment is permitted and sometimes essential. Occasionally it proves almost impossible to correct the thoracic joint when there is an associated rib torsion except by a combined thrust technique, described later as technique 5.9.

Owing to the curvature of the rib and its attachments in front and behind, the direction of the twist changes as the rib passes forward through the axilla and is reversed at the anterior end, so that in an internal torsion the upper margin is the more prominent at the anterior end of the rib (Fig. 10.4). If the bone is thought of as the kind of rigid structure that we handle

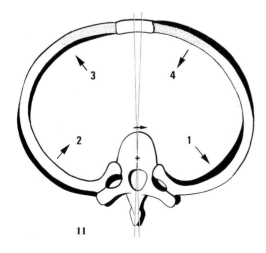

Fig. 10.4 To show the rib torsion caused by rotation of the vertebra above and reversed torsion anteriorly (after Kapandji).

in anatomy classes such torsional changes seem impossible; however, the evidence suggests that living bone is deformable and in some ways plastic in nature. Trained fingers can appreciate the differences in shape before and after treatment but it is fair to say that accurate rib diagnosis demands a degree of palpatory skill and is difficult for a beginner.

Ribs restricted in external torsion are found much more commonly than those restricted in internal torsion.

External torsion diagnosis
There is restriction of respiratory movement of that rib.

The upper border of the rib is prominent posteriorly and the lower border less prominent than normal.

The intercostal space above the rib is wide and that below is narrow.

There is tissue texture change and tenderness at the insertion of iliocostalis at the rib angle and often also in the intercostal muscles in the space below.

The upper vertebra is (was) rotated towards the side of the rib and was probably extended, ERS.

Internal torsion diagnosis
There is restriction of respiratory movement of that rib.

The lower border of the rib is prominent posteriorly and the upper border less prominent than normal.

The intercostal space below the rib is wide and that above is narrow.

There is tissue texture change and tenderness at the insertion of iliocostalis at the rib angle and often also in the intercostal muscles in the space above.

The upper vertebra is (was) rotated away from the side of the rib and was probably extended (ERS).

Laterally flexed rib

This is often a very painful condition in which the rib is elevated acutely. It is usually caused by a sudden sidebending strain of the neck and upper thoracic spine. The rib acts as if it had a fixed pivot in front as well as at the back (and the term 'bucket handle' would be more appropriate for this than for the lateral expansion respiratory rib dysfunction). It is painful at any level but when it affects the second rib there may be severe arm pain from the effect on the brachial plexus and the shoulder will be carried high to avoid pressure on the neurovascular bundle. There will often be paraesthesiae in the arm and hand. Treatment is painful, especially at the 2nd rib.

Diagnosis
The history of injury is very suggestive. A rib will be found with severely restricted respiratory motion most marked in exhalation. In the axilla the rib will be found elevated with a narrow space above and a wide space below. The rib will be acutely tender. There may be signs of sympathetic dysfunction in the arm and any attempt to lower the shoulder will

cause an increase in the pain. Imaging and EMG studies are normal and the patient is likely to have been suspected of malingering.

Anteroposterior compression

The possibility of the occurrence of this deformity also depends, as does the lateral compression, on the plastic nature of living bone. Anteroposterior compression is not rare in road traffic accidents and is usually caused by a blow on the front of the chest as when the driver hits the steering wheel.

Diagnosis
Both anterior and posterior ends of the rib are less prominent than the neighbouring ribs and the rib is prominent laterally in the axilla. The rib is also tender, particularly in the axilla. Pain may be severe, resembling a rib fracture, but X-rays and bone scans will be negative and these patients have often been accused of malingering.

Lateral compression

This deformity is produced by a blow on the side of the chest and is sometimes seen after a side-on collision. It is usually accompanied by severe pain.

Diagnosis
The signs are the reverse of those in antero-posterior compression; there is a prominent anterior end of the rib and a prominent rib angle with flattening of the lateral aspect of the rib in the axilla. As with antero-posterior compressions, these are painful like a rib fracture, but imaging is negative.

TREATMENT OF RESPIRATORY RIB DYSFUNCTIONS

The most important point in diagnosis is the difference between inhalation and exhalation restriction. The next most important is to identify the key rib. As there can be more than one key rib, re-examination after treatment is always advisable. If present the second key rib should also be treated. Muscle energy is the most frequently used treatment for rib dysfunctions but respiratory ribs are not subluxations and for these thrusting can be used if necessary. Thrusting can also be used for torsions.

Muscle Energy

1. Restrictions of inhalation

Described for right-sided restrictions.
   There are three components to the treatment:
   (a) inhalation effort by the patient;

(b) muscle effort by the patient resisted by the operator;

(c) rib elevation assistance by the operator.

Operator resistance is used to stabilise one end of the muscle in order to make the other end move. As in all muscle energy procedures, some of the gain takes place when the slack is taken up after relaxation.

Help from the operator in elevating the rib is given by him pulling laterally and caudad medial to the angle of the rib(s). Because the rib angle is behind the axis of motion, pulling caudally on the angle will elevate the anterior end.

The position with the arm elevated helps by stretching any tight fascial tissue that may be restricting inhalation. The alternatives are required for those with stiff shoulders.

Ribs 11 and 12 are treated differently and both inhalation and exhalation restrictions will be dealt with under the latter section.

1.1. Ribs 1 and 2

Diagnostic points. The first, or second rib is the uppermost rib of a group, or the only rib, which stops moving on inhalation before the rib on the other side.

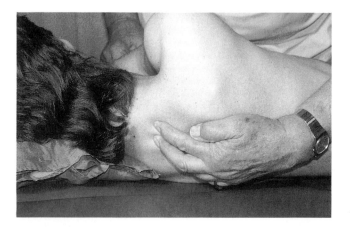

a

b

Fig. 10.5 Treatment of inhalation restriction ribs 1 and 2. (a) Finger tips hooked over posterior shafts ribs 1 and 2; (b) position for patient effort, the forearm on the table.

Both ribs can be treated at the same time. Isotonic contraction of the scalene muscles is used.

1.1.1. The patient is supine with the operator at her left side. He lifts her right shoulder with his right hand and hooks the terminal phalanges of his left index and middle fingers over the superior edge of the medial end of the posterior shaft of rib 1 and at or medial to the angle of rib 2 (Fig. 10.5a).

1.1.2. Her shoulder is then returned to the table with his left arm under her, and his forearm resting on the table top.

1.1.3. The patient's head is rolled 15–20° to the left; this also sidebends the neck, putting the scalenes on stretch. Her right forearm is then placed over her forehead and held there by the operator (Fig. 10.5b).

1.1.4. The patient then inhales fully and attempts to lift her head against the operator's resistance. If the shoulder is not mobile the operator can give the counterforce with his hand on her forehead directly without elevating her arm.

1.1.5. After 3–5 seconds she is told to relax and, as she does so, the operator 'takes up the slack' by pulling the rib angles laterally and caudad.

1.1.6. Steps 1.1.4 and 1.1.5 are repeated two to four times while the operator maintains the pull with his left hand.

1.1.7. After a slow release of his pull, the operator should re-examine the position.

1.2. Ribs 3, 4 and 5

Diagnostic points. One of these ribs is the uppermost rib of a group, or the only rib, which stops moving on inhalation before the rib on the other side. The pectoralis minor muscle is used.

1.2.1. The patient lies supine with the operator at her left. He hooks the tips of his left index, middle and ring fingers over the shafts of the 3rd, 4th and 5th ribs, medial to the angles so that, with his forearm on the table, he can pull laterally and caudad. As detailed in steps 1.1.1 and 1.1.2 above.

1.2.2. Her right arm is raised so that it lies beside her head. His right hand controls the front of her right elbow (Fig. 10.6a). If the shoulder is not sufficiently mobile, the arm can be allowed to rest at her side and the resisting force applied with the thumb to the inferomedial aspect of the coracoid process (Fig. 10.6b) or with the palm of his hand over the front of her shoulder joint (Fig. 10.6c).

1.2.3. The patient inhales deeply and tries to elevate her right arm, anteriorly for a pump handle restriction, more laterally if the restriction is of the bucket handle type. If the operator's resistance is on the front of the shoulder the patient's effort is to bring the shoulder anteriorly and a little medially for a pump handle restriction or more laterally if the restriction is of bucket handle type.

1.2.4. After 3–5 seconds the patient relaxes and, as before, the slack is taken up by pulling laterally and caudad on the medial rib shafts.

1.2.5. The process is repeated two to four times with the operator maintaining the new position after each effort.

1.2.6. Re-examine.

Fig. 10.6 Treatment of
inhalation restriction ribs 3 to 5.
(a) With arm beside the head
and hand on elbow; (b) with
the thumb on the coracoid
process; (c) with the hand on
the front of the shoulder.

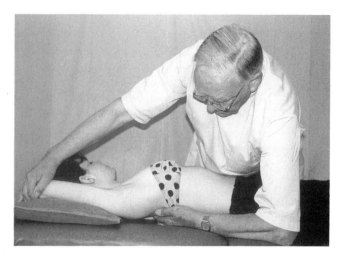

a

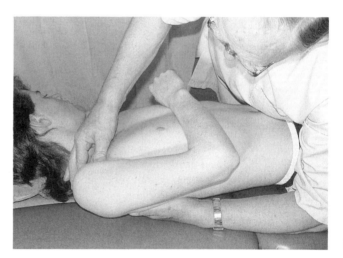

b

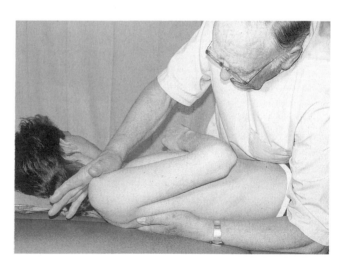

c

1.3. Ribs 6 to 10

The main muscle is the serratus anterior.

Diagnostic points. One of these ribs is the uppermost rib of a group, or the only rib, which stops moving on inhalation before the rib on the other side.

1.3.1. The patient is supine with the operator at her left. He hooks the tips of his left index, middle ring and little fingers over the shafts of ribs 6 to 9, medial to the angles, once again with his forearm resting on the table. Rib 10 can also be treated this way but it is not often the key rib.

1.3.2. Her arm is elevated as before but her forearm is brought to the left above her head and her wrist is grasped by the operator's right hand to give the resistance (Fig. 10.7a). If the shoulder is too stiff to permit this movement, the scapula can be stabilised by the operator's right hand pushing backwards and medially on the humeral head and acromion (Fig. 10.7b), or, if the shoulder is sufficiently mobile, it may be flexed to a right angle and the resistance applied to the elbow while the patient attempts to push it upwards (anteriorly).

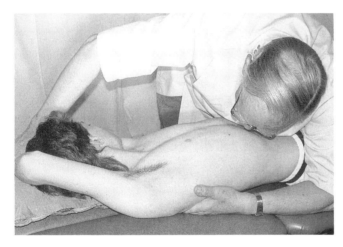

a

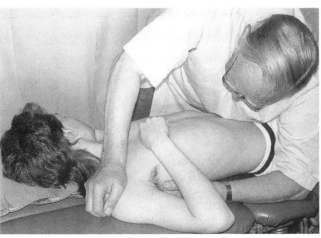

b

Fig. 10.7 Treatment of inhalation restriction ribs 6 to 10. (a) With the arm over the top of the head; (b) with the hand on the front of the shoulder.

1.3.3. For the more common bucket handle restriction, the patient's effort at the top of forced inhalation should be to pull her right arm to the right. If there is more pump handle component the direction of pull should be more anteriorly. In each case the effort is resisted by the operator. If the resistance is on the front of the shoulder the patient's effort is to bring the shoulder anteriorly and caudad.

1.3.4. After 3–5 seconds the patient should relax and the operator takes up the slack as before. The process is repeated two to four times with the lateral and caudad pull maintained by the operator.

1.3.5. Re-examine.

2. Restriction of exhalation

Described for right sided restrictions.

There are also three components to the treatment:
(a) exhalation effort by the patient,
(b) patient positioning by the operator,
(c) control of rib motion by the operator.

The exhalation effort and the patient positioning are designed to produce the maximum exhalatory motion in the restricted rib. The operator then holds the rib in that position while the patient inhales and he follows the rib down on the next exhalation. It should be emphasised that the rib is not forced down but is held in position against the inspiratory effort. The costochondral junction must be spanned by the thumb when holding the rib down, otherwise damage to it can occur even with simple patient effort.

2.1. Rib 1
This is a special example because of the anatomy. It is often known as the 'disappearing thumb trick'.

Diagnostic points. On exhalation the first rib stops moving down before that on the other side and the second ribs move evenly.

2.1.1. The patient is supine and the operator sits at the head of the table.

2.1.2. To relax the tissues, the operator lifts her head with his left hand to produce flexion and a slight right sidebend.

2.1.3. His right thumb finds the rib. For the common pump handle restriction, the anterior end of the rib is found from above, deep to the medial end of the clavicle and immediately lateral to the sternomastoid insertion; for those who have a wide sternomastoid it is often easier to approach the rib between the sternal and clavicular heads (Fig. 10.8a). For a bucket handle restriction contact is made with the shaft of the rib posterolateral to the neurovascular bundle (Fig. 10.8b).

2.1.4. The patient exhales and the operator follows the downward motion of the rib with his thumb. At the same time he increases the forward flexion of the neck, adding more sidebending for the bucket handle restriction.

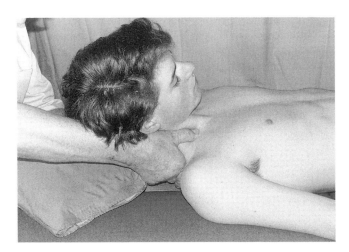

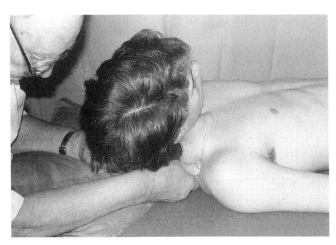

2.1.5. During the inhalation phase the operator keeps the rib down by holding the position with his thumb.

2.1.6. The cycle is repeated two or more times and after the last exhalation the patient is asked to push her head back to the table, against slight resistance. The rib is held down until after the end of an inhalation phase.

2.1.7. Re-examine.

2.2. Ribs 2–10

The technique is the same for all these ribs except that for the upper ribs with more pump handle restriction the head and neck should be raised forwards. The lower ribs require more sidebending to help to correct the bucket handle restrictions.

Diagnostic points. The rib to be treated is the lowest (key) of a group, or is the only rib that on exhalation stops moving before those on the other side.

2.2.1. The patient is supine and the operator stands or sits at her head. Using the right thumb and thenar eminence (1st metacarpal) the operator contacts the upper border of the dysfunctional rib *so that he spans the costochondral junction*. For bucket handle restrictions the contact should be more lateral and for pump handle more medial but the junction must always be protected (Fig. 10.9a).

2.2.2. With his left hand reaching down so that his finger tips are under the upper thoracic vertebrae, the operator lifts her head and neck down to the point where the tissue tension just reaches his right thumb (Fig. 10.9b).

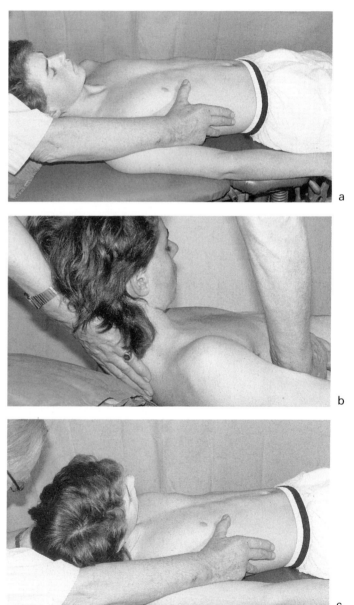

Fig. 10.9 Treatment of exhalation restriction typical ribs. (a) Protecting the costochondral junction; (b) lifting head forwards for pump handle restriction; (c) lifting head sideways for bucket handle restriction.

2.2.3. The patient exhales fully and the operator follows the movement with his right thumb, and by further lifting her head and neck to bring the flexion down to the new point of tension.

2.2.4. On inhalation, the operator maintains the position. The cycle is repeated two or more times and the patient then pushes her head and trunk back to the table top against light resistance and the operator's thumb control is released after the end of an inhalation phase.

2.2.5. Re-examine.

3. Ribs 11 and 12, inhalation and exhalation restrictions

The treatment for these two is similar; the main muscles used are the quadratus lumborum and those of the abdominal wall. The differences are in the patient positioning and the direction of the operator effort. The effectiveness appears to be the result of this positioning and direction, the desired movement being the only one permitted when the muscle effort is made.

Diagnostic points. The 11th or 12th rib does not open the calliper as widely on inhalation or close it as tightly on exhalation as on the other side. There is likely to be tissue texture change on the restricted side.

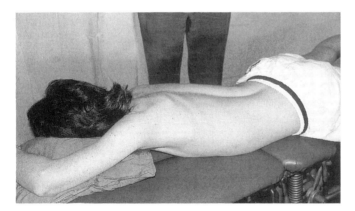

a

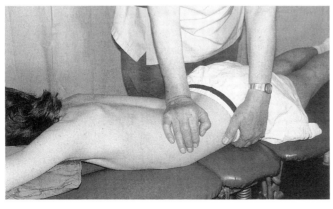

b

Fig. 10.10 Treatment of inhalation restriction ribs 11 and 12. (a) Sidebent position on the table; (b) position for patient effort (or for thrust).

3.1. Restriction of inhalation
Described for the left side.

3.1.1. The patient is prone and, to assist the inhalation movement on the left, she is sidebent to the right and her left arm should be above her head. The operator stands at her right (Fig. 10.10a).

3.1.2. With the heel of his right hand the operator contacts the medial ends of the 11th and 12th ribs so that he can 'scoop' them away laterally. His arm should point laterally and *craniad*.

3.1.3. With his left hand under her anterior superior iliac spine he lifts the left side of her pelvis (Fig. 10.10b).

3.1.4. The patient takes a deep breath *in* and, while holding her breath, attempts to pull her pelvis back to the table.

3.1.5. After 3–5 seconds she relaxes and breathes out. When she has fully relaxed the slack is taken up by the operator's left hand.

3.1.6. Two to four repetitions are made and the position re-examined.

3.2. Restriction of exhalation
Described for the left side.

3.2.1. The patient is prone and, to assist the exhalation movement on the left, she is sidebent to the left. Her left arm should be by her side (Fig. 10.11a). The operator stands at her right.

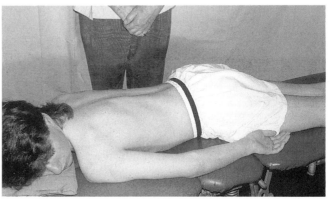

a

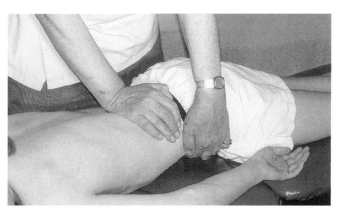

b

Fig. 10.11 Treatment of exhalation restriction ribs 11 and 12. (a) Sidebent for exhalation restriction; (b) position for patient effort (or for thrust).

3.2.2. With the heel of his right hand the operator contacts the medial ends of the 11th and 12th ribs so that he can 'scoop' them away laterally. His arm should point laterally and *caudad*.

3.2.3. With his left hand under her anterior superior spine he lifts the left side of her pelvis (Fig. 10.11b).

3.2.4. The patient breathes *out* deeply and, while holding her breath, attempts to pull her pelvis back to the table.

3.2.5. After 3–5 seconds she relaxes and breathes in. When she has fully relaxed the slack is taken up by the operator's right hand.

3.2.6. Two to four repetitions are made and the position re-examined.

4. Thrust

4.1. Typical ribs supine techniques

These techniques can all be used for treatment of inhalation or exhalation restrictions. They are useful for ribs 3–9 but are easier at the 4–7 levels. They are variants of the supine thoracic techniques, the chief difference being in the position of the fulcrum at the back. The patient's arm positions described in Chapter 9 can be used but a thrust through the elbow of the ipsilateral side is usually better.

Described for the 6th left rib, inhalation or exhalation restriction.

Diagnostic points. The 6th left rib is the key rib of a group that stops moving earlier on inhalation or exhalation than the rib on the other side (or it is the only restricted rib).

4.1.1. The position is similar to that in the supine thoracic techniques. The patient is supine and the operator stands to her right side. She should cross her left arm (*one arm only*) over her chest and hold her right shoulder with her left hand.

4.1.2. The operator lifts her left shoulder with his left hand so that he can insert his right hand under her with the base of the thenar eminence in contact with the posterior shaft of R6. For inhalation restriction the thenar eminence should be above the rib shaft near the angle, for exhalation restriction it needs to be below. His fingers are used to support the right side of her spine (Fig. 10.12a). For the lower ribs some flexion of the spine may be needed to allow the rib angle to come close to the table top in the presence of the thoracic kyphosis.

4.1.3. After she is returned to the supine position the operator leans over her and with his chest or upper abdomen directs the thrust against her elbow towards his right thenar eminence (Fig. 10.12b).

4.1.4. The thrust is given at the end of a deep respiratory effort in the appropriate phase of respiration and at the same moment the operator makes a rotatory movement with his right thenar eminence; for inhalation restriction on the left side the rotation is clockwise, as seen from the front, so that the posterior rib shaft is taken caudad (Fig. 10.12c), and for exhalation restriction counterclockwise, to take the posterior shaft craniad (Fig. 10.12d).

4.1.5. Retest.

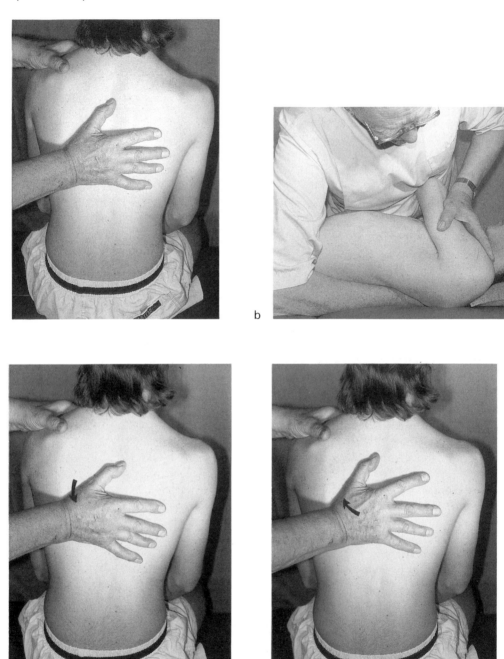

Fig. 10.12 Thrust treatment for typical ribs. (a) The hand position shown sitting for clarity; (b) position for elbow thrust on one arm; (c) showing hand rotation for inhalation restriction; (d) showing hand rotation for exhalation restriction.

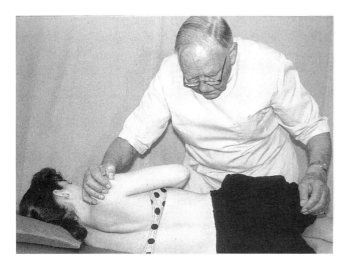

a

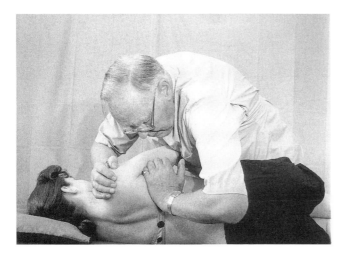

b

4.2. Middle ribs, sidelying

Described for the 5th right rib.

4.2.1. The patient lies on her left side with her spine in neutral and the operator stands in front of her (Fig. 10.13a).

4.2.2. With the pisiform of his left hand the operator contacts the 5th rib at the angle. For an inhalation restriction the contact needs to be above (craniad) the angle and for an exhalation restriction it is below (caudad).

4.2.3. With his right hand the operator rotates her upper trunk to the right by backward pressure on her shoulder until the tension reaches the level of the 5th rib as felt by his left hand.

4.2.4. After the slack has been taken out the thrust is given at the end of the appropriate phase of respiration in a direction that is anterior and craniad for exhalation and anterior and caudad for an inhalation restriction (Fig. 10.13b).

4.2.5. Retest.

4.3. Rib 1. Supine technique

Described for the left side.

Diagnostic points. The 1st left rib stops moving before that on the opposite side in either inhalation or exhalation. With inhalation restriction it may be the uppermost of a group. For exhalation restriction, if rib 1 is to be treated, it will be the only restricted rib.

4.3.1. The patient is supine and the operator stands at her right side. He slides his right hand diagonally under her upper trunk so as to grip the 1st left rib with his fingers (Fig. 10.14).

Fig. 10.14 Position for supine thrust for rib 1, in- or exhalation.

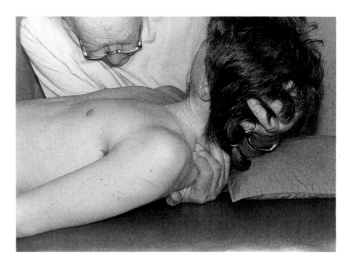

4.3.2. With his finger tips he pulls back the edge of the trapezius muscle to find the back of the rib. For exhalation restriction his fingers are used to roll the rib forwards and down while for an inhalation restriction they roll the rib backwards and up.

4.3.3. With his left hand the operator sidebends her head and neck to the left and rotates it to the right until the tension comes to the rib.

4.3.4. The thrust is with the left hand on the back of her head at the end of the appropriate phase of respiration (inhalation for a restriction of inhalation and exhalation for an exhalation restriction). The head is turned further to the right which rotates T1 to the right and pushes forward on the back of the rib while the fingers of the operator's right hand guide it into the corrective position.

4.3.5. Retest.

4.4. Rib 1. Sitting technique

Described for the left side.

Diagnostic points. See technique 4.3.

4.4.1. The patient sits up tall with legs over the side of the table, and the operator stands behind her with his right foot on the table top close to her right side. She drapes her right arm over his knee, giving him ability to change her sidebending position through his right leg.

4.4.2. The operator places the web of his left hand over the inner part of her left first rib and with his right forearm and hand he controls her head and protects her neck. Because he will use a thrust with his left hand his elbow needs to be raised to bring the forearm into line with the thrust direction (Fig. 10.15). For inhalation restriction the left hand contacts the posterior part of the rib. For exhalation restriction the side of the index finger is used to contact the shaft of the rib laterally but behind the neurovascular bundle.

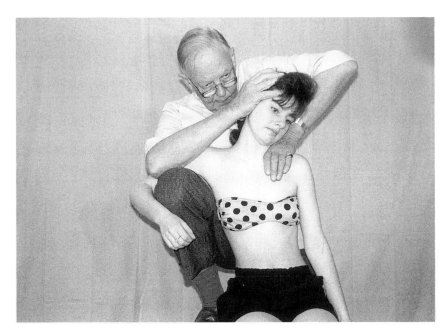

Fig. 10.15 Sitting thrust for rib 1, inhalation, for exhalation the index finger is more lateral. Note use of knee to control translation sideways of the trunk.

4.4.3. The operator monitors with his left hand while he introduces left sidebending by translation, using his right thigh from below and forearm from above.

4.4.4. The high velocity, low amplitude thrust is given in the direction of the right nipple by his left hand with slight exaggeration of the left sidebend from above through his right forearm.

4.4.5. Retest.

4.5. Rib 2
Described for the 2nd right rib, inhalation or exhalation restriction.

4.5.1. The patient sits on a table or stool with her upper spine in neutral and the operator stands behind her.

4.5.2. The operator places his right thumb against the back of the shaft of the 2nd right rib so that he can push either up (craniad) or down (caudad) as required (Fig. 10.16a).

Fig. 10.16 Sitting thrust for rib 2, in- or exhalation. (a) Thumb contact on the rib posterior shaft; (b) thrust position, (operator to the side for clarity).

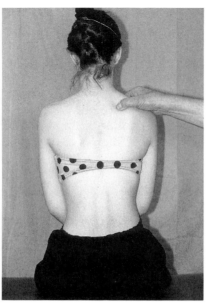
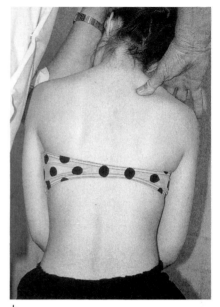

a   b

4.5.3. With his left hand he takes her head into right sidebending and left rotation until the tension reaches the upper edge of the rib.

4.5.4. At the end of the appropriate respiratory phase and when all slack has been taken out the thrust is given on the rib by his right thumb. The direction should be anterior and craniad for an exhalation restriction but anterior and caudad for restriction of inhalation (Fig. 10.16b).

4.5.5. Retest.

Ribs 11 and 12
The thrust techniques are very similar to those using muscle energy activation.

Described for the left side.

Diagnostic points. The 11th or 12th rib does not open the calliper as widely on inhalation or close it as tightly on exhalation as on the other side. There is likely to be tissue texture change on the restricted side.

4.6. For restriction of inhalation
4.6.1. The patient is prone and, to assist the inhalation movement on the left, she is sidebent to the right and her left arm should be above her head. The operator stands at her right.

4.6.2. With the heel of his right hand the operator contacts the medial ends of the 11th and 12th ribs so that he can 'scoop' them away laterally. His arm should point laterally and *craniad*.

4.6.3. With his left hand under her anterior superior spine he lifts the left side of her pelvis (Fig. 10.10a and b).

4.6.4. When all slack has been taken out by lifting the pelvis, the patient takes a deep breath in and the operator gives a high velocity, low amplitude thrust laterally and craniad.

4.6.5. Retest.

4.7. *For restriction of exhalation*
Described for the left side.

4.7.1. The patient is prone and, to assist the exhalation movement on the left, she is sidebent to the left. Her left arm should be by her side. The operator stands at her right.

4.7.2. With the heel of his right hand the operator contacts the medial ends of the 11th and 12th ribs so that he can 'scoop' them away laterally. His arm should point laterally and caudad.

4.7.3. With his left hand under her anterior superior spine he lifts the left side of her pelvis (Fig. 10.11).

4.7.4. When all slack has been taken out by lifting the pelvis, the patient breathes out deeply and the operator gives a high velocity, low amplitude thrust laterally and caudad.

4.7.5. Retest.

TREATMENT OF STRUCTURAL RIB DYSFUNCTIONS

These are likely to be associated with intervertebral dysfunctions and the general rule is that the intervertebral joint is treated first. Indeed, many rib dysfunctions will return to normal if the intervertebral problem is corrected.

Accurate diagnosis is important as the treatment varies widely depending on precisely what is wrong. Diagnosis depends on finding that the rib position is out of the normal line, usually both in front and behind, and that there is tissue texture abnormality. The latter is most commonly found in the insertion of the iliocostalis at the rib angle. The rib angle and the costochondral junction are usually tender and all these treatments are likely to be painful. It will often be found that the anterior tenderness is immediately less following treatment of a subluxation.

Muscle Energy

5.1. *Anterior subluxation*
Diagnostic points. The rib angle is anterior to the expected position in the anteroposterior curve and medial to that in the lateral curve. The respiratory excursion of the rib will be much diminished. The insertion of iliocostalis is tense, often oedematous and tender. It may be necessary to assess the position with the patient sitting because of the effect of pressure on the ribs by the table top in either supine or prone lying.

Described for the 4th left rib.

5.1.1. The patient sits with her spine in neutral and the operator stands behind her. She holds her right shoulder with her left hand and the operator grasps her left elbow with his right hand (Fig. 10.17a).

Fig. 10.17 Treatment of anterior subluxation of a typical rib. (a) Position from in front; (b) from behind, rib angle and direction marked; (c) alternative for lower ribs, pushing on the other fist.

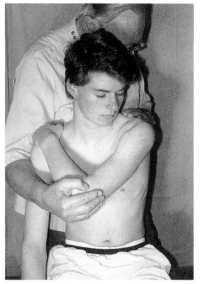

a

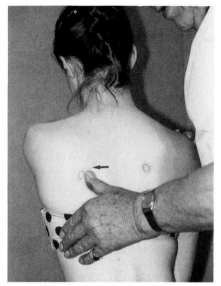

b

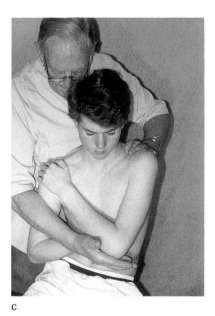

c

5.1.2. With his left thumb, the operator contacts her 4th left rib medial to the angle and prepares to pull it laterally. He should adjust the elbow position so that the tension in the tissues at the back reaches his left thumb (Fig. 10.17b).

5.1.3. If there is restriction of inhalation, the next step is done in inhalation. If the restriction is of exhalation, the treatment is done in that phase. In the correct phase of respiration, he *pulls* the rib angle to the left while she *pulls* her elbow to the left against the operator's resistance.

Alternatively for the lower ribs, she may pull her elbow down against resistance and in that case she can insert her right fist between her left elbow and the front of the rib to help to push it back (Fig. 10.17c).

5.1.4. After 3–5 seconds she should relax but the operator retains his pull on the rib angle.

5.1.5. Steps 1.3 and 1.4 are repeated two to four times and after the operator relaxes his pull the position is re-examined.

5.2. Posterior subluxation

Diagnostic points. The rib angle is posterior to the expected position in the anteroposterior curve and lateral to that in the lateral curve. The respiratory excursion of the rib will be much diminished. The insertion of iliocostalis is tense, often oedematous and tender. It may be necessary to assess the position with the patient sitting because of the effect of pressure on the rib by the table top.

Described for the 4th left rib.

5.2.1. The patient sits with her spine in neutral and the operator stands behind her. She holds her right shoulder with her left hand and the operator grasps her left elbow with his right hand as in Fig. 10.17a.

5.2.2. With his left thumb, the operator contacts her 4th left rib lateral to the angle and prepares to push it medially. He should adjust the elbow position so that the tension in the tissues at the back reaches his left thumb (Fig. 10.18a).

5.2.3. If there is a major restriction in one phase of respiration, the treatment is done in that phase.

5.2.4. The patient is then instructed to *push* her elbow to the right against the operator's resistance at the same time as he *pushes* the rib angle

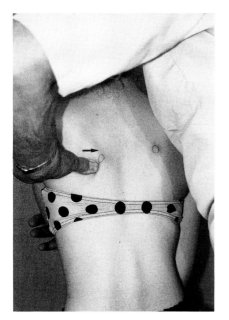

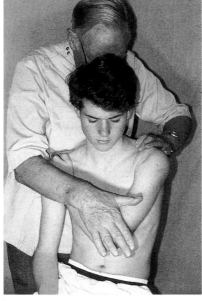

Fig. 10.18 Treatment of posterior subluxation of a typical rib. (a) From behind, rib angle and direction marked; (b) alternative resistance to raising elbow.

a b

to the right. Alternatively, she may raise her elbow against resistance (Fig. 10.18b).

5.2.5. After 3–5 seconds she should relax but the operator maintains his push.

5.2.6. Steps 1.4 and 1.5 are repeated two to four times and after the operator relaxes his pull the position is re-examined.

5.3. Superior subluxation of the 1st rib

Described for the left side.

The medial end of the rib is not less than 6 mm (¼ inch) higher on the dysfunctional side and it will be tender. The C7–T1 and T1–2 joints should always be checked and, if necessary, treated before this diagnosis is made.

5.3.1. The patient sits and the operator stands behind her.

5.3.2. The operator places his right foot on the table top beside the patient and drapes her right arm over his thigh to give him lateral control of her trunk.

5.3.3. With the index and middle fingers of his left hand he palpates the posterior end of her 1st left rib in front of the trapezius muscle, pulling the muscle back so that he can reach the superior surface of the rib (see Fig. 10.3). With his thumb he finds the posterior aspect of the rib, feeling through the trapezius.

5.3.4. With his right hand he sidebends her neck to the left to relax the tissues around the rib and adjustment of his knee position helps to keep her balanced (Fig. 10.19).

5.3.5. The patient then pushes her head to the right against the operator's resistance to contract the right scalenes and, by reciprocal inhibition, make the left scalenes relax. The pressure must be controlled because, although easy pressure causes the antagonists to relax, if she

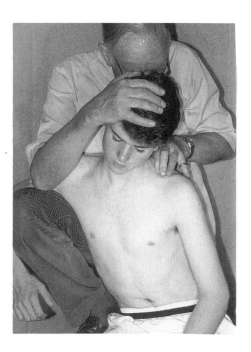

Fig. 10.19 For superior subluxation of rib 1.

presses too hard they will tighten again to stabilise the cervical spine. A few pounds pressure is all that is required.

5.3.6. When the tissues on the left are relaxed the operator pushes the rib down into position. Often, however, the rib will have 'hitched' on the top of the transverse process and, in this event, firm forward pressure by the thumb is necessary to disengage it, before the rib can descend.

5.3.7. Re-examine.

5.4. External torsion

Diagnostic points. This will nearly always be associated with an intervertebral dysfunction. The vertebra forming the upper half of the costovertebral joint will be (or will have been) rotated to the side of the dysfunctional rib and will have limited flexion. The rib shaft at the back has a prominent upper margin and the lower margin will be difficult to feel. The intercostal space above is wide and that below is narrow. The intercostal muscles in the narrow space are likely to be tense and tender. Described for a left rib.

5.4.1. The patient sits and holds her right shoulder with her left hand.

5.4.2. The operator stands behind her and puts his right hand on her left elbow so that he can resist a lifting effort (Fig. 10.18b).

5.4.3. The operator puts his left thumb against the upper border of the dysfunctional rib at the angle and positions the elbow so that the tension just reaches his thumb.

5.4.4. He then pushes forward on the superior border of the angle of the rib while the patient attempts first to elevate and then to depress her left elbow through a number of cycles against the operator's resistance (Fig. 10.20).

5.4.5. Re–examine.

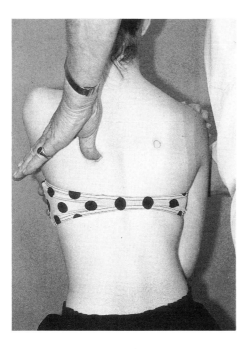

Fig. 10.20 For external torsion showing position and mark at angle.

5.5. *Internal torsion*

This dysfunction is less common than external torsion.

Diagnostic points. It will nearly always be associated with intervertebral dysfunction. The vertebra forming the upper half of the costovertebral joint will be rotated away from the side of the dysfunctional rib and will probably have limited flexion. The posterior rib shaft has a prominent lower margin. The upper margin is less prominent than usual. The intercostal space above is narrow and will probably be tense and tender. That below is wider than usual.

Described for a left rib.

5.5.1. The patient sits and holds her right shoulder with her left hand.

5.5.2. The operator stands behind her and puts his right hand on her left elbow so that he can resist downward pressure.

5.5.3. The operator puts his left thumb against the lower border of the dysfunctional rib at the angle and positions the elbow so that the tension just reaches his thumb.

5.5.4. He then pushes forward on the inferior border of the dysfunctional rib at the angle while the patient attempts first to elevate and then to depress her left elbow through a number of cycles against the operator's resistance (Fig. 10.21).

5.5.5. Re-examine.

5.6. *Lateral flexion*

Often a most painful and incapacitating condition, especially if in the 3rd or, worse, the 2nd rib.

Described for the 3rd left rib.

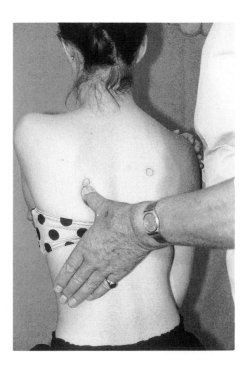

Fig. 10.21 For internal torsion showing position and mark at angle.

Diagnostic points. The rib is prominent and very tender in the axilla and its respiratory excursion is much limited particularly in exhalation. The intercostal space above is narrow with the muscle very tight and tender. The origin of the pectoralis minor muscle from the rib will also show tissue texture change and will be tender. There will be a history of an acute lateral flexion strain.

5.6.1. The patient is supine and the operator stands at her left side.

5.6.2. The operator must reach high enough to hook the terminal phalanges of his index and middle fingers over the superior border of the rib. This is not easy at the 3rd and more difficult still at the 2nd; it is done by repeated movements in which the operator places his right hand on her ribs in the left axilla and works his hand up while he sidebends the patients head to the left and has her repeatedly reach down with her left hand towards her knee and then relax (Fig. 10.22a).

5.6.3. The final step can be very painful especially at the second rib level and must be performed rapidly and firmly. The rib is held down while the head and neck are straightened by the operator's left hand (Fig. 10.22b).

5.6.4. Re-examine.

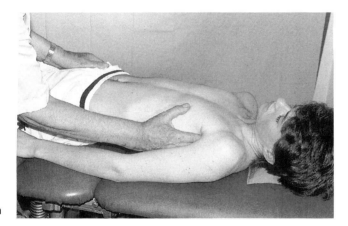

a

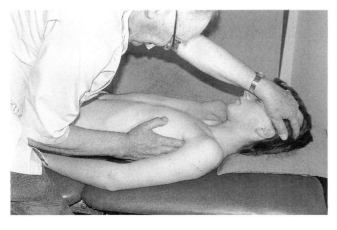

b

Fig. 10.22 For laterally flexed rib. (a) Starting to reach fingers over top of rib; (b) final position, correction by holding rib down while head and trunk are straightened.

5.7. Anteroposterior compression

Diagnostic points. The anterior and posterior ends of the rib are less prominent than the expected position in the curves. The rib is prominent in the axilla but intercostal spaces above and below are even.

5.7.1. The patient stands and the operator stands at her normal side. For the higher ribs she should have her arm over his shoulder; for the lower ribs she should have her arm by her side.

5.7.2. With his middle fingers the operator circles the dysfunctional rib pulling her trunk against his, with the finger tips putting medial pressure over the rib in the mid axilla (Fig. 10.23).

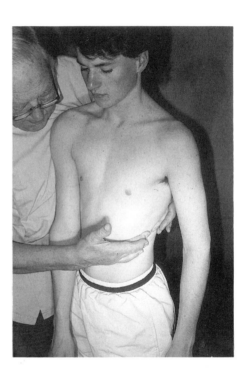

Fig. 10.23 For anteroposterior compression of a left rib.

5.7.3. She should breathe in and out for the operator to find the point of minimal tissue tension at the rib.

5.7.4. Using that phase of respiration she is asked to bend her trunk toward the operator while he maintains the medial compression on the rib.

5.7.5. After two to four repetitions the rib is re-examined.

5.8. Lateral compression

Diagnostic points. The anterior and posterior ends of the rib are prominent but the rib is 'missing' in the axilla. Intercostal spaces are even. The condition is uncommon but painful.

5.8.1. The patient stands and the operator stands at her affected side. She should raise her affected arm and place it over his shoulder.

5.8.2. He places one hand over the costochondral junction and the other over the angle of the dysfunctional rib.

5.8.3. While the operator compresses the rib front to back, the patient inhales deeply and pulls her arm down on to his shoulder (Fig. 10.24a and b).

5.8.4. This is repeated two to four times if necessary and the position rechecked.

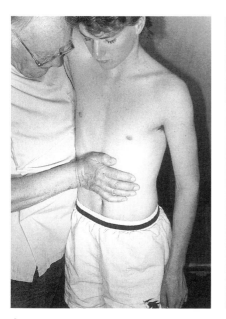 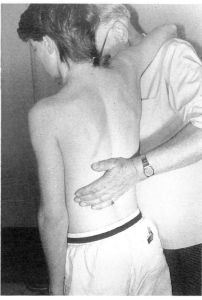

a   b

Fig. 10.24 a and b For lateral compression of a right rib.

Thrust

5.9. Combined treatment for external rib torsion and ERS dysfunction
This is performed by an addition to the supine technique used for ERS dysfunctions in the thoracic spine. It is valuable for ERS dysfunctions associated with external torsion of the rib because sometimes successful treatment can be achieved only by doing both together. Described for the right 8th rib with T7–8 ERSrt.

Diagnostic points. The 8th right rib has a prominent upper border with a wide interspace above and the lower border is difficult to feel. T7 is rotated to the right and will not go into full flexion. There is marked tissue texture change around the spinal and costovertebral joints.

5.9.1. The patient is supine and the operator stands to her left (opposite the most posterior transverse process). She should cross her arms over her chest so that her right elbow is directly in front of her left with her hands in her opposite axillae.

5.9.2. The operator reaches across and lifts her right shoulder with his right hand so that he can insert his left hand under her. In this technique the lower segment vertebra (T8) is supported by the operator's left thumb and fingers. He uses his thenar eminence to contact the inferior part of the angle of the dysfunctional rib so that by rotation of his hand, he can correct the rib torsion at the same time as the main thrust corrects the vertebral problem (Fig. 10.25a).

5.9.3. The operator then reaches down her neck with his right hand to support her head and he flexes and sidebends her to the left until movement just begins at T7. Rotation is introduced by turning her head to the left, again until motion just begins at T7 (Fig. 10.25b).

5.9.4. Bringing his chest or upper abdomen over the patient's elbows, the operator gives a high velocity, low amplitude thrust dropping his weight on to her elbows in the direction of his left thumb while twisting his thenar eminence clockwise as seen from the front (for the right side) to raise the rib angle.

5.9.5. Retest.

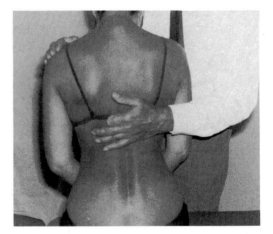

a

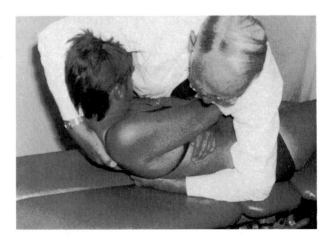

b

Fig. 10.25 For combined external rib torsion and ERS at the superior vertebra. (a) Hand position and direction of twist; (b) head and trunk position

Treatment of the cervical spine

The most serious accidents caused by manipulation without anaesthesia have been from treatment of the upper cervical spine in extension and nearly full rotation. This position is not necessary and it is important to avoid the risk which it involves. The problem is caused by interference with the vertebro-basilar arterial circulation and it has recently been shown that the mechanism is usually an intimal tear leading to dissection rather than direct obstruction. Thrusting manipulation is not the only cause; it has even been recorded as happening when the person has held his own neck voluntarily in that position for a period of time without external force of any kind.

There has not been any record of an accident of this nature occurring with muscle energy treatment and the techniques described here do not involve the adoption of the dangerous position. Sometimes, however, the nature of the joint restriction is such that it is useful to be able to use thrust techniques. In the fourth edition the thrusting techniques which had been described in the earlier ones were omitted; one of the authors still uses those techniques occasionally but it is less easy to be fully specific than with the ones now described. Neither involve the use of the dangerous position and the ones described here are among those regularly taught at the postgraduate manual medicine courses at Michigan State University College of Osteopathic Medicine.

The cervical spine is unique in that there are no neutral dysfunctions although the small amount of rotation which occurs at the occipitoatlantal joint is to the side opposite to the sidebending. For the beginner there appears often to be a difficulty in locating the barrier, especially after the first patient effort. The caution is that it is more than ever important not to go beyond the barrier when positioning the joint for either muscle energy or thrusting treatment.

1. TYPICAL CERVICAL VERTEBRAE, C2–7

Muscle energy

1.1. Restriction of extension
Described for restriction of rotation and sidebending to the left at C5–6, FRSrt, a very common dysfunction.

   Diagnostic points. There is tissue texture change at the segment. With the neck flexed C5 will translate easily from right to left and from left to right. With the neck extended there is restriction of translation from left to right but that from right to left remains free.

1.1.1. The patient is supine and the operator sits or stands at her head.

1.1.2a. The operator uses his left index finger to contact the posterior aspect of the left lateral mass (articular pillar) of C6, the lower vertebra of the motion segment. With that contact he fixes C6 and extends the C5–6 joint until the tension just reaches his finger. Note that to produce extension the lift must be at the lower vertebra and to produce flexion it is at the upper (Fig. 11.1a and b).

1.1.2b. Alternative operator position. This concerns the placement of the fingers only. In the variant the index fingers of each hand are used to contact the vertebra by gripping the spinous process between the tips and using the sides of the proximal phalanges, instead of the finger tips, to contact the lateral mass of the vertebra. The remainder of the technique is the same (Fig. 11.1c).

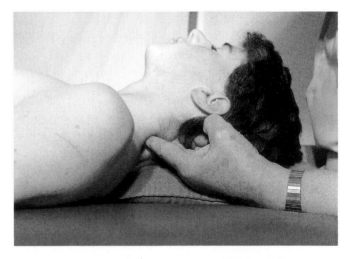

a

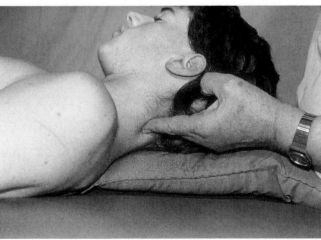

Fig. 11.1 Treatment for FRSrt of typical cervical vertebrae. ME. (a) Finger under lateral mass of C6 to extend C5–6 joint; (b) finger under lateral mass of C5 to flex C5–6 joint.

b

1.1.3. With his right hand on the right side of her head he introduces left sidebending and left rotation until the tension reaches his finger (Fig. 11.1d).

1.1.4. The patient is then asked to attempt gently to push her head to the right or to lift it off the table. The effort is maintained for 3–5 seconds while the operator resists so that she does not move and she is then asked to relax.

1.1.5. When she has relaxed fully, the operator increases slightly the lift with his left hand and the rotation and sidebending with his right hand, to reach the new barrier.

1.1.6. Steps 1.1.4 and 1.1.5 are repeated two or more times depending on response and if the response is poor, it may be wise to try the other available direction for the patient's effort (flexion instead of sidebending or vice versa).

1.1.7. Retest.

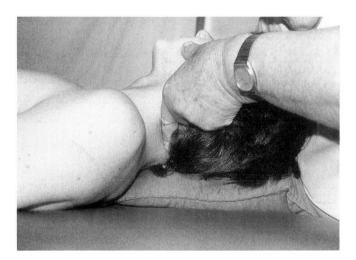

c

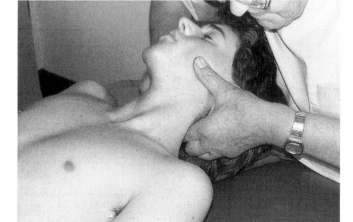

d

Fig. 11.1 (continued) (c) Using the finger tips on the spinous process; (d) position of patient effort (sidebend is not well shown).

1.2. Restriction of flexion

Described for restriction of left rotation and sidebending at C4–5, ERSrt.

Diagnostic points. There is tissue texture change at the segment. With the neck extended C4 will translate easily from right to left and from left to right. With the neck flexed there is restriction of translation from left to right but that from right to left remains free.

1.2.1. The patient is supine and the operator sits or stands at her head.

1.2.2. In order to introduce left sidebending the operator controls her head with his right hand. With the palm of his left hand he supports her occiput and with his left index finger and thumb respectively he contacts the right and left articular pillars of C4 (Fig. 11.2a).

1.2.3. He flexes her neck until he feels the tension reach his left finger and thumb and then introduces left sidebending with his right hand. At the same time he translates C4 to the right to sidebend from below to the barrier (Fig. 11.2b).

1.2.4. The patient is then asked to make a gentle effort to sidebend her head to the right or to press it back into the table. The effort is maintained for 3–5 seconds and the operator resists so that she does not move. She is then asked to relax.

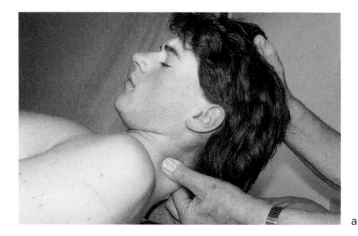

a

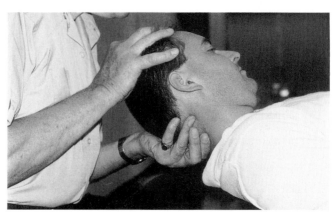

b

Fig. 11.2 Treatment for ERSrt of typical cervical vertebrae. ME. (a) Position of monitoring hand seen from the left; (b) position for patient effort seen from the right.

1.2.5. When relaxation is complete the operator takes her to the new barrier in all three planes by a slight increase in flexion, sidebending and rotation.

1.2.6. Steps 1.2.4 and 1.2.5 are repeated two or more times, if necessary asking the patient to make the effort in the alternate direction.

1.2.7. Retest.

Thrust

1.3. Restriction of extension
Described for restriction of rotation and sidebending to the left at C5–6, FRSrt.

1.3.1. The patient is supine and the operator sits or stands at her head.

1.3.2. The operator controls her head with his right hand and brings the second metacarpophalangeal joint of his left hand against the left lateral mass (articular pillar) of C5, the superior vertebra (Fig. 11.3a).

1.3.3. Using the metacarpophalangeal joint of his left index and the tips of his right fingers as monitors, the operator introduces extension and left sidebending until the movement is localised to the barrier (upper

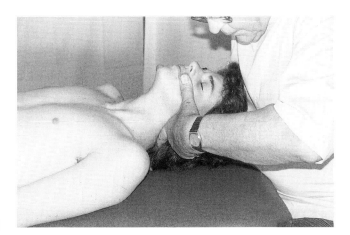

a

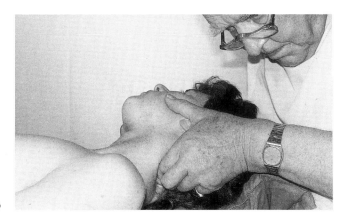

b

Fig. 11.3 Thrust treatment of FRSrt at C5–6. (a) Lateral aspect of index 1st MP joint against the lateral mass of C5 (upper vertebra); (b) position for thrust towards SP of Ti.

border of C5 from above and lower border of C6 from below). It is sometimes helpful to rotate the head a little to the right to 'get it out of the way' (Fig. 11.3b).

1.3.4. When all the slack has been removed by extension, left sidebending and left rotation of C5 a high velocity, low amplitude thrust is given by the operator's left hand on the lateral mass of C5 in the direction of the spine of T1. The force should be directed toward the spinous process of T1 from any of the typical cervical levels.

1.3.5. Retest.

1.4. Restriction of flexion, first technique, using sidebending
Described for ERSlt at C4–5.

1.4.1. The patient is supine and the operator sits or stands at her head.

1.4.2. The operator controls her head with his left hand and brings the second metacarpophalangeal joint of his right hand against the right facet joint at C4–5.

1.4.3. Using his right hand as monitor, the operator introduces flexion and right sidebending until the movement is localised to the barrier (upper border of C4 from above and lower border of C5 from below) (Fig. 11.4).

Fig. 11.4 Sidebending thrust for ERSlt at C4.

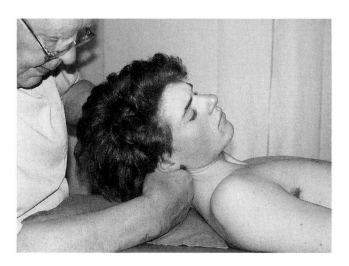

1.4.4. When all the slack has been removed by right sidebending and right rotation, a high velocity, low amplitude thrust is given by the operator's right hand against the C4–5 joint directly to the left. This 'opens' the left facet joint.

1.4.5. Retest.

1.5. Restriction of flexion, second technique, using rotation
1.5.1. The patient is supine and the operator sits or stands at her head.

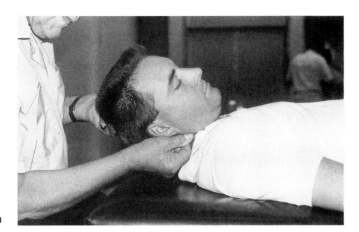

a

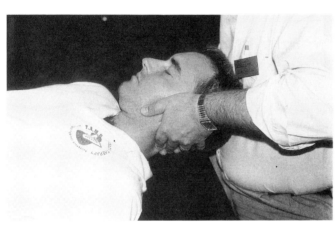

b

Fig. 11.5 Rotatory thrust for ERSlt at C4. (a) Blocking the right fact joint with index and thumb; (b) index 1st MP joint behind the lateral mass of C4.

1.5.2. The operator controls her head with the palms of both hands and 'blocks' movement at the right facet joint of C4–5 with his right index and middle fingers (Fig. 11.5a).

1.5.3. His left second metacarpophalangeal joint is brought against the posterior aspect of the left lateral mass of C4 (Fig. 11.5b).

1.5.4. Using both hands to monitor, the operator introduces flexion, right sidebending and right rotation until the movement is localised to the barrier (upper border of C4 from above and lower border of C5 from below).

1.5.5. When all the slack has been removed by flexion, right sidebending and right rotation, a high velocity, low amplitude thrust is given by the operator's left hand against the posterior aspect of the lateral mass of C4 to produce rotation to the right.

1.5.6. Retest.

2. THE ATLANTOAXIAL (C1–2) JOINT

At this joint rotation is the significant motion, there is a small amount of sidebending and flexion and of craniad to caudad translation.

Described for restriction of rotation to the right.

Diagnostic points. There is tissue texture change at the segment. With the neck flexed as far as it easily goes (but without flexion of the head on the neck) the range of rotation of the head to the right is less than to the left.

2.1. Muscle energy

2.1.1. The patient is supine and the operator sits or stands at her head.

2.1.2. The operator supports her head with the palms of both hands and flexes her neck as far as it will easily go, usually about 45°.

2.1.3. Monitoring on the lateral aspects of the axis (C2), the operator turns her head to the right until C2 just does not move (Fig. 11.6).

Fig. 11.6 For atlantaxial joint, axis rotated left. ME.

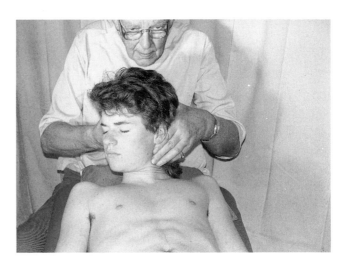

2.1.4. The patient is then asked to turn her head gently to the left and the effort is maintained for 3–5 seconds while the operator resists movement.

2.1.5. The operator then rotates her head to the new barrier and steps 2.1.4 and 2.1.5 are repeated two or more times.

2.1.6. Retest.

2.2. Thrust, first technique

2.2.1. The patient is supine and the operator sits or stands at her head.

2.2.2. The operator supports her head with the palms of both hands and flexes her neck as far as it will easily go, usually about 45°.

2.2.3. The operator uses his left second metacarpophalangeal joint against the left posterior arch of her atlas to monitor and localise the force. He then rotates her head to the right to reach the barrier, i.e. until C2 just does not move.

2.2.4. When all rotatory slack has been taken out the thrust is given by both hands turning her head to the right. The force is localised to C1–2 by the contact with his left index (Fig. 11.7).

2.2.5. Retest.

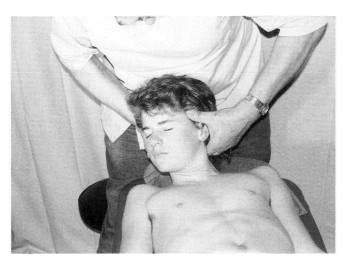

Fig. 11.7 For axis rotated left. Thrust with index finger.

2.3. Thrust, second technique
Steps 2.3.1 and 2.3.2 are as steps 2.2.1 and 2.2.2.

2.3.3. With both hands on the sides of her head, fingers pointing caudad, the operator takes up any slack by turning her head to reach the barrier.

2.3.4. The thrust is given by a rotatory movement of both hands while maintaining the flexion (Fig. 11.8).

2.3.5. Retest.

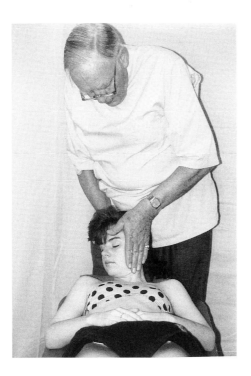

Fig. 11.8 For axis rotated left. Thrust with both hands.

3. THE OCCIPITOATLANTAL JOINT

At this joint the major motion is flexion and extension but there is also a small amount of sidebending. Sidebending is used both in treatment and the more usual diagnostic tests because, being the smaller amplitude motion, it is easier to assess. The sidebending is accompanied by a very small range of rotation which is always to the opposite side.

Muscle energy

3.1. For restriction of extension and sidebending to the right. FSlt
   Diagnostic points. There is tissue texture change at the segment. The head does not translate as far to the left as to the right when extended. Translation may be equal when the head is flexed; the joints of the lower cervical spine are free to sidebend. Anteroposterior translation will show restriction of forward translation on the right.
   3.1.1. The patient is supine and the operator stands or sits at her head.
   3.1.2. The operator holds her occiput with his right hand so that the web of his hand is under the posterior cervical muscles just below the nuchal line, not in contact with the posterior occipitoatlantal membrane. With his left hand he controls her chin and his forearm is against the left side of her skull. Because the tendency will be for the chin to be depressed, control needs to be on its inferior aspect.
   3.1.3. The extension movement is introduced by both hands rotating her head until the barrier is reached. This is extension of the skull on C1 NOT extension of the cervical spine (Fig. 11.9).

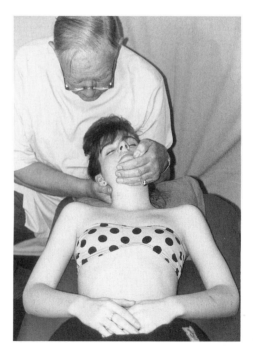

Fig. 11.9 For OA joint FSlt, position for patient effort. ME.

3.1.4. Fine tuning is by sidebending to the right by the operator's left forearm. If the chin is allowed to remain in the midline, the left rotation is automatic and can be neglected.

3.1.5. From this position the patient is asked to look down to her feet or, if more force is thought necessary, to push her chin down gently. Either of these will activate the neck flexors and the eye movement is almost always sufficient.

3.1.6. After 3–5 seconds she is asked to relax and, even when it was eye movement only, the anterior muscles will 'let go'. When eye movement is being used a useful instruction is 'look up above your head'. When she has relaxed fully the operator takes up the slack by sidebending and extension of the head to the new barrier and steps 3.1.5 and 3.1.6 are repeated two or more times.

3.1.7. Retest.

3.2. For restriction of flexion and sidebending to the left. ESrt
   Diagnostic points. There is tissue texture change at the segment. The head does not translate as far to the right as to the left when flexed. Translation may be equal when the head is extended; the joints of the lower cervical spine are free to sidebend. Anteroposterior translation will show restriction of posterior translation on the right.

3.2.1. The patient is supine and the operator stands or sits at her head.

3.2.2. The operator holds her occiput with his left hand so that the web of his hand is under the posterior cervical muscles just below the nuchal line, not in contact with the posterior occipitoatlantal membrane. With his right hand he controls her chin and his forearm is against the right side of her skull. Because the tendency will be for the chin to be elevated the operator needs one finger on its anterior aspect (Fig. 11.10).

3.2.3. The flexion movement is introduced by both hands rotating her head until the barrier is reached. This is flexion of the skull on C1, NOT flexion of the cervical spine.

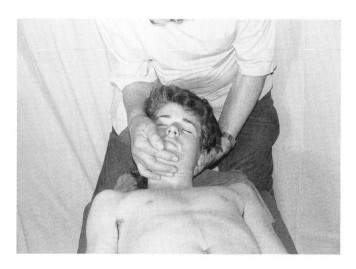

Fig. 11.10 For OA joint ESrt, position for patient effort. ME.

3.2.4. Fine tuning is by sidebending to the left by the operator's right forearm. If the chin is allowed to remain in the midline, right rotation is automatic and can be neglected.

3.2.5. From this position the patient is asked to look up above her head or, if more force is thought necessary, to lift her chin gently. Either of these will activate the neck extensors and the eye movement is almost always sufficient.

3.2.6. After 3–5 seconds she is asked to relax and, even when it was eye movement only, the posterior muscles will 'let go'. When eye movement is being used a useful instruction is 'look down to your feet'. When she has relaxed fully the operator takes up the slack by sidebending and flexion of the head to the new barrier and steps 3.2.5 and 3.2.6 are repeated two or more times.

3.2.7. Retest.

Thrust

3.3. For restriction of extension
Described for restricted sidebending to the right. FSlt

3.3.1. The patient is supine and the operator stands or sits at her head.

3.3.2. The operator holds her occiput with his right hand so that the web of his hand is under the posterior cervical muscles just below the nuchal line, not in contact with the posterior occipitoatlantal membrane. With his left hand he controls her chin and his forearm is against the left side of her skull.

3.3.3. The extension movement is introduced by both hands rotating her head until the barrier is reached. This is extension of the skull on C1, NOT extension of the cervical spine (Fig. 11.9).

3.3.4. Fine tuning is by sidebending to the right by the operator's left forearm. If the chin is allowed to remain in the midline, the left rotation is automatic and can be neglected. In order to have the required force available for the thrust the operator should move to the right side of the patient's head so that he can thrust mainly with his left hand on the occiput.

3.3.5. When all slack has been removed, the thrust is given by a high velocity, low amplitude movement with both hands in a craniad direction.

3.3.6. Retest.

3.4. For restriction of flexion
Described for restricted sidebending to the left. ESrt

3.4.1. The patient is supine and the operator stands or sits at her head.

3.4.2. The operator holds her occiput with his left hand so that the web of his hand is under the posterior cervical muscles just below the nuchal line, not in contact with the posterior occipitoatlantal membrane. With his right hand he controls her chin and his forearm is against the right side of her skull.

3.4.3. The flexion movement is introduced by both hands rotating her head until the barrier is reached. This is flexion of the skull on C1, NOT flexion of the cervical spine.

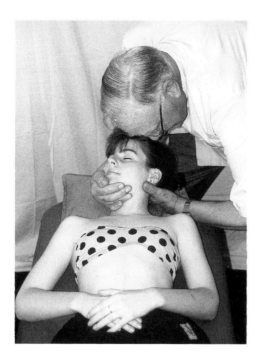

Fig. 11.11 For OA joint, thrust, shown for ESrt.

3.4.4. Fine tuning is by sidebending to the left by the operator's right forearm. If the chin is allowed to remain in the midline, right rotation is automatic and can be neglected.

3.4.5. When all slack has been removed, the thrust is given with both hands by a high velocity, low amplitude movement in a craniad direction (see Fig. 11.11).

3.4.6. Retest.

Chapter 12

The plan of treatment

While this text is only concerned with treatment of the musculoskeletal system, it is important to remember that manual treatment should be given only in the context of total patient care. Many of the referred pain syndromes with which the practitioner of manual medicine has to concern himself can also be caused by visceral disorders. Continuing abnormal discharge of nerve impulses from a viscus (of any kind) can produce a segmental facilitation with changes in the soma including abnormal tissue tensions and joint dysfunctions. In a similar manner, somatic dysfunction can cause visceral changes. *The nerve connections are all two way streets.* Although details will not be given in this book it is important in each patient to examine and assess more than just the musculoskeletal system.

Patients who seek help from practitioners of manual medicine most commonly do so because of pain. While it is of first importance to relieve the pain, it is vital to find from whence it comes rather than to assume that, because the pain is felt at point A, it is necessarily caused by a structure at point A. 'Pain is a liar' is a favourite expression of Dr Fred Mitchell jr, DO, son of the man who developed the muscle energy concept. 'It is no use chasing the pain' is another which the authors particularly associate with Dr Philip E. Greenman, DO. The message in either case is that a structural examination to find the dysfunctional areas in the musculoskeletal system is needed for diagnosis, not just a local examination of the part which is the site of the symptoms.

Each practitioner of manual medicine will develop his own plan of examination. The scheme outlined in earlier chapters is similar to that used by many. It is clear that it would require a long time to examine in detail every joint in the spinal column, let alone in the rest of the musculoskeletal system. An overall screening examination can help by pointing out areas which require more detailed testing and a scan will further define those levels that must be examined in full detail. A scheme for screening and scanning examinations is described in Chapter 3. The most important part of the musculoskeletal examination is the segmental definition, and when this is complete the operator will know, for each joint examined, the precise direction of the restrictions to motion so that he can plan a specific treatment.

RECOMMENDED ORDER OF TREATMENT

The normal approach to treatment is to start with dysfunctions of the pubis, because if the rotation about the transverse axis through the symphysis is restricted the motion of the entire pelvic mechanism is altered. The next priority, as mentioned in Chapter 7, is innominate shear dysfunctions, when they are present, because these also prevent the normal operation of the pelvic joints. From this point on there is more flexibility in the order of treatment but as a general rule the lumbar spine is treated before the rest of the pelvis, the more so if the lumbar spine does not show normal adaptation to the sacral position.

The order in which the pelvis is treated is of some importance. After the pubis and innominate shears have been treated and as much of the lumbar spine as is necessary, the sacroiliac (torsions and sacral nutations) and then the iliosacral dysfunctions are dealt with, of which the last should be iliac flares if they are present.

Any dysfunctions in the thoracic spine should be treated before the cervical region unless the necessary technique causes an increase in pain from the cervical lesions. It is common to find that the symptom of neck pain is more the result of dysfunctions in the upper thoracic region than in the neck itself. This may partly be due to the posture which the cervical spine is forced to adopt when there are the very common FRS dysfunctions in the upper thoracic region. The 'dowager's hump' is caused by upper thoracic FRS dysfunctions and when these are present the neck has to extend in order to keep the face pointing forwards.

In dysfunctions of the thoracic spine in which there is restriction of extension (FRS), some techniques use neutral mechanics to introduce the rotation first. This is done because the facets are in close apposition in the flexed position and gapping the joint makes restoration of extension easier. A technique that restores rotation first is described in Chapter 9. This preliminary approach is not needed for the ERS dysfunctions.

When it comes to the neck itself opinions are divided as to the order of treatment. Sidebending, by translation, is the standard movement for examination of the occipitoatlantal joint for restriction, but this movement can also be restricted by stiffness lower down. That may result in a false positive test if the lower cervical joints are not treated first. For this reason the authors prefer to treat the occipitoatlantal joint last. Below that level it matters less and there is sometimes good reason to treat first the joint with the most intense tissue texture abnormality. If treatment is started at other than the lowest dysfunctional joint, it is important to remember that in positional diagnosis a vertebra is always assessed with reference to the structure next below.

CHOICE OF METHOD

'If all you have in your tool box is a hammer, it is funny how many things look like nails.'

There are many reasons for having a variety of treatments for spinal joint dysfunctions, and indeed for any medical condition. One is because not all patients are alike. Treatment may need to be tailored to suit an 80-year-old frail person or, at the other end of the scale, a near 300 lb dock worker or farm labourer. The patient may have other medical problems which would prevent the use of some forms of treatment. Not all operators are alike, a six-foot operator (of either sex) will be able to use techniques that are difficult for those of short stature. Sitting lumbar and lower thoracic techniques are easier for the small operator who must work on a large patient, but even more important is that the short operator should have a low table. If only one table is available it is much better that it should be adjustable in height; if this is not possible the table needs to be low enough so that the operator can get on top of a large patient even if this tends to produce backache from bending low enough to do some of the other techniques. The idea that the correct height is so that, when standing, the operator's finger tips just touch the surface leads to a table that is difficult for a small person to use when faced with a large patient. At times it may be necessary to treat a patient on a bed, either in hospital or at home. Without a firm surface some of the techniques are very difficult.

MULTIPLICITY OF DYSFUNCTIONAL LEVELS

It has been inferred but not explicitly stated that, in almost all patients, the dysfunctions are multiple. The primary lesion is probably solitary in many people; however, the asymmetry introduced into the axial skeleton requires a compensatory adjustment to maintain the forward pointing attitude of the eyes and to level the vestibular apparatus. These secondary asymmetries may become fixed so that when the causative lesion is treated they become self perpetuating. It seems probable that most dysfunctions are originally caused by injury and this is true even in those who deny a history of injury. So many patients, when challenged, come back at a later visit having remembered a fall or other injury some time before the symptoms started.

Two recent cases in the practice of one of the authors are illustrative. A school teacher in his forties was seen with unusual symptoms but he had several levels in his spine that were dysfunctional. The X-rays showed degenerative changes and a history of earlier injury was suspected. It was originally denied but later he telephoned to say that at the age of 13 he had been concussed when he had an accident on his bicycle. This could quite clearly have been the original cause. Apparently the memory had been suppressed. The second was a woman in her late twenties with somewhat similar findings. When challenged about childhood injury, this was strongly denied but on her second visit she admitted that she had had horses in her teens and had had several falls.

In schoolchildren's orthopaedic clinics one of the authors saw many primary school children with symptoms arising from lumbar dysfunctions. In most of these a parent would remember an injury when specifically asked, but the history had to be searched for before it was mentioned. Unless they are treated, by the time these children have reached adulthood, the compensatory asymmetries will almost certainly have become fixed and themselves require treatment. When something then occurs to produce symptoms it may well be that the immediate source is a joint which was originally part of the compensation. In that event the causative joint will, of course, need treatment but, unless the original primary dysfunction is found and treated, the recent one is likely to recur quickly. This sequence of events may be repeated giving a third, fourth (or more) generation of dysfunctions. Patients with this type of problem are common in any manipulative practice and it is often difficult to find all the joints requiring treatment.

Examination of the spine in any patient who has a history of back problems of more than a few weeks' duration is likely to reveal a number of levels where there is restriction of motion, often with palpable changes in tissue feel. In such patients the most important level may be difficult to find and the level which is immediately important, as symptom producer, may not prove to be the one that ultimately unlocks the puzzle. How many levels one ought to treat at the first session will depend on a number of factors.

The best guide is the acuteness of the condition. If the patient is in great pain and hardly able to move, it would be less than kind to do a full examination and treat every dysfunctional joint that one found. Such patients are not easy to examine; it may be impossible to get them into the position in which the examination is usually made and, for instance, the available range of forward bending may be so small that the forward flexion tests do not mean anything. These are the very people that are crying out to be helped but if it is not possible to make a diagnosis it will not be wise to 'do something regardless'. In patients whose condition is very acute the question that should be considered as of first importance is which is the most acute dysfunction? This should then be treated gently, by muscle energy or functional indirect methods and the patient seen again within a few days. Subsequent treatments will become more like those for the less acute patient as improvement occurs.

Treating the wrong level, or treating the correct level in the wrong direction, will often cause an increase in pain; fortunately it is usually only temporary. Increased pain can also occur after the correct treatment; it usually happens during the first day after treatment and is probably the result of an inflammatory reaction. Because both these happen it is important to perform a careful re-examination on anyone who has increased pain, the more so if it has lasted more than 24 hours. The abnormal findings with which we work are often subtle and even those with long experience can find that their assessment was apparently wrong. This can be due to faulty observation or faulty interpretation of the findings, but equally it may be due to the removal, by correct treatment, of the superficial 'layer' of dysfunctions and the exposing of what lies under them.

For the patient who comes with a more chronic problem, even if the reason for the visit is a recent acute episode, the approach can be more thorough. Here what is first required is to find the level from which the immediate symptoms are coming, remembering that pain is almost more commonly referred than local to the place complained of. The examination should not stop there. A full structural examination is needed to find the associated dysfunctional levels and any that show significant tissue changes should be treated. If there are many levels needing treatment the number that are addressed on any one occasion will depend on the age and state of health of the patient (and on the patience and time available to the operator!), but the principle is that the primary dysfunction will probably need treatment before lasting relief can be obtained. If many levels are treated at one time a non-steroidal anti-inflammatory drug may be required as reactions do sometimes occur.

The primary dysfunction may have very little tissue texture change over it if it is old, as so often it is, and it may be difficult to find. The question as to whether to treat a restricted level over which the tissues feel normal may have to depend on whether recurrences of dysfunction at other levels seem to happen sooner than expected. The decision will be based on whether, on the one hand, the recurrences appear to be the result of asymmetrical tension caused by the apparently silent joint having an effect on the others or, on the other hand, the adaptation to the asymmetry is old and silent and does not appear to be the cause of the recurrences.

It will very often be found that, on the second or subsequent visit, examination will show a different set of findings, almost as if there were new layers of dysfunctions being uncovered. In some patients it will not be possible to find the original lesion until some of the more recent things have been treated. This is one of the reasons why it is essential to examine the patient again at each visit rather than continue to treat what was first found. If the treatment has been effective, the situation will not be the same and a full examination, at least of the part concerned, is essential before giving another treatment.

TREATMENT OF PATIENTS WITH A POSSIBLE DISC PROTRUSION

As will be pointed out in Chapter 13, there are circumstances which make surgery very urgent but this is only so when there is evidence of cord or increasing peripheral nerve compression. There is no doubt that surgery is occasionally the only satisfactory treatment for those with unequivocal signs of protrusion, and the more so with extrusion of disc material. There is also ample evidence in the experience of most manual medicine practitioners to show that, even in the presence of such unequivocal evidence, relief may be obtained by conservative measures including manual intervention. The word 'unequivocal' is possibly out of place because it seems that the only certain signs are those of a space occupying lesion and that even these signs may be absent in those for whom surgery proves to be essential. Fortunately one or a few treatments by manual means can be safely used in almost all such patients and these can be continued so long as improvement goes on. Manual treatment will often serve as a diagnostic test in that if the condition improves surgery is unlikely to be needed.

There are numerous examples in the literature of those with myelographically proved protrusions in which complete resolution of the symptoms has been achieved with manual treatment only. One example in the practice of one of the authors had the myelogram reproduced in

Fig. 12.1 Myelogram showing filling defect on right side at L5–S1.

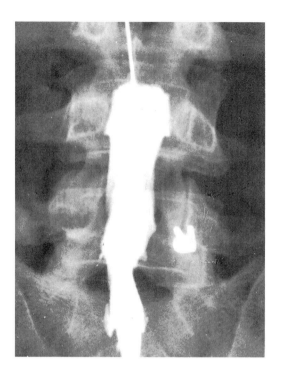

Fig. 12.1. He had been seen by a neurosurgeon and advised to try a period of bed rest before having surgery. The author saw him because after the suggested period of bed rest he was no better and the neurosurgeon was on holiday. While the L5–S1 level was clearly the site of a right sided protrusion the treatment which started his improvement on his first visit was to the right sacroiliac joint. He returned to work in 2 weeks but received a total of 12 treatments over 2 months and with these the straight leg raising gradually returned. A minor recurrence 3 months later required two further treatments. Manipulative treatment can certainly be tried in those who decline surgery, provided that there is no evidence of increasing neurological deficit or of cauda equina pressure. If patients still wish to avoid surgery, in spite of increasing neurological deficit, it is wiser to stop any manual treatment and to try to persuade them to have surgery before the damage to the nerve structures is irreversible.

There is another possible diagnosis in those whose symptoms remain after biomechanical balance has been achieved and which may require surgery for relief. This is the condition known as internal disc disruption which is described in Chapter 13.

THE PROBLEM OF THE PATIENT WHO HAS HAD SURGERY

There is a difference in one's approach to the patient whose surgery was initially successful and the one who had little or no benefit. The surgical approach is almost always limited to one joint or to two neighbouring levels. This does not take into account any of the secondary dysfunctions in other parts of the spine. As has been said before, a recurrent pain can feel exactly the same to the patient but be arising from a different joint or muscle. The bank manager mentioned in Chapter 13 who had had successful surgery on a low lumbar disc some years previously returned with what, to him, was the same pain. Treatment to the thoracolumbar junction was what he needed to relieve his recurrent symptoms.

There are a number of dysfunctions that are frequently found in the 'failed back' population, the most common is pubic symphysis dysfunction, followed by sacral base unlevelling, whether due to leg inequality or some other cause, and imbalance of length or strength of the long hip and thigh muscles. Also common are fixed posterior (superior) nutation, posterior sacral torsion, innominate shear dysfunctions and lumbar mechanics that are non-adaptive to whatever sacral dysfunction is present.

In the post-surgical patient posterior nutation and posterior torsion are common as is imbalance of length and strength in the hip and thigh muscles. The symptoms produced by a posterior nutation or posterior sacral torsion combined with an FRS dysfunction at L5 or L4 can easily be mistaken for those of a disc protrusion. This is probably part of the reason for the frequency with which they are found; other reasons may be the coexistence of disc protrusion with these dysfunctions and perhaps the fact that the surgery is usually performed in nearly full flexion.

THE PROBLEM OF THE SHORT LEG

As a consequence of the tendency of the pelvis to twist with one innominate rotating forwards and the other backwards, serious errors are introduced in any attempt to measure differences in leg length from the anterior superior spine to the medial malleolus and it is recommended that that method should be abandoned. Clinical and radiological methods that are more accurate were described in Chapter 3.

The change in apparent leg length can be illustrated by a diagram (Fig. 12.2). With the subject erect, an alteration in the angular position of the sacroiliac joint will result in a change in the angle made by a fixed line on the innominate with the horizontal. The only alternative would be for the spine to tilt but that does not happen when the subject remains erect. This must cause a change in the angle θ which is that between the vertical and a line joining the centre of motion of the hip joint with the supposed axis of the SI joint (it makes no difference to the argument if a different point is chosen). Simple geometry tells us that the distance A–D in Fig. 12.2a is not the same as that in Fig. 12.2b if θ has been changed.

The change in relative rotation of the innominates resulting from asymmetry of their position relative to the sacrum will affect apparent leg length. The leg will appear short on the side on which the innominate is in the posterior position. However, a change in the angle θ will also occur if there is pubic asymmetry. If the pubis is elevated, the rotation

Fig. 12.2 Diagram to show effect of innominate rotation on apparent leg length.

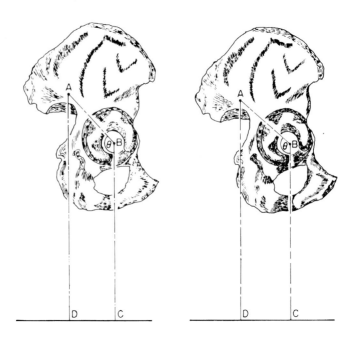

of the innominate about the femoral head will be posterior (tending to make the leg appear longer) even although a superior pubis is usually associated with a posterior innominate.

Structural differences in the length of the legs are not uncommon. Sometimes as the result of malunion of a fracture, sometimes as a consequence of limb overgrowth, sometimes for no known reason. Differential limb growth may result from increased circulation associated with a vascular anomaly, overuse of one side, chronic infection, or from decreased circulation after poliomyelitis affecting one side more than the other. Leg inequality is familial is some instances and these often have differences of 12 mm (½ inch) or more. A natural tendency of the human body is to preserve the forward pointing attitude of the head and to level the eyes and the vestibular apparatus. One of the ways in which the body may attempt to do this, in presence of a leg inequality, is by a torsional movement of the pelvis so that, on the long leg side, the innominate is in the posterior position and on the short leg side it is anterior. This does not cause any trouble unless the pelvis becomes dysfunctional but, as the innominate position will recur as soon as the patient stands up, if dysfunction starts there will be a tendency for it to recur.

Unlevelling of the sacral base is most commonly due to a difference in leg length but is also found when there is a congenitally small hemipelvis and when there is an innominate shear or it may be due to fixed (dysfunctional) pelvic torsion. There are also other factors involved because the sacral base tilt does not always follow or be equivalent to the difference as measured to the top of the femoral head. If the base is not level the spine has to develop a scoliotic curve to keep the eyes and vestibular apparatus level, this in turn requires compensatory adjustments higher up and is a predisposing cause to the development and maintenance of dysfunctions.

In those with a leg length difference or structural asymmetry a raise in the shoe can be very helpful. In patients with dysfunctional pelvic torsion there is similarly a sidebend of the sacrum but, if the legs are equal, correction of the torsion is the treatment of choice, not levelling of the sacral base by a shoe lift. Differences of less than 7 mm ($\frac{1}{4}$ inch) do not always require correction but, if the difference is greater than that, a raise in the heel of the shoe may be very helpful. Opinions differ as to whether a raise should be prescribed as soon as a difference of more than 10 mm ($\frac{3}{8}$ inch) is found. Some practitioners feel that it will help and should be prescribed immediately; others like to try the effect of adequate manipulative treatment first and prescribe the raise if recurrences occur quickly or frequently. An excellent review of the subject with suggestions is given by Greenman[1]. In a recent (1991) personal communication Dr Greenman gave a figure of 60% as the frequency of sacral base unlevelling of 6 mm or more in the 'failed back' patients that he sees in his practice.

A difference of up to 19 mm ($\frac{3}{4}$ inch) can usually be accommodated by raising the heel of one shoe and, if the difference is more than 12 mm ($\frac{1}{2}$ inch), lowering the other. More than that needs a sole raise as well for comfortable walking. Recent experimental work on the problem of the short leg was referred to in Chapter 3 (Irvin[2]). An example of the importance of correcting inequality was a male of about 40 wearing a prosthesis for a high thigh amputation. Initially it was difficult to examine him fully because of his amputation but it became clear that he had an iliosacral dysfunction on the amputated side. Treatment made him much more comfortable but only for a few days at a time. A standing X-ray while wearing the prosthesis showed that the limb was 26 mm (1 inch) too long. In spite of the prosthetist's protests he was persuaded to shorten the limb and the problem did not again recur.

THE MYOFASCIAL PAIN SYNDROME

There appear to be three different mechanisms for the production of pain in muscle (Simons[3]); the myofascial pain syndrome characterised by Travell trigger points (TrPs), fibromyalgia characterised by tender points (TePs) which are found in specific locations and are symmetrically distributed in the body and pain associated with joint dysfunction. In much of the literature there is confusion over the precise meaning of these terms; fibromyalgia is probably the one most frequently called fibrositis in the past. The classification given by Simons will be adopted in this edition.

THE TRAVELL TRIGGER POINT

This is the characteristic finding in the myofascial pain syndrome (MPS) and has been described in detail for the whole of the body in Travell and Simons[4]. The description and the treatment were developed by Dr Janet Travell with encouragement from her physiatrist father and her first published paper on the subject is dated 1952[5]. This has been followed by many other papers, of which those recommended for anyone interested in the development of the treatment are (in chronological order)[6,7,8,9] as well as the book referred to above. Simons gives an excellent review of the extensive literature on muscle pain syndromes and in the papers in the *Journal of Manual Medicine* referred to above[3] the latest work is discussed. These papers were originally part of volume 17 of *Advances in Pain Research and Therapy*[10]. Mennell[8], in the journal of the American Osteopathic Association, describes many of the more important triggers and the charts of their patterns of referred pain. He also describes treatment by cooling spray.

The true trigger point (TrP) is described as predictable in location in any one muscle, although there is often more than one site in a muscle. Each site in each muscle has its own predictable pattern of referred pain which, when known by the operator, tells him where to look for the TrP. The point is a small circumscribed area of thickening in a taut band in the muscle and the patient is usually unaware of its existence until someone finds and presses on it when it may be exquisitely tender. TrPs are always tender and pressure will usually reproduce the referred pattern of pain, sometimes eliciting the cry from the patient 'that's my pain'. When the TrP is stimulated by snapping the finger across it or by direct needling, the muscle will twitch. After successful treatment the tenderness, the taut band in the muscle and the twitch will have disappeared.

There can be TrPs in almost every skeletal muscle in the body, some are of much greater interest than others to those treating patients with back pain, either because they are more common or because they mimic pain patterns from other sources and are likely to be overlooked. They appear to be more common in muscles that are overused or those weakened and stretched by tightness of the antagonists.

Travell lists the most common TrPs associated with:

1. back pain, the quadratus lumborum and the longissimus dorsi;
2. lower limb pain, the glutei and the adductor group, to which the authors would add the piriformis;
3. pain in the head and neck, the sternomastoid, the trapezius, the suboccipital muscles and the muscles of mastication;
4. pain in the shoulder, the trapezius, the levator scapulae, the scalenes and the posterior cervical muscles;
5. pain in the upper limb below the shoulder, the spinati, the scalenes, the deltoid, the subscapularis and the pectoralis major and minor.

In the care of patients with musculoskeletal pain the operator will find sometimes that treatment of the TrP results in apparent total resolution of the problem. This, unfortunately, is the exception rather than the rule. In most patients the original cause of the TrP is still operative and, if that is not found and treated, the TrP will recur however well itself was treated. In such patients there may be temporary relief of pain followed by recurrence. When that happens it will often be found that the TrP has once again become active. The finding of a TrP does not relieve the necessity of looking for other causes of pain. In the authors' experience there is almost always a spinal or pelvic joint dysfunction associated with a TrP which suggests that the skeletal dysfunction may often be the cause of the TrP. In some of those where treatment of the TrP alone gives lasting relief there is a history of other treatment which had not fully relieved the symptoms. The possibility arises that the original treatment had removed the skeletal cause but that the TrP had maintained the symptoms. It is true that referred pain from a TrP can mimic that from spinal or pelvic joint dysfunction. Untreated TrPs can also be the cause of recurrence of skeletal joint dysfunction, usually at the same level as the one which caused the TrP. The nerve connections to these structures all seem to act as two-way rather than one-way streets.

It is of great importance to remember that the patient may feel and complain of precisely the same pain, but the origin of the pain is not necessarily the same on two different occasions. Nor is it rare to find that more than one cause of any given pain may be operating at the same time. From this follows the advice that the examination of the patient with pain is not complete until TrPs have been excluded in the appropriate areas of muscle, nor even when another cause has been found is it wise to omit the structural examination of the appropriate part of the skeleton. Simons[3] gives five major and four minor clinical criteria for the diagnosis of myofascial pain syndrome due to trigger points as well as criteria for defining a trigger point for research purposes.

Treatment of trigger points

The treatments advised by Dr Travell are a cold spray on the skin accompanied by stretching, injection or dry needling. There are several important details.

First, the cold must not be too intense. The object is to obtain reflex relaxation of the muscle by cooling the skin, not to chill the muscle which by causing shivering may actually increase the hypertonus.

Second, the application of the spray should be from a sufficient distance away that the spray itself has begun to evaporate and is cold.

Third, the spray should start over the trigger point and continue over the reference zone in roughly parallel lines.

Fourth, the stretch should be applied during or immediately after the spray.

Fifth, if injection is to be used it should be of plain local anaesthetic without either adrenalin, which tends to tighten the muscle, or steroid which has no additional benefit over the local anaesthetic. Dr Travell uses procaine because of its general analgesic effect, but many people use lidocaine as being less likely to cause a sensitivity reaction. The injection needs to affect the small trigger point itself and the more accurately it is given, the smaller the amount needed; $\frac{1}{2}$ or 1% is all that is required for the purpose.

Sixth, If the exact trigger point can be penetrated dry needling is enough to abolish it.

Following any of these treatments muscle re-education is helpful to make recurrence less likely and it is important to look for causes. Trigger points are often caused by dysfunction in spinal joints, usually in myotomal relation to the trigger but they themselves can cause satellite triggers. Satellites are likely to be found in the pain reference zone of the primary trigger but may be in close relation to the primary trigger point. Details of location, reference zones and treatment of trigger points in muscles are given by Travell and Simons[4]. Trigger points will also respond to isometric exercise followed by stretching as described in the following section.

THE FIBROMYALGIA SYNDROME

This corresponds more to what in the past has often been called fibrositis. It has recently (1990[11]) been defined as a chronic pain condition and is associated with multiple symmetrical tender points and widespread complaints characteristic of the chronic pain syndromes. It is commonly accompanied by sleep disturbances, depression and chronic fatigue. Simons quotes experimental work suggesting that fibromyalgia is in fact a systemic disease and a disorder of serotonin function has been advanced as a possible cause.

TREATMENT FOR ASSOCIATED LONG MUSCLE PROBLEMS

In the diagnostic process the tight muscles with which the operator is mainly concerned are the short, fourth layer group, the multifidi, the rotatores and the intertransversarii. The more superficial, longer muscles may act as restrictors and, although they will affect several levels, they may have enough effect on an individual joint to prevent resolution of its dysfunction until they are treated. Long restrictors will be found on the concave side of a neutral group but they will also affect the non-neutral dysfunction which is so commonly found at one or both ends of such a group.

Treatment of long restrictors is part of the soft tissue treatment mentioned in Chapter 6; for the thoracic and lumbar regions it is usually done with the patient prone, but the technique in which the muscle mass is pulled towards the operator can also be used in side lying. If the patient is prone and the operator is standing on the opposite side to the tight muscle, the treatment is given with the heel of the hand or with the thumb or thumb and thenar eminence and the muscle is steadily pushed away. If the operator stands on the same side the finger tips are used to put traction on the muscle mass. With those differences, the principles of the treatment are the same prone pushing, prone pulling or side lying pulling. The principles are to get hold of the muscle mass either with the finger tips or the heel of the hand and press in such a way that the muscle is stretched sideways. For the longissimus the point of initial application of the stretch should be in the medial gutter. For the iliocostalis it should be in the lateral gutter. The movement must be deliberate and care must be taken to avoid the fingers slipping over the muscle mass. After one part of the muscle has been stretched in this manner the contact can be moved up or down to stretch any other tight areas. Some muscles require special techniques; the quadratus lumborum is an example. Because of its depth it is not possible to stretch the quadratus lumborum in the same way as the longissimus, but if the treatment table has a swinging leaf so that the lower limbs can be swung from side to side, it can be done prone with the level localised by a thumb against each lumbar spinous process in turn. In this position the cold spray can also be used. Without a swinging leaf it is necessary either to lift both legs and swing them, or with the patient lying on her side, to lift the limbs vertically first on one side then on the other. Both techniques are hard work but the quadratus is an important muscle in the maintenance of lumbar and pelvic dysfunctions.

In the neck the same type of stretch can be applied but is most easily done with the patient supine and the operator standing or sitting at her head. The finger tips are used and, with the general mobility and smaller muscles in this region, it is easier to give more specific attention to individual levels. Flexion, extension and side bending can be added if it is wanted to make the treatment more localised. The basic principle of stretching is the same but in this region traction can also be added. Traction may be in the long axis of the spine or combined with sidebending, with or without flexion or extension when the effect on the muscle is often known as 'separation of origin and insertion'. It is important in this region also to avoid allowing the fingers to slip over the muscle mass.

Areas of tight muscle for which this kind of stretching is difficult, or when the muscle is too uncomfortable for it to be possible to perform a stretch properly, may be treated as if they were the more localised special variety described as trigger points.

Epidural injections

There are two main varieties of epidural injection, local and caudal; they are not used in quite the same way. The local injection is given beside or as close as possible to the nerve root that appears to be involved. This is a technique requiring special skill and at least in North America it is regarded as part of the specialty of the anaesthetist. The caudal injection is given into the sacral hiatus and is easier, not requiring special expertise.

Local epidural injections are given for a variety of reasons but the effect that appears to help most is the anti-inflammatory action. For this reason the usual injection is a mixture of local anaesthetic with a steroid. Such injections can be very helpful when there is evidence to suggest that inflammation plays a significant part in the maintenance of the problem. It must be recognised that there is an inflammatory factor in many spinal joint dysfunctions. However, local epidural injections do not remove the mechanical aspect of the spinal joint dysfunction and in patients where this is the important factor they may have a very short benefit or none at all. Wyke[12] states that irritation of the nerves and their receptors may be either mechanical or chemical. The latter may be inflammatory but more often results from sustained muscle contraction. He says 'Muscular pain may become superimposed on and actually become more important than the primary spinal pain'. Later he also adds 'Contrary to the traditional opinions of many doctors, inflammatory disorders of the back muscles and their related connective tissues are seldom the cause of back pain except as a complication of some acute febrile illness'.

Caudal epidural injections can be helpful, either by themselves or in the expectation that they will allow a manipulation to be performed by reducing the muscle spasm. In the authors' experience they become less necessary as the palpatory skill and general ability of the operator increases. The effect seems to be more one of blocking impulses in nerve than in reducing inflammation and in accord with this there does not appear to be any advantage in using steroid in addition to the local anaesthetic. Quantities as large as 50 ml have been advocated[13] but one of the authors (JFB) has never used more than 20 ml of 1% or even ½% lidocaine.

THE PROBLEM OF THE 'NEUROTIC' PATIENT

In the past there has been, in the medical profession, a tendency to brand as neurotic any patient who did not respond to the treatment offered. It is interesting to watch the changes in one's own attitude as one's experience increases. The unexpected resolution of a problem by some means other than what was expected can open one's eyes to the possibility that the patient was right after all!

This does not mean that there is no difficulty with those whose psyche is disturbed. Whether it is the main cause of pain is immaterial; there is in all back pain patients an element of muscle tightness and it is not unreasonable to assume that anything that tightens muscle further would make that worse. The angry, the anxious, the depressed and the fearful all suffer from 'tension'. Why do we call it that? Electromyography can demonstrate the actual increase in motoneuron firing in these people. In practice these are the very patients that respond poorly to treatment.

There is a great difference between those whose anxiety is the result of long unrelieved back pain and those who have unrelated causes for their tension. In the former, as soon as the operator shows the patient that there is something that can be located as a cause the tension starts to abate. So many have been insulted with the 'it's all in your head' attitude (or actual statement) that it is small wonder that they suffer from tension. As soon as improvement starts with proper treatment their problem largely resolves.

For those with depression or anxiety from unrelated causes the problem remains and, for some, psychological or spiritual help may be needed before treatment will do more than temporary good. Such patients tend to take up the time of a practitioner of manual therapy because, for many, the only relief that they get even if temporary is from manual treatment.

There is another special class, those who do not respond as well as expected because of pending litigation after an accident and the advice sometimes given by lawyers. The first thing is that these people are much less common that has been thought but it would be foolish to deny that they exist. Sometimes it is necessary to refuse to do any more until after the case has been settled. The confirmation that most patients are genuine is in the finding that even after a favourable settlement the pain remains and the patient clearly needs treatment.

OSTEOARTHRITIS

It seems strange that it is necessary to remind physicians and others that the term osteoarthritis is a specific term referring to a type of degenerative change occurring in synovial joints. There are many synovial joints in the axial skeleton but the discs themselves are not parts of synovial joints and the disc narrowing with spur formation that is so common is not osteoarthritis.

The synovial joints in the spine are subject to true osteoarthritis and in some of them this can lead to symptoms that are resistant to treatment by manual means but this seems only to be true when there is a major productive reaction around the joint. In both the facet joints and the uncovertebral joints of the cervical spine productive changes can cause nerve impingement with weakness and loss of sensation. There is usually associated pain but this is probably due to another cause; pressure on nerve does not cause pain except at the moment of application of the pressure and then only if it is rapid. In the lumbar spine osteoarthritic changes with osteophyte formation can cause narrowing of the available space in the canal, one of the causes of spinal stenosis. The same is probably true of the thoracic spine especially in its lower half.

It is fairly common to see osteoarthritic changes in facet joints without evidence of narrowing of the canal or pressure on nerves. In these patients treatment by manual methods is usually no less successful than in those without the changes, but their presence does mean that it is likely that the original injury was a long time ago. The longer the history the more likely it is that several treatments will be needed to achieve maximum relief.

DISC MARGIN SPURS

It is quite common to see large spurs at the anterior and lateral margins of discs that have normal depth as well as with those that are narrowed. It seems that these spurs are the result of traction on the ligamentous tissues bridging the bones and the most likely cause of this would appear to be a change in the elasticity and thickness of the disc itself, in spite of the fact that they can occur with normal disc height. Sometimes it only needs a little imagination to 'see' that the spurs have formed round an anterior disc protrusion. There is little mention, in the literature, of anterior protrusions of disc material. Judging by the X-ray appearances, they are not rare but they do not seem to be associated with any pattern of symptoms other than those of somatic dysfunction at the same level.

Overlapping spurs will sometimes look as if they were solid pieces of bone bridging the two vertebrae but close examination of other projections will almost always rule out ankylosis. It is not wise to assume that a joint showing such spurs is fused (and therefore not likely to be the cause of symptoms) without careful motion testing and, if necessary, extra X-rays in different projections. *It is the authors' opinion that anterior and lateral spurs are not of themselves sources of symptoms.*

Posterior and postero-lateral marginal spurs are different in that they are in a location that makes possible pressure on a nerve and sometimes repeated minor trauma to the dura which may cause cord damage. In the presence of such spurs it is important to assess both spinal cord and peripheral nerve function before considering treatment by manual means other than indirect or gentle muscle energy techniques.

DANGERS AND CONTRAINDICATIONS

This was the subject of a workshop held in Denmark in February 1990. Several of the presentations and their conclusions are published in the *Journal of Manual Medicine*, 1991, volume 6, No. 3, to which those interested in the details are referred.

The recommendations include careful diagnosis and, in particular, avoidance of treatment by high velocity thrusting in the upper cervical spine when it is extended and rotated.

There is scarcely a treatment in medicine that is without its attendant danger. There is the possibility of doing harm by almost any active treatment, and this is certainly true of manipulation. Fortunately, the danger is small and with care it can be avoided. Suitable manipulative procedures are less frequently associated with complications than almost any other treatment. It has been said, but the authors have no figures, that the frequency of vertebro-basilar circulatory catastrophe is less than that of significant adverse reactions to aspirin. It is of the utmost importance, however, that the dangers should be recognised because, although rare, the complications can be serious.

The dangers fall into three groups:

1. Those caused by the manipulation doing damage to a bone weakened by some pathological process, with possible dissemination of that process.
2. Spinal cord or cauda equina pressure caused by a massive disc extrusion.
3. Circulatory disturbance caused by damage to a vessel or by reflex arterial spasm.

DANGERS IN MANIPULATING A WEAKENED BONE

It should be recognised that, in each of the following categories, to have used manual treatment of a type that could cause danger is a failure of judgement based on improper diagnosis.

Bone may be weakened by a small number of pathological processes, all of which will in time be visible in X-rays. It may well be, however, that the patient comes for help at an early stage before any radiographic change is visible even in high quality films. This makes it necessary to maintain a high index of suspicion and is one of the advantages of the referral system of specialist medical practice. The real advantage is only obtained if the referring physician gives the operator an adequate history.

The commonest causes of weakening of bone are osteoporosis, infection and neoplasms.

Osteoporosis is the most common and will always be visible in good X-rays before the bone is weakened enough to be a source of danger. Although osteoporosis is common, pain caused by it is relatively uncommon. Many patients with significant loss of bone density will have back pain due to somatic dysfunction which can be treated by manual means and it would be sad to refuse them help just because care and gentle technique are necessary.

Infection is now uncommon and because of the widespread muscle spasm around infected lesions, it is less likely to be missed. The spasm around an infected joint will usually prevent movement with any test and this should alert the examiner. The intensity of the muscle spasm may be enough to protect the area from damage and make it unlikely that a single manipulation of the type described would do any significant harm. The patient is usually ill, but while the patient with dysfunction may be in severe pain, she is not ill. Early infective lesions may not show on X-ray films and a negative film is not evidence against infection.

One of the authors was sent, by his family physician, a patient who had received 20 thrust type treatments in 21 days without any benefit. That history was a warning and by the time he was seen, he did appear to be ill. X-rays were taken which showed a partial collapse of L5 from a probable infection, although the films that had been taken 3 weeks before appeared normal. The biopsy proved the infection to be staphylococcal and the patient made a good recovery. Interestingly, there did not seem to be evidence to prove that significant harm had been done by the manipulations.

Neoplasms may not show on X-rays until the bone is weakened enough to be a danger. Simple growths in bone are not often of sufficient size to cause weakness; they will usually have been there long enough to be visible radiologically and they are not common. Primary malignant neoplasms are also uncommon in bone but secondaries are common and may be large enough to be a danger before they are suspected. Patients are often reluctant to admit that they have, or have had, malignancies and it is in this field in particular that a history from the family physician may be very helpful. Even if the bone can be weakened seriously before X-rays show anything, the growth will usually, by this time, have resulted in a detectable disturbance of the general body economy. Pelvic growths can also be the cause of back pain and must be remembered in the differential diagnosis.

Danger of massive disc extrusion

This is a real danger but the only iatrogenic case known to the authors resulted from a manipulation done under general anaesthetic and the movements included full flexion. The patient, a doctor's wife, had a permanent cauda equina paresis (it happened before Mixter and Barr had published their original paper) and the physician who performed the manipulation was very concerned when he heard that one of the authors (JFB) was starting to do this work. The same author has had a similar accident happen to two of his patients but neither appeared to have been iatrogenic. In one the accident was caused by bending to pick up a pencil and in the other by sitting up in bed and coughing. The one who reported the accident at once was on the operating table within 2 hours and did very well, about a 95% recovery. The other was not on the table until the following day and had only a partial recovery. Clearly the matter is of extreme urgency.

The danger seems to lie in the forcing of flexion. During his postgraduate training the author referred to above worked under an orthopaedic surgeon who used manipulation under anaesthetic with many good results; he never allowed forced flexion under anaesthetic and never had an accident with this treatment. The same author has had similar experiences using manipulation under anaesthetic but since he has learned to be specific he has ceased to use general anaesthesia which can actually be a hindrance because localisation becomes more difficult.

Danger of an accident to the arterial supply to the brain and spinal cord

Millions of high cervical manipulations using high velocity techniques are performed every year and the number of accidents is very small. Unfortunately when an accident does happen the results are serious and may be fatal; in those that survive permanent paresis is common and may be severe. An excellent review of the data up to 1980 is given by Kleynhans[14]. The precise cause of the circulatory difficulty has been a matter of argument and more recent research has shown that a dissecting aneurysm is often present. Levin[15] reports a personal case in which the patient suffered a stroke while being positioned on the table prior to examination. In her case bilateral dissecting aneurysms were found in the vertebral arteries and, in the hands of a vascular surgeon, she made a good recovery. The majority of the accidents reported have been associated with high velocity (and often high amplitude) manipulation of the upper cervical spine in the fully extended and rotated position. That the accident can happen even in the absence of externally applied force is clear. There are several recorded cases in which the victim merely put his head in the extended and rotated position and held it there for a time.

Asymmetry of size of the vertebral arteries is common and stroke from vertebral artery blockage was thought to be more likely if the circulation in the other vessel is reduced from lack of development. It has been shown by angiography that the artery is narrowed if the head is turned fully to the opposite side in maximal extension. In the cadaver, but not in the living subject, complete obstruction has been found in this position.

A test ascribed to De Kleyn is quoted by Lewit[16] as being useful for determination of vertebral artery insufficiency. The test is performed by having the patient supine with her head extended over the end of the table. The operator rotates the head first to one side and then to the other watching for the development of nystagmus or a complaint of dizziness or nausea. Unfortunately ischaemic catastrophe has been recorded recently following use of the De Kleyn test and in the opinion of the authors it should not be used. This in spite of the fact that the test has been mandatory in Germany before cervical manipulation is performed. Observations of several practitioners suggest that *anxiety, rather than nystagmus, is the earliest sign of cerebral anoxia and it is recommended that, if the patient becomes anxious during any procedure on the upper cervical spine, the procedure should immediately be abandoned.*

A safer test can be performed during the examination of the active range of motion. The patient is asked to extend the head on the neck and in that position to rotate first to one side and then to the other without being touched by the operator. The rotated position is maintained for 5 seconds and the patient carefully watched for anxiety, dizziness or nystagmus. The test is stopped immediately if any such sign appears. If the test is positive it does not necessarily mean that it is impossible to treat the occipitoatlantal or atlantoaxial joint but it indicates the need for special care.

The number of accidents occurring in Switzerland up to about 1980 from thrusting manipulation of the cervical spine was found to be 1 in 400,000 cases with 'reactions' in 1 in 40,000[17]. Most, but not all, of the cases have involved the vertebro-basilar axis and have resulted in thrombosis of this or its branches. In the same paper Dvorak and Orelli report a case of tetraplegia after manipulation of the neck which was ascribed to ischaemia. In 1982 after a presentation by Dr Philip E. Greenman, DO, the muscle energy approach has been adopted and according to a personal communication there have been no further accidents when this approach has been used. The authors have reason to believe that the gentle high velocity, low amplitude treatments included in this edition are safe and they find that something more than muscle energy or indirect treatment is occasionally required.

Regrettably high velocity, and sometimes high amplitude treatment in the extended and rotated position of the head is still taught in some reputable schools. It is hoped that this will not continue because, as long as it does, there will be a likelihood of further accidents of this nature.

The hypermobile joint

It is essential to distinguish between those people who have greater mobility in all their joints from the patient who for some reason has one or a few joints which are more mobile than the rest. Those who have been active in acrobatics or dancing from an early age always tend to have a greater than usual range of motion in most, if not all, of their joints. This overmobility is no contraindication to treatment even by thrusting. There is a difficulty, however, because the excess mobility makes localisation more difficult and great care is required both in diagnosis and treatment.

Hypermobility is one of the contraindications to thrust treatment, but, although hypermobile joints may be the source of symptoms and may require treatment before the patient obtains relief, it will often be found that the basic cause is a *hypomobile* joint in the neighbourhood but of which the patient is not aware. It is as if the stiff joint were making the loose one do all the work until it objects and becomes the source of symptoms. That picture is not uncommon and does lend itself to relief by manual methods. If the restricted joint is very close, it may be felt that thrusting should be avoided but this may still be used if localisation is accurate. The alternative is to use a muscle energy or indirect treatment. In these patients it will very often be found that as the restricted joint regains its motion, the hypermobility of the other joint disappears.

Joints that have been pushed beyond the anatomical barrier into subluxation may become restricted there; for example, anterior or posterior (structural) ribs and innominate shears. Reduction is needed before they can begin to operate in their normal manner but, as the joint ligaments have already been stretched, any thrusting force should be avoided. Reduction can almost always be achieved by muscle energy treatment without putting any extra strain on the ligaments. Some form of protection may be needed after reduction like the cinch type SI belt used after treatment of a superior innominate shear.

Spinal joints above or below a fusion, or above or below a section of the spine that has restricted motion because of degenerative change will often be hypermobile. In this case the cause cannot be removed as it can with simple dysfunction; it may still be possible to give relief by treating the hypermobile joint to restore as much symmetry as possible. Again this is a contraindication to thrusting. Such hypermobility can sometimes be inferred from ordinary X-ray films and an example is reproduced in Fig. 12.3. Both C5–6 and 6–7 are narrowed and show spur formation posteriorly; there is no doubt that they would have restriction of motion. C4 has slid forward slightly on C5 and the upper half of the body of C5 is less in A–P diameter than C4 and much less than C6. This suggests that C4 is hypermobile and has been 'eroding' the anterosuperior surface of C5.

There is another type of hypermobility, which may be the result of repeated injury or sometimes anatomical anomalies such as spondylolisthesis (or are these stress fractures?), sometimes with facet joint arthritis and sometimes with no obvious cause. Diagnosis presents difficulty; it is much easier to feel restriction than to be sure that a joint is more mobile that it ought to be. This is a different problem from the one posed by the subluxated rib or sacroiliac joint, which are restricted outside their normal range and restoration of symmetry in the normal range is what is required. Anatomical anomalies such as the very rare absence of the odontoid process cause a special type of hypermobility.

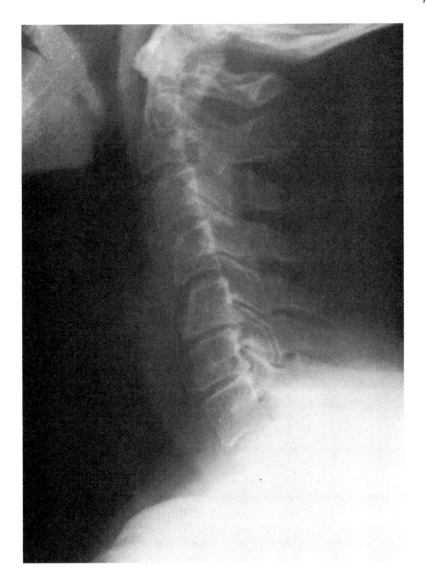

Fig. 12.3 Plain lateral X-ray of cervical spine suggesting hypermobility of C4–5, see text.

The difference between the wide range of normal mobility found in acrobats and dancers and true hypermobility is quite small. In examining a patient, with this in mind, it is necessary to make allowance for the range of motion in joints that are considered normal when assessing those that are in question. It helps to remember that in the generally overmobile patient, the excess mobility is found in almost all joints that are not the site of somatic dysfunction. Excess mobility of joints is a feature of the Marfan group of syndromes and here again the excess motion is present in all joints. Patients with Down's syndrome may have instability of the occipitoatlantal junction and need extra care, so do those with recent acute pharyngeal infections. For these patients diagnosis is relatively simple if a high index of suspicion is maintained as it should be for other general conditions at all times.

One of the factors in diagnosis of hypermobility is the 'end feel', the tissue changes which the operator senses when the joint under examination gets close to the barrier. In a hypermobile joint there is a sensation of lack of restriction throughout the range and the normal tightening towards the end of the range is less marked so that the joint comes up to the barrier more abruptly. This is also true of the overmobile joint of the acrobat and the dancer but the difference is unlikely to be as great and the finding of similar end feel in other joints confirms the diagnosis of functional overmobility.

Translation anteroposteriorly or in sidebending, and rotation are useful in making the diagnosis of hypermobility. With the patient lying on one side with hips and knees bent the operator can control her knees with his abdomen or thigh, and feel with both hands for the movement between the spinous processes when he presses her thighs back and then releases the pressure. The level being tested can be changed by introducing more or less flexion or extension of the patient's hips. In this way the joint in question can be compared with neighbouring ones and its motion assessed. A similar test of sidebending and rotation can be performed starting from the same position. This test has to be assessed with one hand because in order to control the sidebend the operator needs to lift or depress the patient's feet. Sidebending in one direction is tested by raising the feet; in the other direction by depressing them.

The definitive diagnostic test is by having stress X-ray films of the level in full flexion and extension and in right and left sidebending but because of the exposure to radiation it is wise only to do this when clinical evidence suggests hypermobility of the particular level.

It must be remembered that patients with hypermobility from any cause may present with back pain which does not arise from the unstable level and in that event treatment of the dysfunctional joint by manipulation may be needed. In such patients care must be taken to protect the hypermobile segment.

REFERENCES

1. Greenman Philip E. (1979). Lift therapy; use and abuse. *JAOA*; **79**:238–250.
2. Irvin R.E. Reduction of lumbar scoliosis by use of a heel lift to level the sacral base. *JAOA*; **91**:36–44.
3. Simons D.G. (1991). Muscle pain syndromes. *J. Manual Medicine*; **6**:3–23.
4. Travell J.G., Simons D.G. (1983). *Myofascial Pain and Dysfunction*. Baltimore: Williams and Wilkins.
5. Travell J., Rinzler S.H. (1952). The myofascial genesis of pain. *Postgrad. Med.*; **11**:425–434
6. Travell J. (1952). Ethyl chloride spray for painful muscle spasm. *Arch. Phys. Med.*; **33**:291–298.
7. Travell J. (1960). Temporomandibular joint dysfunction. *J. Prosthetic Dentistry*; **10**:745–761.
8. Mennell J. McM. (1975). The therapeutic use of cold. *JAOA*; **74**:1146–1158.

9. Simons D.G. (1975). Muscle pain syndromes. *Am. J. Phys. Med.*; **54**: 289–311, **55**:15–42.
10. *Myofascial Pain and Fibromyalgia.* (Fricton J.R. and Awad E., Eds.) (1990) Raven Press: New York
11. Wolfe F. *et al.* (1990). In *Arthritis Rheum.*; **33**:160–172.
12. Wyke B. (1980). The neurology of low back pain. In *The Lumbar Spine and Back Pain*, 2nd edn. (Jayson M., ed.) pp. 265–339. Tunbridge Wells: Pitman Medical.
13. Cyriax J. (1975). *Textbook of Orthopaedic Medicine*, 6th edn. vol. 1; London: Ballière Tindall.
14. Kleynhans A.M. (1980). Complications of and contraindications to spinal manipulative therapy. In *Modern Developments in the Principles and Practice of Chiropractic.* (Haldeman S., ed.), pp. 359–389. East Norwall, Connecticut: Appleton-Century-Crofts.
15. Levin S. MD, FACS, personal communication.
16. Lewit K. (1986). *Manipulative Therapy in Rehabilitation of the Motor System.* London: Butterworth.
17. Dvorak J., Orelli F.v. (1982). The frequency of complications after manipulation of the cervical spine (in German). *Schweitz. Rundschau med. (praxis)*; **71**:64–69.

Chapter 13

What causes the pain and what does manipulation do?

The precise nature of the changes which take place in an intervertebral joint which cause it to give rise to symptoms are still the subject of many conflicting theories. Nor is it known for certain why those symptoms, once started, so often tend to be recurrent in spite of treatment. As stated earlier, there is no 'little bone out of place' nor is there a dislocation to be reduced although there are some joint dysfunctions where there is technically a subluxation. These latter are joints which have become hypermobile and then restricted in motion outside their normal range. They are treated rather differently from the usual dysfunctions which are restricted within their normal range and need to be made to move more freely.

There are relatively few basic physical signs which can be elicited in a sufficient proportion of back pain patients to justify the belief that they are fundamental to the condition. Two objective signs are almost always present, and indeed, if one looks in the right places, it is probably true to say that they are always present. These are loss of mobility and localised changes of tension and texture in the soft tissues. To be of real diagnostic value the loss of motion should be localised to the individual joint, the tissue changes are expected at the same level.

The tissue changes almost always include hypertonus in muscle in the same segment as the loss of mobility. It is impossible for a patient, at will, to make a single segment stiff, nor can localised hypertonus or other tissue texture abnormalities be produced voluntarily. These changes are, therefore, truly objective and of great value in medico-legal assessment.

Subjective signs are notoriously unreliable but in this work there is one that may be of value. It is the tenderness often complained of by a patient when the operator is palpating over an area of tissue texture change in a spot that was unexpected by the patient. Because much of the pain associated with spinal joint dysfunction is referred, the patient is often unaware of the level from which it arises. In such circumstances the tenderness elicited by palpation can be a useful confirmatory sign that the level being palpated is at least part of the cause of the symptoms. This unexpected tenderness may be seen, for instance, in patients with low back pain; in such patients there may well be dysfunction needing treatment in the low lumbar region but, at least in those who have had previous attacks, there is likely to be another joint near the thoracolumbar junction that is a major part of the cause. The patient is unlikely either to be aware of, or to expect, something that high up and a surprised complaint of tenderness when such a joint is found may be a valuable confirmatory sign. Lewis and Kellgren's work referred to later[38] should lead us to expect thoracolumbar dysfunctions in cases of 'lumbago'.

Localised loss of mobility

In the acute phase, soon after an injury, loss of mobility may be widespread but when that phase is over there is likely to be a remaining loss of motion in one or more spinal joints, or in part of the pelvic mechanism, or both. It is important to remember that there may be no loss of overall range of movement because neighbouring joints tend to compensate by developing increased mobility[1]. Techniques for clinical assessment of this loss of mobility have been described in Chapters 3, 4 and 5; it can be demonstrated radiographically but requires special projections which were described. *This is the basic reason why it is wrong to perform only an overall examination of the range of a part and conclude that there are no restrictions.* Unfortunately that is what is done all too often by medical examiners, and as one would expect it is done chiefly by those acting for the defence or for the compensation organisations. One of the authors has seen many patients who have had that kind of report and he has been saddened to hear the patient say that the examining physician had never even touched the patient's back during the examination!

Localised hypertonus

In the acute phase the muscle spasm is very obvious and no one will deny its existence. In the more chronic patient, careful examination may be required in order that localised tension abnormalities are not overlooked. Obesity makes it more difficult to detect subtle abnormalities of tissue tension and texture but the more difficult ones are the people who have the dense, almost fibrous type of subcutaneous tissue. They are not easy to palpate even when they are not obese. Such patients are disheartening to the beginner and there is no easy answer to feeling through their tough layers. Fortunately there are many patients with soft and often thin subcutaneous tissue, easy to feel through and much better for the beginner to practise on.

In this examination it is most important to localise the abnormalities. In most simple dysfunctions the tissue changes are found very largely on one side of the joint. If changes feel the same on both sides it is a suggestion that there may be underlying pathology rather than simple dysfunction.

THE NATURE OF THE DYSFUNCTION

In editions before the fourth emphasis was placed on the muscle changes almost to the exclusion of other tissue abnormalities. This is not the whole story; new methods of treatment have shown that relief can result even when nothing is done directly to the muscles. Even so, the concept of tight muscle as the cause has its uses. Patients appreciate that their own muscles are in spasm, or at least hypertonic, and they are aware of the pain that a cramping muscle will give. Many are also aware that tension from any cause will tighten their muscles and can understand that this might be the truth in the still too common slanderous statement 'it is all in your head'. The authors do feel that it is proper to explain that tight muscle is not the whole cause.

Persistent neck and arm pain, with or without upper back pain, is often associated with upper thoracic dysfunctions more than problems in the neck itself. These may easily be missed by those unfamiliar with manual medicine and, because of the frequency of this problem, the examination for hypertonus in the upper thoracic spine with the patient sitting and the operator standing in front can be very useful (see Chapter 3, Fig. 3.24). It is often easy to find a dysfunction by the presence of hypertonus in the deep spinal muscles which will always be tender, so that the patient knows that the operator has found something. A remark like 'a funny place to keep your head' is sometimes appropriate and helps to break the ice. This method of examination also helps to get the patient to relax because she will at once sense that the operator knows something more than some of her previous advisers. A patient who has not got confidence in the operator will not relax well. When she finds that he can quickly put his finger, unprompted, on one of the sore places, confidence is immediately improved, the more so when she did not even know that that spot was tender. For those who have not had the experience, it is a very happy thing to watch the obvious relief shown by the patient when a previously unrecognised dysfunction is found and the threat of it 'being all in her head' is over. As pointed out in Chapter 6, the success of muscle energy, indirect and myofascial treatment point strongly to the conclusion that soft tissue is the main restrictor. On the other hand the occasional sudden 'snap' (with ensuing disappearance of the signs) during a gentle muscle energy treatment suggests that there must be a mechanical block of some kind in at least those dysfunctions. This raises several questions:

1. What causes the snap that sometimes happens during a muscle energy treatment?
2. What is it that happens in the muscle in a dysfunction?
3. Why should high velocity treatment work?
4. What part does the disc play?

1. The snap

This is common in high velocity treatment and is supposed to be due to sudden release of nitrogen from the joint fluid. Whether or not that is the correct explanation is uncertain, but this is not the question with which we are now concerned. Sometimes, during the patient contraction phase of an isometric technique, the joint will release with an audible (and palpable) snap. Testing thereafter shows a return of mobility but it is difficult to believe that gently contracting muscle can produce a 'snap', and the operator force is only enough just to prevent motion. It seems that, in addition to other restrictors, there must be some sort of block in the joint, or to motion of the joint, which, by moving out of the way, can result in a sudden release.

2. What is the trouble in the muscle?

Examination by the techniques described will show that the muscle is palpable. The small fourth layer muscles are only palpable when contracted. The fact that they are tight may itself be palpable and this is certainly true of more superficial muscles when they are giving the same kind of trouble. However, the motoneurons are apparently silent at least when the patient is relaxed, although the restriction is still present.

Resting muscle length is controlled by specialised muscle fibres called spindles which are themselves 'set' by the tone in the gamma motoneuron system. This setting of the resting length is physiological; certain types of muscle action require a preliminary tight setting of the tension, for instance when exerting near maximum power over a small range. Other actions must start with the muscle relaxed and movements with a wide range, such as a golf swing, are examples.

Guarding after injury is well recognised and appears to be due to a resetting of the 'gamma gain' so that the spindles become shorter, causing the main muscle fibres to shorten as well. This also is a normal reaction, apparently to protect the part from further injury, but the trouble arises when the circumstances for which the muscle guarding is useful are over. The pain of cramp is well recognised as coming from muscle; this is not the same phenomenon and for a variety of reasons. In cramp the whole muscle appears to contract and often very tightly, if not maximally. In cramp the pain is felt more in the muscle than at a distant point and it can often be relieved by passive stretching and sometimes actually by use of the muscle. Muscle in a state of cramp will not contract normally. Muscle with a shortened resting length will contract normally when stimulated and when the contraction is over it will relax back to its shortened resting length. The problem is that it is unable to relax enough to allow full movement of the joint concerned.

The Travell trigger point (the eponym is used to distinguish it from the other conditions to which the term trigger point has been applied from time to time) is a localised area of tightness in muscle which causes pain. The pain is commonly referred and often to an area which may not be in dermatomal, myotomal or sclerotomal relation to the trigger point itself. Trigger points in relatively superficial muscles have been investigated in ways that cannot easily be done for fourth layer spinal muscles. Travell and Simons[2] say that the mechanisms

> . . . remain controversial. Electromyographic, clinical and experimental evidence all suggest that a myofascial TrP, which begins with a muscular strain, becomes the site of sensitised nerves, increased metabolism and reduced circulation. This initial neuromuscular dysfunction phase, if untreated, may progress to a dystrophic phase that causes demonstrable histological change in the muscle.

There is marked similarity between the trigger point and what we find in muscle over dysfunctional spinal joints. This is not necessarily to identify the two as one and the same process but some of what has been proved about trigger points is likely to be applicable to spinal joint dysfunction. The area is tender when palpated but often the patient is unaware of the location of the dysfunction until the operator presses on it; it is of the reference zone that the patient complains. The reference zone itself is tender on palpation and it is important not to confuse the two. The spinal muscle also may cause referred pain that does not always follow the expected distribution. At least certain treatments have been shown to be helpful for both conditions, isometric contraction followed by stretching being the most generally accepted.

Is the condition of the muscle in a spinal joint dysfunction similar to that described by Travell and Simons for a trigger point? The increased metabolism and decreased circulation would fit to account for pain and the metabolic changes would have to have an effect on other soft tissues very soon. The muscle could well be tight enough to limit motion. Wyke, whose work is referred to both in the last chapter and later, describes what he thinks may be the mechanism of pain production in spinal joint dysfunction and it is essentially similar to Travell and Simons as quoted above.

But why should the neuromuscular dysfunction phase persist beyond the time for which protection is needed to allow healing? The precise changes that are the cause of memory are still matters of research but it seems possible that the barrage of abnormal impulses entering the spinal cord after an injury could not only produce local facilitation (so that any other incoming impulse will trip a second order neuron more easily), but also could leave a memory behind and a tendency for the facilitation to persist. The effect could be as if a faulty program had got into the central computer not allowing the muscle to return to normal. Is the need for repeated treatment in so many patients due to a persistent 'rogue' program that has been entered into the central computer by the injury?

The concept of muscular origin of the pain would lead to the suggestion that 'muscle relaxants' could be a useful answer. Unfortunately experience tells us that this is not often the case. The relaxants may help a little but rarely do they act in a way that gives significant relief. This may be because the so-called muscle relaxants all appear to act as central depressants rather than having any direct action on muscle, even when one allows that there is evidence of a central factor in somatic dysfunction. There does not yet seem to be anything that has a selective effect on the gamma system. Maybe that would have the wrong kind of side effects anyway.

3. Why should high velocity thrusting do good?

Why, indeed, should muscle energy treatment help? This seems to be the easier to understand. Post-isometric relaxation is a known part of muscle physiology and, at least in so far as the symptoms are caused by dysfunction in muscle, isometric exercises would be expected to help.

For those treatments that are not isometric, the principle of relaxation of the antagonist can be used to explain the improvement although most such treatments have an isometric factor at work as well. Both these physiological principles are known to be useful in designing treatment for peripheral muscle, whether it be for tightness or for weakness.

There is no doubt that high velocity treatment can help. It has been one of the main tools of the manual practitioner, whether medically qualified or not, for hundreds of years. There are also records of how unskilled thrusting and thrusting for the wrong diagnosis has been disastrous. The question being asked is why is it often helpful? The problem of the dangers was discussed in Chapter 12. It is easy to take the results of research, construct a theory without proof and present it as a fact. Remembering this, and as we do not have proof, the suggestions which follow must be regarded as nothing more than working hypotheses.

We do have some facts from which to start. The diagnosis is made primarily on the objective findings of ART, asymmetry, restriction of motion and tissue texture change. When a successful manual intervention is made, these signs change. The asymmetry may have gone, the motion returned and the tissues may feel almost if not quite normal. These are facts which are verifiable by other observers, but here is one of the difficulties. (The authors are aware of the possibility that this will sound a little as if they considered themselves to be 'superior'; far from it, there are many who are very competent at palpation, none so much as the blind.) Those would-be observers who have not had experience in the kind of examination required to find these signs may feel so little that they deny their existence. When teaching a class how to feel each other, that difficulty can be overcome because in the class there will be some students whose tissues are difficult to feel and others who are relatively easy. A student, trying to feel one of the less easy ones will find it very helpful to examine one of the easier ones first.

The other fact that is pertinent is that following a high velocity thrust, there seems to be proprioceptor silence in the area for a short time[3,4].

Traditionally the old manipulators were 'putting a little bone back in place'. This went down well with the patients, it sounded like it, it felt like it and it was different afterwards. The public have always liked to 'go one better' than their doctors and one wonders if this also contributed to their ready belief, on the basis of 'the doctor didn't find it'. It is unfair not to admit that in those cases there was something that the doctor had not found! Modern research and modern imaging have shown that in the large majority of patients there is no little bone out of place but that the joint has restriction of motion.

Many of those doing anatomical research have concentrated on trying to find a basis for mechanical derangement of spinal joints similar to the meniscus in the knee. Meniscoids have been found in some spinal joints but the architecture is such that it seems to need a stretch of the imagination to suppose that these tiny structures could be the major source of such a common problem.

Nerve or nerve root compression has been blamed for many of the symptoms and it is as well to remember that pressure on nerve causes paralysis and numbness, even if at the moment of application of the pressure there may be transient pain. Pressure on nerve undoubtedly does occur and often needs surgery for its relief but that is a rarity compared to the common spinal joint dysfunction.

There is evidence that an inflammatory reaction around nerve or nerve root may cause persistent pain and, when this happens, thrusting manipulation is unlikely to be helpful. Anti-inflammatory medication or epidural injection is often of great value in such cases.

It is not difficult to imagine that a well directed thrust would restore motion to a restricted joint but if it is the soft tissues that are the trouble why does it help? Would not the insult to those tissues tend to make them tighten further? Those beginning to learn techniques of thrusting manipulation will often move the joint too far when trying to find the barrier. This makes the manipulation more difficult because, if the joint is pushed against the barrier, the muscles tend to become even tighter. When the barrier is correctly engaged and the thrust is sudden that does not happen. If the force is applied slowly the muscles will tighten and the manipulation is likely to fail. As well as being high velocity (sudden) the thrust must be of restricted amplitude so that the anatomical barrier at the joint is not violated, as Dr John Mennell says, 'less than an eighth of an inch at the joint'. If the muscle spindle is stretched its reaction is to cause the muscle to tighten; this may be part of the reason that a low velocity thrust is not of much value. High velocity thrusting does apparently overcome that tendency and part of its effectiveness may be from the sudden lengthening of the spindles.

It seems that we are brought back to the observation that there is a short period of proprioceptor silence after a high velocity thrust. Is this enough to change the tone in the gamma system to allow the muscle spindles to resume their normal length? Whatever the final answer will turn out to be, it must take into account that the common spinal joint dysfunctions can be relieved by a wide variety of treatments. At the present time it is fair to say that all the usually successful treatments probably have the capability of influencing the muscle spindle length either directly or indirectly.

4. The disc, villain or troublesome complication?

In the past the paucity of clinical signs and the diversity of the symptoms that may arise from disorders of spinal joints led to doubt as to whether they were of spinal origin. The work of Mixter and Barr[5] stimulated interest in the intervertebral disc as a cause of symptoms. Since that time an immense amount of work has been done, but it appears that many of the pieces of the puzzle are still missing. There can be no doubt that actual protrusion and extrusion of disc material occurs and can cause physical pressure on nerve roots or on the cord itself. Such protrusion or extrusion in fact produces a space occupying lesion in the spinal canal and may have to be distinguished from other such lesions. Even in this connection, however, there are a number of factors that require explanation.

First, as mentioned above, pressure on nerve causes paralysis but no pain. An excellent example of this in the practice of one of the authors was a young man who had been sailing. He leaned against the side of the dinghy to balance it on a long reach lasting for more that half an hour. When he moved he found that he had a complete wrist drop with sensory as well as motor changes. The pressure on the radial nerve had been sufficient that it took more than 8 weeks to recover. He insisted that at no time did he have any pain.

The dural sleeve of the nerve root is sensitive to certain kinds of stimulus. The anterior aspect of the dura is particularly sensitive and the nociceptor endings can be stimulated mechanically or chemically[6]. It appears, however, that the pain produced would be in the back, not in the leg.

Secondly there is the observation that, in many cases, symptoms of back and referred pain have been present for a long time before there is any evidence of an actual disc protrusion. When a true protrusion is found, a careful evaluation of the history will often fail to reveal any dramatic change in symptoms until there is sufficient pressure on the nerve to produce the different signs of a space occupying lesion. Charnley[7] was clearly unsatisfied that the disc was the primary cause of symptoms when he wrote:

> One of the most surprising things about acute lumbago is that the amount of pain does not seem to be proportional to the amount of organic change within the disc . . . We rarely find convincing protrusions in these cases but what is cogent to the present argument is that the material removed appeared more often to be normal than fibrous and stringy.

Friberg and Hult[8] found symptoms of sciatica in patients who did not have detectable herniation of discs, and Pedersen *et al.*[9] considered that they had evidence that back pain and sciatica could arise from stimulation of sinuvertebral nerve fibres.

There have been many who have thought that actual pressure from disc material was the main cause of the pain. Cyriax[10] maintained that he reduced protruded disc material by his manipulations; Armstrong[11] actually gives diagrams of how a manipulation might move a nuclear sequestrum but goes on to condemn manipulation in any form. The older medical manipulators referred to the lesion as a fixation or strain without specifying a cause.

Anyone with experience in disc surgery will know that the nuclear material in a disc protrusion is not normal. Instead of being a firm, almost rubbery substance, it is composed of a softened sticky material that tends to be stringy in consistency. From the anatomy of the disc we know that protrusion cannot take place until the nucleus is softened and a tear is made in the annulus through which the nuclear material can be forced. Except in the most superficial layers of the annulus, the intervertebral disc has no blood supply and, even if reduction were possible, it does not seem that an avascular tissue could almost instantly heal a track through which nuclear material had protruded.

If one tries hard enough, it is possible to suck excess toothpaste back into the tube; if then you tread on the tube with the top off, it all comes out again. Nachemson and Morris[12] recorded the pressure inside intervertebral discs with the subjects in various positions. Their figures vary from a minimum of 50 kg/cm² standing, to a maximum of 100–127 kg/cm² when seated. This pressure would surely cause softened material to protrude again if there were a preformed track down which it could go. These theoretical considerations suggest that continuous traction would be more likely to be effective in both securing and maintaining reduction. In practice it does not seem to happen that way. Traction is sometimes of value in treatment, especially of those with very acute pain and spasm, and there is some experimental evidence to suggest that partial reduction of protruded disc material may occur[13,14].

The above evidence suggests that the pain is often coming from somewhere other than the disc and the clinical evidence of relief from certain manual procedures does appear to confirm that concept. On the other hand there is now strong evidence that the disc itself may be the source of pain, at least when abnormal. The pain produced when contrast material, or even normal saline is injected into an abnormal disc is often the same as the pain of which the patient complains. If the disc were abnormal enough to allow the pressure to affect surrounding structures, it might be thought that the pain came from those structures but this does not seem always to be likely.

That the disc must play some part in the production of symptoms is shown by work done by Lindblom[15] and Perey[16]. They showed that when a needle is introduced into a disc in order to perform a discogram, the posterior longitudinal ligament is sensitive. The pain was only severe if the disc was abnormal. When the solution was injected into a normal disc it produced a mild pain in the low back. In a disc which was abnormal, but not ruptured, both the back pain and the sciatica were reproduced. This happened even when the solution contained 1% of novocaine, which suggests that the effect was in some way connected with pressure on the annulus or the surrounding structures rather than any effect on the nucleus itself.

Bogduk[17] describes annular tears in the outer layers of the annulus resulting from rotational injury in the lumbar spine and suggests that the radial tears found in the annulus in some cases may be the result of repeated injury causing progressive tearing of more layers. Wyke[18] maintains that the nerve fibres present in the annulus of the disc in the new born disappear as the child develops so that, in the adult, there is no nerve supply to the annulus itself. There have been many investigators[19,20] that have demonstrated nerve tissue in the outer layers of the annulus and some, at least, of the nerves have what appear to correspond to nociceptor endings. Rotational injury in the lumbar spine is common and the range of available rotation appears to be no more than 3°, suggesting that some of the lumbar pain syndromes may be discogenic. In his paper Bogduk[17] does not mention pain from structures other than the disc but he does discuss the development of internal disc disruption, blaming its development largely on contact of nuclear material with vascular tissue as a result of vertebral end plate fractures caused by compression injuries. He gives a bibliography for the evidence that compression injuries tend to cause end plate fractures rather than extrusion of nuclear material into the spinal canal.

INTERNAL DISC DISRUPTION

This condition was first described as such in 1970. It presents with some characteristics that differ from the more common back pain associated with somatic dysfunction. In particular the pain is mainly in the back and is much worse when the joint is loaded. Leg pain is not well localised by the patient and is usually of a deep aching character. Alteration of body posture is awkward and often assisted by the arms, e.g. when standing up from a stoop. The pain is eased by lying down and gets worse as the day goes on. For someone engaged in a manual medicine practice these patients may present as those in whom any biomechanical dysfunctions have been corrected, but the pain remains unchanged or only modified.

In addition to the back and leg pain there will often be a general reaction which may include loss of energy, marked weight loss, headache, and serious psychiatric disturbances[21]. Crock goes on to say that these patients will have normal findings on neurological examination, X-ray, myelogram and CT scan. The diagnosis is made on the symptoms and MRI scan, and can only be confirmed by discogram. There is new experimental evidence[22] that prone springing on the spinous processes can correlate closely with the discographic findings and perhaps a non-invasive test may be developed. Plain X-ray films are only of value if they show clear evidence of instability. Awake discography has been shown to be of great value in that injection into a symptomatic, abnormal disc reproduces the patient's pain[23]; this correlates more closely with the symptom-producing levels than does MRI with or without the contrast medium. According to Bogduk[17] the transverse view that can be provided by CT scanning after discographic injection is very helpful.

There has often been prolonged suffering before the diagnosis is made and this may be part of the reason for the emotional changes but it appears that there is a general effect on the whole person and this is ascribed to an autoimmune reaction to the material of the disc nucleus. Crock[24] describes some of the evidence for this and says that the lower lumbar discs are the most commonly affected. The probability that the nuclear material of the disc can cause antigenic reactions has been discussed for more than 20 years but the work had been mainly concerned with material protruded into the spinal canal. Gertzbein[25] describes the evidence for an autoimmune mechanism in degenerative disc disease in the human. The experimental evidence for an inflammatory effect from injection of homogenised nuclear material into the spinal canal in dogs is described by McCarron *et al*[26].

The treatment advised by Crock is total removal of the disc material and combined anterior and posterior fusion, the so-called '360° fusion'.

More recently an outpatient treatment for disc decompression has been developed and it appears that it may have great promise in this condition[27]. The treatment was developed as an alternative to percutaneous discectomy and consists of laser vaporisation of the disc material under local anaesthetic. The patient has a discogram and if the findings are positive a fine laser fibre is introduced through the same needle and the disc is vaporised under fluoroscopic control. When the procedure is complete the patient is allowed to return home and fusion is reported to be likely. The pain experienced is significantly less than with percutaneous discectomy[28]. In experimental animals the vertebrae have been shown to fuse by bone after the procedure. If further experience shows that this treatment is successful with internal disruption as well as with other disc pathology, the patient's post-operative period is likely to be much less unpleasant.

Symptoms from joints that have no intervertebral disc

As was pointed out earlier, there are two joints in the spine that have no intervertebral discs, but which can still be the source of symptoms strictly comparable to those seen in joints in other parts of the spine. Reference has also been made to the fact that similar symptoms can arise from the sacroiliac joint.

The concept that the sacroiliac joint could be the cause of symptoms was put forward in 1911 by Goldthwaite[29] and again in 1938 by Gray[30]. Both authors recorded instances of dramatic relief following manipulation of the sacroiliac joint. In spite of this, the medical profession has commonly exhibited blank disbelief (once shared by at least one of the authors!) at the idea that the sacroiliac joint could be the cause of symptoms and, more particularly, of referred symptoms. This disbelief almost certainly stems from the teaching of the medical schools and the not unnatural blind acceptance of this teaching by the student. The attitude of the teachers appears to have resulted from the medical profession's preoccupation with the intervertebral disc as the cause of the trouble, and the belief that for the production of referred pain, actual pressure on nerves or nerve roots was required. There is, of course, no nerve of any size on which pressure can conceivably be brought by a minor movement of the sacroiliac joint.

Three specific instances of relief of pain by manipulation of the sacroiliac joint from the practice of one of the authors follow.

1. Pain in the low back
A 34-year-old female presented with a 4-year history of intermittent back pain. There had been a further acute attack 2 weeks before. She had had a below knee amputation of the right leg 10 years previously. Examination showed that, when standing, the right side of the pelvis was significantly higher than the left and the dysfunction was localised to the sacroiliac joint. Measurement of the difference in leg length by the X-ray technique showed that the limb was more than 25 mm (1 inch) too long. Treatment of the sacroiliac joint on a total of seven occasions resulted in marked relief, even before the length of the limb was corrected.

2. Pain referred to the heel

A girl aged 7 gave a history of having jumped from a roof 2.4 metres (8 feet) high, about 10 days before. She complained of being unable to bear weight on her left heel. Examination did not show any abnormality in the heel and X-rays were normal. Examination of the low back showed a sacroiliac strain which required two treatments by manipulation to give complete relief. There had been no back pain and no pain in the leg except at the heel.

3. Pain referred to the knee

A girl aged 13 complained of pain in the front of the knee and said that she had fallen on it 2 weeks before. The only abnormality in the knee was a very tender prepatellar nodule, but examination of the low back did show a sacroiliac strain. There was no history of previous back trouble and she did not admit to having any back discomfort. One treatment of the sacroiliac joint by manipulation stopped the pain but she attended once more, 2 months later, for a recurrence caused by a further fall.

The evidence from the effects of local anaesthetic injection

Injections of local anaesthetic can relieve pain in a way that makes it clear that it is not, in those cases, due to some change in the disc itself, with or without the production of nerve or nerve root pressure.

Occasionally a patient comes with acutely tender areas in peripheral muscle, whether they are true trigger points or the more generalised condition mentioned in Chapter 12. In some of these patients, injection of the tender areas may result in dramatic relief not only of the local symptoms but also of both the referred pain and the back pain. In those in whom the relief is not that dramatic or long lasting, there may be enough change in the symptoms to show that the peripheral muscle is acting as a secondary focus for symptom production. It is probable that this situation is often started by a spinal joint dysfunction, causing the changes in the peripheral muscle which become self-perpetuating and then maintain the symptoms even when the causative spinal joint dysfunction has settled or has been treated.

In an occasional patient, the caudal epidural injection of a weak solution of local anaesthetic will relieve both the local and the referred pain before there is any evidence of change in either sensory or motor function of the low lumbar nerves. This suggests that the mechanism involves the sinuvertebral nerves or the plexus of nerves that surrounds the paravertebral venous system, or even the articular and periosteal branches of the posterior primary division of the spinal nerve roots, all of which have fibres with thin myelin sheaths. The fibres in the spinal nerve roots are less easily accessible to the solution and most have thicker myelin sheaths so that they would be affected less quickly.

The importance of the true disc protrusion must not be overlooked. The dramatic relief which can follow surgical removal of a large disc protrusion is most gratifying to both patient and surgeon. Unfortunately surgery for back pain with or without referred pain is not always so satisfying, and cases which are initially successful will sometimes have further acute recurrences or may develop less acute symptoms that can be enough to prevent the patient doing certain types of work. A typical case in the practice of one of the authors was a bank manager who had had very successful surgery for a disc protrusion 7 years before. The pain had begun to return a week before he was seen. It had come on without known cause and had quickly become severe. When seen there were no abnormal neurological signs but straight leg raising was much reduced. He responded very well to treatment by manipulation and became pain free in about five treatments. The pain was described as being the same as before his surgery and this appears to be an example of a pain referred from a different structure but felt in the same place as in the previous episode.

The changes in the intervertebral disc in those who have actual protrusions are accepted as being due to degeneration. The cause of the degeneration has not been agreed but it is assumed by many to be due to trauma. Roaf[31] said: 'Prolapse of a normal disc either never or hardly ever occurs. It is only when the nucleus pulposus has lost its normal characteristics – probably through poor nutrition subsequent to ischaemia, secondary to infection or trauma – that prolapse of the disc material takes place.'

Major protrusions of disc material requiring surgery for their relief are uncommon in the young but by no means unheard of. The youngest known to the authors was a girl of 11. She had signs of a space occupying lesion which proved at surgery to be a large protrusion and she made an excellent recovery after the surgery. It is difficult to believe that a child of 11 could be suffering from idiopathic degeneration of her discs. Could it be due to loss of mobility at that joint?

The neurological evidence

Wyke[32] has shown that there are three routes by which pain fibres reach the dorsal root ganglion from the spinal canal: the sinuvertebral nerves, the plexus around the paravertebral venous system and branches of the posterior rami which supply the apophyseal joints, the periosteum and the related fasciae of the surface of the vertebral bodies and their arches, the interspinous ligaments and the blood vessels.

According to Wyke, the receptor endings of these nerves (and the nerves themselves) can only be caused to discharge by either mechanical or chemical irritation. Mechanical causes can be:

1. abnormal postural stress;
2. local oedema, from either direct trauma or acute inflammation;
3. direct compression;
4. excessive distension of veins in the paravertebral plexus;

Chemical irritants may be:

1. irritants associated with inflammation or with sustained muscle activity;
2. much less commonly, iatrogenic (contrast media etc.).

Stimulation of these pain receptor systems causes reflex contraction of related muscles which, if sustained, can itself give rise to chemical irritation of the receptor endings, closing the circle. In this way Wyke says that *muscular pain may become superimposed on and actually become more important than the primary spinal pain.* He also points out that the reflex spasm produced by a visceral lesion can cause a spinal pain–spasm–pain cycle which can become self perpetuating. It was reported in Chapter 2 that as a result of his research into the anatomy Wyke deduces that denervation by transcutaneous procedures is not possible. He also says: 'Contrary to the traditional opinions of many doctors, inflammatory disorders of the back muscles and their related connective tissues are seldom the cause of back pain except as a complication of some acute febrile illness.'

Experimental work on the subject of referred pain

The problem of referred pain is one which has received much attention from neurologists, anatomists and physiologists. Kellgren[33] reports work started by Lewis and carried on by himself in which an irritant solution of 6% saline was injected into volunteers at various sites. He showed that by injecting the irritant beside the spinous process of the 1st sacral vertebra, he could produce the typical pain of sciatica with radiation all down the leg. The injection was basically into muscle but the manner in which it was given suggests that the interspinous and flava ligaments and the periosteum on the posterior aspect of the vertebra may have been involved. A similar injection at the 1st lumbar level produced a typical attack of lumbago. Similar experiments have been done by others including Sinclair *et al.*[34], Feinstein *et al.*[35] and Hockaday and Whitty[36]. Many of the workers in this field have observed that referred pain is associated with hyperalgesia in the reference zone and often there is cutaneous hypoaesthesia in the same area. It has been suggested that there is both a central and a peripheral mechanism in the production of referred pain, and that the central mechanism involves both the spinal cord and higher centres.

The evidence is that it is not necessary to have actual damage to the segmental nerve root in order to have referred pain and, indeed, these experiments have shown that the referred pain from the injections is not necessarily confined to the dermatome, myotome or sclerotome of that level (Hockaday and Whitty[36]).

Inflammation has been cited as causing pain and clinical observations appear to support this. The clinical evidence comes from the observed benefit of measures designed to counter inflammatory reactions, such as steroid injections in the epidural space and administration of anti-inflammatory medication. That there will be an inflammatory reaction after injury is clear, but why should it tend to persist long after? Wyke's suggestion that the reaction, originally mechanical, could be maintained chemically by the metabolites of continuing muscle hypertonus may offer an explanation.

Is tight muscle the main cause of the pain?

The theory that, in spinal joint derangements, the immediate cause of pain is the tight muscle is an attractive one in many ways. There cannot be many people who have not experienced muscle pain from cramp. The chemical irritation of muscle by hypertonic saline is known to produce referred pain. One of the most significant common factors in the wide variety of available treatments, whether manipulative or not, appears to be their ability to promote relaxation in muscle. That peripheral muscles can cause specific patterns of referred pain has been demonstrated clearly by Travell, Mennell, Simons and others in publications previously referred to. They have also shown that, if the abnormally tight portion of the muscle is made to relax, the pain diminishes. It has also been shown that irritation of deep muscles, and other mesodermal tissues around the spinal joint, will cause referred pain similar to clinical syndromes[17–20,37,38].

Korr[39] gives experimental evidence for the existence of spindle dysfunction with overaction of the gamma system in the dysfunctional muscles. The concept of a muscle in which the resting length adjustment has been turned up to near maximum tightness appears to fit with clinical observations. The joint stiffness is rarely absolute. Movement away from the painful direction is nearly always possible but there remains a barrier to movement, usually most marked in one direction. It seems reasonable to argue that this is what would happen if the muscles on one aspect of the joint were abnormally tight.

The precise means whereby the sensation of pain is produced is not clear. It is tempting to blame it an accumulation of pain-producing metabolites resulting from the overactivity that keeps the muscle tight. On the other hand it is difficult to see how the circulation in the muscle could be significantly compromised by the degree of tightness required to produce even the maximum shortening of its resting length. It may be that the explanation will be found to be an overflow of the continuing afferent discharge in the gamma system, although Wyke's work, referred to above, did cause him to favour the metabolite explanation.

Perhaps the question should be: Is the cause of the dysfunction a faulty program introduced by some means into the muscle control mechanism?

REFERENCES

1. Froning E.C., Frohman B. (1968). Motion of the lumbar spine after laminectomy and spinal fusion. *J. Bone Jt Surg.;* **50**:879–918.
2. Travell J., Simons D.G. (1983). *Myofascial Pain and Dysfunction*, p.5. Baltimore: Williams and Wilkins.
3. England R., Deibert P. (1972). Electromyographic Studies. Part I: Consideration in the evaluation of osteopathic therapy. *JAOA;* **72**:162–169.
4. Grice A.A. (1974). Muscle tonus changes following manipulation. *J. Can. Chiropractic Ass.;* **19**:29–31.
5. Mixter W.J., Barr J.S. (1934). Rupture of the intervertebral disc with involvement of the spinal canal. *New Engl. J. Med.;* **211**:210–215.

6. Wyke B. (1970). The neurological basis of spinal pain. *Rheumatol. Phys. Med.;* **10**:356–366.
7. Charnley J. (1958). Physical change in the prolapsed disc. *Lancet;* **ii**:43–44.
8. Friberg S., Hult L. (1951). Comparative study of the abrodil myelogram and operative findings. *Acta Orthop. Scand.;* **20**:303–314.
9. Pedersen H.E., Blunk C.F.J., Gardner E. (1956). Anatomy of the lumbo-sacral posterior rami. *J. Bone Jt Surg.;* **38A**:377–391.
10. Cyriax J. (1955) *Textbook of Orthopaedic Medicine,* 5th edn. London: Cassell.
11. Armstrong J.R. (1965). *Lumbar Disc Lesions.* 3rd edn. London: Livingstone.
12. Nachemson A., Morris J.H. (1964). *In vivo* measurements of intradiscal pressure. *J. Bone Jt Surg.;* **46A**:1077–1092.
13. Onel D., Tuzlaci M., Sari H., Demir K. (1989). Computed tomographic investigation of lumbar disc herniations. *Spine;* **14**:82–90.
14. Mathews J.A. (1968). A study of lumbar traction. *Ann. Phys. Med.* **9**:275–279.
15. Lindblom K. (1951). Technique and results of diagnostic disc puncture and injection. *Acta orthopaed. Scand.;* **20**:315–326.
16. Perey O. (1951). Contrast medium examination of the intervertebral discs. *Acta Orthopaed. Scand.;* **20**:327–334.
17. Bogduk N. (1990). Pathology of lumbar disc pain. *J. Manual Med.;* **5**:72–79.
18. Wyke B. (1987). In *The Lumbar Spine and Back Pain.* (Jayson M., ed.), 3rd Edn. Edinburgh: Churchill Livingstone.
19. Bogduk N., Tynan W., Wilson A.S. (1981) The nerve supply to the human lumbar intervertebral discs. *J. Anat.;* **132**:39–56.
20. Yoshizawa H., O'Brien J., Smith W.T., Trumper M. (1980). The neuropathology of intervertebral discs removed for low back pain. *J. Pathology;* **132**:95–104.
21. Crock H.V. (1986). Internal disc disruption. *Spine;* **11**:650–653.
22. Bookhout M. personal communication.
23. Simmons J.W., Emery S.F., McMillin J.N., Landa D., Kimmich S.J. Awake discography. *Spine;* **16**:S216–S221.
24. Crock Henry V. (1983) *Practice of Spinal Surgery.* New York: Springer-Verlag.
25. Gertzbein S.D. (1977). Degenerative disk disease of the lumbar spine. *Clin. Orthop.;* **129**:68–71.
26. McCarron R.F., Wimpee M.W., Hudkins P.G., Laros G.S. (1987). The inflammatory effect of the nucleus pulposus. *Spine;* **12**:760–764.
27. Isaacs Edward A. personal communication.
28. Brochure from Humana Hospital, Richmond, Va. U.S.A.
29. Goldthwaite G. (1911). The lumbo-sacral articulation. *Boston Med. Surg. J.;* **164**:365–372.
30. Gray H. (1938). Sacro-iliac joint pain. *Int. Clin.;* **2**:54–69.
31. Roaf R. (1958). Physical changes in the prolapsed disc. *Lancet;* **ii**:265–266.
32. Wyke B. (1980). The neurology of low back pain. In *The Lumbar Spine and Back Pain,* 2nd edn. (Jayson M., ed.), pp. 265–339. Tunbridge Wells: Pitman Medical.
33. Kellgren J.H. (1949). Deep pain sensibility. *Lancet;* **i**:943–949.
34. Sinclair D.C., Feindel W.H., Weddell G., Falconer M.A. (1948). The intervertebral ligaments as a source of referred pain. *J. Bone Jt Surg.;* **30B**:514–521.
35. Feinstein C., Langlin J.N.K., Jameson R.M., Schiller F. (1954). Experiments in pain referred from deep somatic structures. *J. Bone Jt Surg.;* **36a**:981–997

36. Hockaday J.M., Whitty C.W.M. (1967). Patterns of referred pain in normal subjects. *Brain;* **90**:481–496.
37. Kellgren J.H. (1939). On the distribution of pain arising from deep somatic structures. *Clin. Sci.;* **4**:35–46.
38. Lewis T., Kellgren J.H. (1939). Observations relating to referred pain. *Clin. Sci.;* **4**:47–71.
39. Korr I.M. (1975). Proprioceptors and somatic dysfunction. *JAOA;* **74**:638–650.

Chapter 14

Examination and treatment of muscle imbalances

Manual treatment of spinal dysfunction has traditionally focused on mobilisation of joints with little attention paid to the surrounding soft tissue structures. Normal spinal function is dependent not only on passive joint mobility, but also on normal muscle activity and central nervous system regulation of movement patterns[1]. The focus of this book in previous editions has been towards restoration of joint mobility. This chapter will emphasise examination and treatment of muscle imbalances involving both the upper and lower quarters which have particular influence on the trunk and the pelvis. Attention will be paid not only to muscle length and strength, but also to the observation and correction of faulty movement patterns which can perpetuate recurrent and chronic musculoskeletal dysfunction.

Much of our present-day understanding regarding muscle imbalances and neuromotor retraining comes from the work of Janda[1,2] and Lewit[3]. Janda has observed that certain muscle groups respond to dysfunction (i.e. pain or impaired afferent impulses from the joint) by tightening and shortening, while other muscle groups react by inhibition, atrophy and weakness. This is not a random occurrence but is fairly predictable from joint to joint and from patient to patient. Until recently, evaluation of muscle function was concerned primarily with strength testing, with little attention paid to muscle tightness or resting muscle length. Janda believes that normalisation of length of a tight (hypertonic) muscle plays an important role in a therapeutic exercise programme and that the importance of muscle tightness has been underestimated. According to his clinical experience, to try to strengthen a weakened muscle first is futile as it will be inhibited by its shortened antagonist. The muscle groups that respond by tightening and shortening are characterised as postural muscles, or muscles which are usually active in maintaining postural balance and are readily activated in most movement patterns. Muscles that respond by inhibition, atrophy and weakness are referred to as dynamic or phasic muscles. This is a clinical observation with the physiological basis for the differentiation remaining unclear. There has as yet been no correlation of postural and dynamic muscles to fibre typing or histological studies.

Janda believes that there are two major body regions in which muscle imbalances are more evident or in which they begin to develop:

1. The shoulder girdle (upper quarter)
2. The pelvic girdle (lower quarter).

Upper quarter

Janda has identified the following muscle groups as showing a tendency to hyperactivity or increased tone (postural function) in the upper quarter: levator scapulae, middle and upper trapezius, sternocleidomastoid, pectorals and the flexors of the upper extremity.

The muscles with a phasic (dynamic) function in the upper quarter which tend to be weak (inhibited) are the lower part of the trapezius, serratus anterior, supra and infraspinatus, deltoid, the deep neck flexors and the extensors of the upper extremity.

In addition to length and strength considerations, patterns of participation of various muscle groups during functional activities must also be evaluated as faulty movement patterns may lead to joint strain and osteoarthritic changes. Janda has noted a particular syndrome of the upper quarter which he has called the 'upper crossed syndrome', defined as an imbalance of the following muscle groups: tight and shortened pectoralis major, upper trapezius and levator scapulae accompanied by weakness of the lower stabilisers of the scapula, lower trapezius and serratus anterior. This muscular imbalance allows a forward head posture, straightening of the cervical lordosis, increased kyphosis at the cervicothoracic junction and internal rotation of the shoulder girdles. Joint restrictions may result from these imbalances, leading to loss of mobility for upper cervical spine flexion, mid cervical spine extension and cervicothoracic spinal extension. In addition, because of the change in position of the shoulder girdle, there will be an alteration in shoulder mechanics which can create a strain of the shoulder joints[1].

Upper quarter evaluation

To evaluate for muscle imbalances in the upper quarter, the following tests can be used:

1. Supine cervical flexion test. The patient lies supine with her knees bent and the feet flat on the table and is asked to raise her head off the table to look towards her feet. The operator should watch for activation of the sternocleidomastoid and scalene muscles which substitute for inhibited deep neck flexors and cause the head to extend on the neck rather than allowing smooth cervical spine flexion (Figs 14.1, 14.2).

2. Bilateral shoulder abduction. The patient is sitting with her back to the operator and is asked to abduct both her arms over her head. Observation is made of scapulohumeral rhythm, looking particularly for premature and excessive abduction of one scapula and elevation of the shoulder (Fig. 14.3). Faulty elevation of one shoulder girdle may be due to imbalance, on that side, between the levator scapulae and upper trapezius muscles which are tight and the lower trapezius, serratus anterior and supraspinatus which are weak. This muscular imbalance typically leads to an impingement syndrome which strains the shoulder and frequently creates a strain in the cervical spine through the hyperactivity of the levator scapulae as it attaches to the upper four cervical segments.

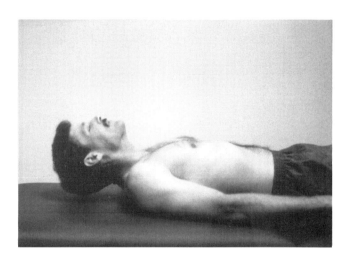

Fig. 14.1 Incorrect movement pattern for cervical spine flexion. Note activation of the sternocleidomastoid muscle.

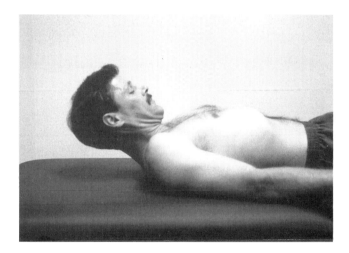

Fig. 14.2 Correct movement for cervical spine flexion.

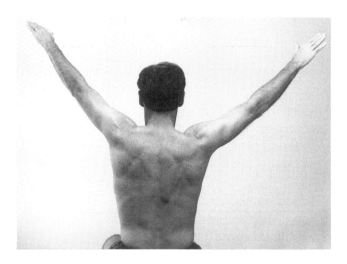

Fig. 14.3 Bilateral shoulder abduction. Note faulty elevation of left shoulder.

3. Scapular stabilisation. The patient is on her hands and knees with her elbows bent enough to hold the shoulders at the same height as the hips. The operator looks for winging of the medial border of the scapula which indicates weakness of and lack of stabilisation by the lower trapezius, serratus anterior or rhomboid muscles (Fig. 14.4).

Fig. 14.4 Scapular stabilisation exercise in the hands and knees position.

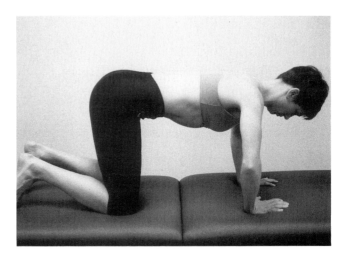

4. Lower trapezius, alternative test. The patient is prone with the arm abducted to 125° and externally rotated. The operator resists scapular retraction and depression at the inferior angle of the scapula (Fig. 14.5).

Fig. 14.5 Test for recruitment of the lower trapezius.

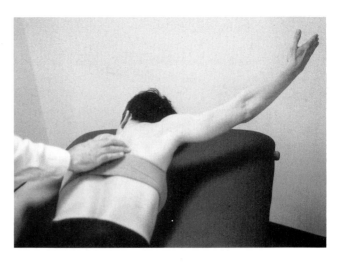

5. For length of latissimus dorsi. The patient is supine with her knees bent and feet flat on the table, and puts both shoulders through a full range of flexion. The operator watches for recruitment of extension of

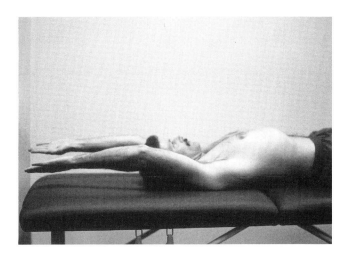

Fig. 14.6 Supine test for length of the latissimus dorsi.

the lumbar spine and/or failure to obtain adequate shoulder flexion (Fig. 14.6).

6. For length of pectoralis minor. With the patient supine the operator observes the relative anteroposterior position of the shoulders. Tightness of the left pectoralis minor is illustrated in Fig. 14.7.

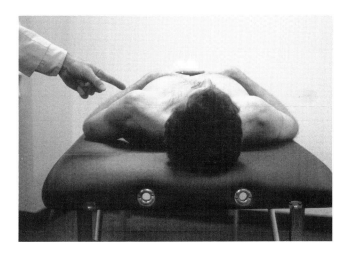

Fig. 14.7 Forward shoulder position created by tightness of the left pectoralis minor.

Upper quarter treatment, stretching

Stretching the commonly tight muscles can be by a static stretch that is held for 20–30 seconds and repeated several times, or by post-isometric relaxation for which an isometric muscle contraction is performed for 5–7 seconds followed by relaxation and taking up the slack to the new motion barrier.

The muscles commonly found to be tight in the upper quarter can be treated by the following exercises:

1. Upper trapezius and levator scapulae. To stretch the right levator scapulae muscle the patient sits and looks forward and to the left with her head tilted to the left. Her left hand may be placed on the top of her head to support the head and neck but she should be cautioned not to pull forcefully with the hand as this could cause an overstrain of the joints of the cervical spine. The patient grasps the edge of the seat with her right hand and leans to the left and slightly forward, giving a passive stretch of the levator scapulae (Fig. 14.8). To isolate the upper trapezius

Fig. 14.8 Self stretch of the right levator scapulae.

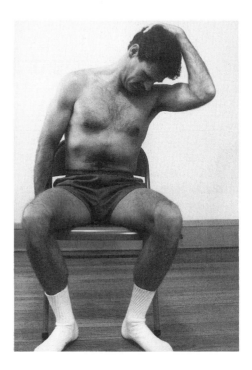

muscle selectively the head is bent to the left and slightly forwards but rotated to the right. Leaning to the left while grasping the edge of the seat with the right hand will stretch the trapezius passively (Fig. 14.9).

2. Pectoralis minor and sternal fibres of P. major. The patient stands facing the wall with the left shoulder abducted to 90° and the palm of her left hand placed against the wall with the elbow slightly bent. The patient then turns her feet to the right to be parallel to the wall while keeping her left shoulder down and back. She presses against the wall with her right hand to turn the upper trunk to the right. Most of the stretch should be felt in the pectorals and anterior shoulder and perhaps the biceps. The stretch may be static or with a series of contract/relax cycles (Fig. 14.10).

3. Latissimus dorsi. Acting with the teres major, the latissimus extends, adducts and internally rotates the humerus. Particularly when tight bilaterally, the latissimus dorsi can restrict extension throughout the thoracic

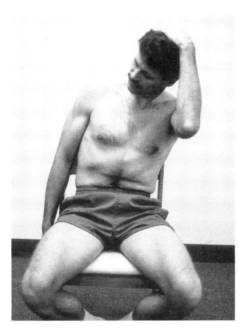

Fig. 14.9 Self stretch of the right upper trapezius.

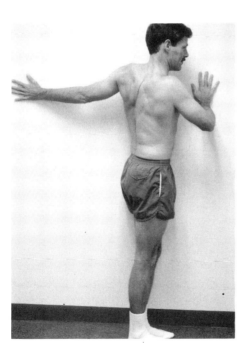

Fig. 14.10 Patient attempting left anterior shoulder stretch. Note patient's inability to correctly depress the left scapula during the stretch.

spine and can therefore have a profound effect on head and neck posture as well as limiting shoulder flexion.

The stretch is done with the patient kneeling with hands and elbows held together and supported on a chair or stool. By sitting back on the haunches elongation is obtained through the thoracic and lumbar areas, straightening the spine as much as possible. To promote external rotation of the shoulders the hands and elbows should be held together throughout the stretch. By moving the pelvis into a posterior tilt, a more selective stretch can be put on the latissimus dorsi (Fig. 14.11). The exercise is best done as a continual movement towards elongation, held for 20–30 seconds and repeated two to three times.

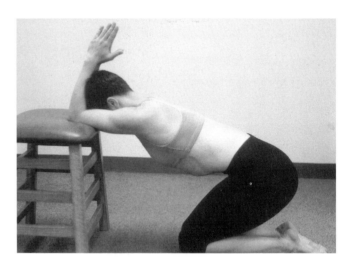

Fig. 14.11 Latissimus dorsi stretch in kneeling.

Upper quarter treatment, retraining

Exercises for strengthening weakened muscles are performed after addressing the tightness found in the antagonistic musculature. In our clinical experience we have found, as reported by Janda, greater success by stretching the tight and shortened muscles prior to attempting strengthening of a weakened muscle group. A shortened and tight muscle appears to be over activated in various movement patterns, and this activation may be so intense that it makes the strengthening exercise of a weakened muscle impossible due to the reflex inhibition[1]. The exercises used for retraining are often simply a modification of the testing procedures mentioned earlier and include the following.

   1. *Deep neck flexors*. Activation of these muscles is first attempted in sitting, asking the patient to nod the chin toward the chest without participation of the superficial neck flexors (Fig. 14.12). The patient should feel a slight stretch in the posterior occipitoatlantal region. The position is held for 5–10 seconds and is repeated five to six times. Once this movement is well controlled, the patient can attempt more aggressive strengthening in the supine (anti-gravity) position, again emphasising smooth cervical spine flexion (see Fig. 14.2).

   2. *Lower trapezius*. Retraining to facilitate the lower trapezius can be done in prone lying with various angles of shoulder abduction. Emphasis is placed on the patient learning to move the scapula medially and inferiorly to activate the lower trapezius (Fig. 14.13).

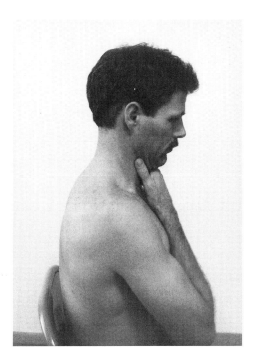

Fig. 14.12 Re-education of the deep neck flexors. Palpation of superficial neck flexors to ensure that they remain relaxed.

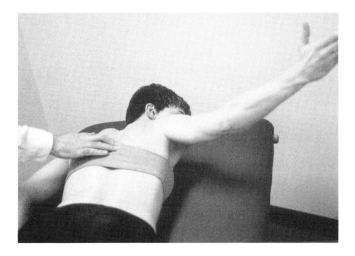

Fig. 14.13 Retraining of the lower trapezius.

3. Serratus anterior. The patient is on hands and knees with elbows bent enough so that her shoulders and hips are at the same height. The thoracic spine is straight and the scapulae are stabilised against the rib cage. Once this is done successfully she is asked to lift one hand off the floor while keeping her shoulders level and avoiding winging of the scapula on the supporting side (Fig. 14.14). The position is held for approximately 10 seconds and repeated five to six times.

Fig. 14.14 Retraining of the right serratus anterior.

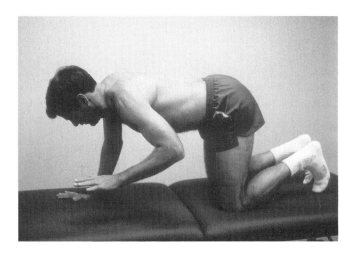

4. Shoulder abduction. Before this exercise is attempted the patient must be able to activate the lower trapezius when prone. She lies supine with her knees bent, her feet flat and her arms at her sides, externally rotated. Bilateral shoulder abduction is initiated while she stabilises the medial border of the scapula in retraction and depression. The patient maintains a posterior pelvic tilt with the lumbar spine flat and should only abduct the arms as far as is possible without elevating the shoulder girdle or losing the contact of the dorsum of the hands with the floor (Fig. 14.15). Once the full range of abduction is achieved supine, the same exercise can be repeated sitting.

Lower quarter

Janda[1] has also identified a common pattern of muscle imbalances which occur in the lower quarter with the hyperactive postural muscles being

Fig. 14.15 Retraining for shoulder abduction when supine. Note the elevation of the left shoulder girdle complex indicating an abnormal movement pattern which must be avoided during the retraining process.

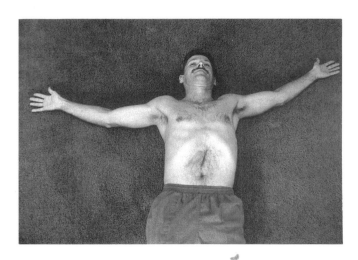

the iliopsoas, rectus femoris, tensor fasciae latae, quadratus lumborum, the thigh adductors, piriformis, the hamstrings and the lumbar erector spinae musculature.

The muscle groups showing a tendency towards inhibition and reflex weakness include the gluteus maximus, medius, and minimus and the rectus abdominis, as well as the external and internal obliques.

Janda refers to a 'lower crossed syndrome' characterised by imbalances between the shortened and tight hip flexors and lumbar erector spinae musculature and the weakened gluteus maximus and abdominal muscles. This imbalance has deleterious effects on the lumbar spine during gait since hip extension will not be performed by an inhibited gluteus maximus and the movement is taken over by the lumbar erector spinae. This in turn causes hyperlordosis and hypermobility in the lumbar spine in the sagittal plane, with strain on the intervertebral discs and ligaments[3].

In the frontal plane an imbalance develops between the weakened gluteus medius and minimus and the tight tensor fasciae latae and quadratus lumborum muscles creating excessive sway in the pelvis during walking[3].

Lower quarter evaluation

To evaluate for muscle imbalances in the lower quarter, the following tests may be used.

1. Iliopsoas. The patient is supine with her hips at the edge (end) of the table. One knee is drawn to the chest to flatten the lumbar spine and the other leg is allowed to hang freely. Assessment is made of the length of the iliopsoas.

By observing if there is 90° of knee flexion the length of the rectus femoris is assessed and by observing whether there is adduction or abduction, the relative tightness of the adductors or tensor fasciae latae are assessed respectively (Fig. 14.16)[4].

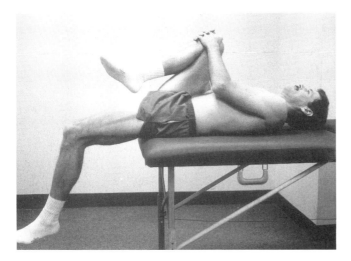

Fig. 14.16 Left iliopsoas length test. Note the visible tightness of the left iliotibial band.

2. Hip extension (gluteus maximus). The patient is prone with her knee straight and she is asked to extend the hip actively. By both vision and palpation the 'firing pattern' of the muscles involved in this movement is observed. The correct order is ipsilateral hamstrings first, then gluteus maximus, contralateral erector spinae and, last, ipsilateral erector spinae[5]. Failure to activate the gluteus maximus may be noted, with a substitution pattern by the hamstrings and erector spinae musculature. This substitution pattern may be strong enough to produce active hip extension with little weakness noted on manual muscle testing. Chronic hamstring tightness may be a response to the substitution pattern for gluteus maximus weakness on that side and will continue to be perpetuated unless this muscle imbalance is corrected. Also to be noted in this test is the tendency for the lower thoracic and upper lumbar spine to rotate towards the contralateral side when the gluteus maximus fails to participate in active extension of the hip and the pelvis is not adequately stabilised (Fig. 14.17).

Fig. 14.17 Abnormal left hip extension firing pattern. Note the hypertonicity of the right thoracolumbar erector spinae and rotation of the thoracolumbar junction to the right.

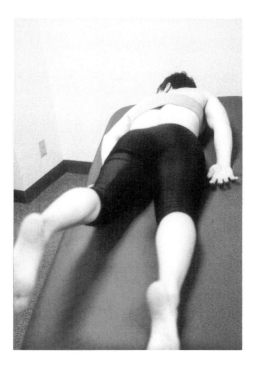

3. Pelvic tilt/heel slide (abdominals). The patient is supine with her knees bent and feet flat on the table and is asked to flatten her low lumbar spine by doing a posterior pelvic tilt. With her back remaining flat the patient is asked to slide one foot along the table and, if this is performed easily, to slide both feet. This assesses the ability of the abdominals to maintain a posterior pelvic tilt while the iliopsoas muscles are activated (Fig. 14.18).

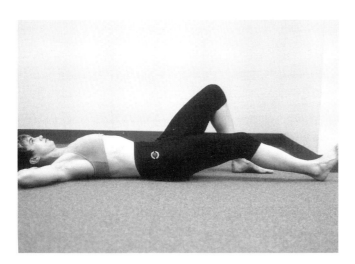

Fig. 14.18 Pelvic tilt/heel slide.

4. Hip abduction (gluteus medius and minimus). The patient lies on her side with her under leg flexed and her upper leg extended. The examiner observes and palpates the firing pattern in the gluteus medius and the tensor fasciae latae while the patient is asked to abduct the upper leg. A common substitution pattern is for the tensor to initiate the movement when the gluteus medius is weak; this produces flexion and internal rotation of the hip during active hip abduction.

5. Straight leg raising (hamstrings). A straight leg raise with the hip in external rotation and abduction tests the length of the medial hamstrings while a straight leg raise with the hip in internal rotation and adduction tests the length of the lateral hamstrings. It is important to monitor for pelvic rotation since an additional 10–15° range of straight leg raising occurs when posterior rotation of the pelvis is allowed. The operator palpates with one hand on the contralateral

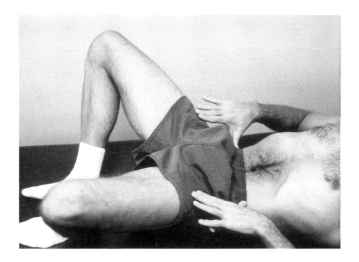

Fig. 14.19 Hip adductor length test.

ASIS to monitor for recruitment of posterior pelvic rotation during straight leg raising, assessing both the medial and lateral hamstrings of each leg.

6. Hip adductors. The patient is supine with her knees bent and feet flat on the table (or floor) and performs a posterior pelvic tilt. She then allows her knees to abduct while the pelvic tilt is maintained (Fig. 14.19). If there is an imbalance on one side, with weak abdominal muscles and tight adductors the posterior pelvic tilt cannot be maintained and the pelvis will rotate anteriorly on that side.

Lower quarter treatment, stretching

Once again the tight muscles are stretched before initiation of any strengthening or movement reeducation programme.

The following muscle groups are commonly tight and can be treated either by sustained stretch for 20–30 seconds repeated two to three times, or by post-isometric relaxation techniques, contracting the muscle against resistance for 5–7 seconds before relaxation and engagement of a new motion barrier.

1. Iliopsoas. The iliopsoas can be lengthened by a supine stretch in the previously described stretch position as in Fig. 14.16, or with a more dynamic exercise in half kneeling which requires active rather than passive stabilisation and recruitment of the gluteus maximus and hamstring musculature as illustrated in Fig. 14.20. In the half kneeling

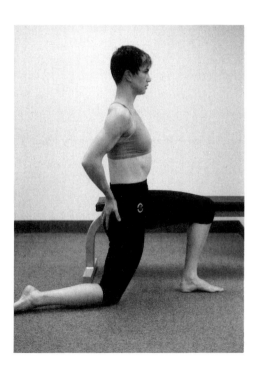

Fig. 14.20 Self stretch of the right iliopsoas muscle in half kneeling.

exercise the side to be stretched is positioned with internal rotation and extension of the hip. There is active contraction of the gluteus maximus muscle on the ipsilateral side and the hamstring muscles on the contralateral side to stabilise and rotate the pelvis posteriorly during the stretch. Restriction in extensibility of the iliopsoas muscle can prevent lumbar spine mobility in all directions and typically needs to be addressed in almost every low back pain patient.

2. Rectus femoris. The rectus femoris muscle can be stretched with the patient in standing. The knee is flexed so that the foot on that side is supported on the back of a chair placed behind the patient. The pelvis is rotated posteriorly and the patient sits back towards the heel maintaining the pelvic tilt and allowing the opposite knee to flex. This stretch is ideal as it teaches dynamic control of the pelvis while isolating the stretch to the rectus femoris specifically (Fig. 14.21).

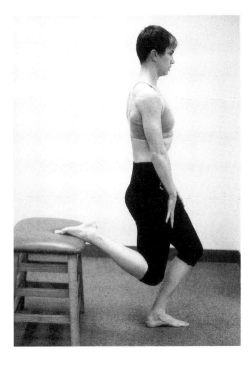

Fig. 14.21 Rectus femoris stretch in standing.

3. Hip adductors. These can be stretched in sitting with neutral lumbar spinal mechanics as in Fig. 14.22 or by a stretch in the supine position described for testing (Fig. 14.19). Both exercises are designed to address the hip adductors specifically while maintaining a neutral lumbar spine and controlling the pelvis dynamically by muscle action, especially of the abdominals.

4. Quadratus lumborum. The stretch is done with the patient on her side with her back at the edge of the table or bed and the muscle to be

Fig. 14.22 Hip adductor stretch in sitting.

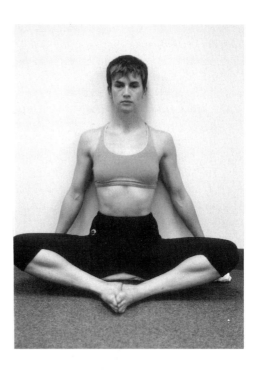

Fig. 14.23 Right quadratus lumborum stretch.

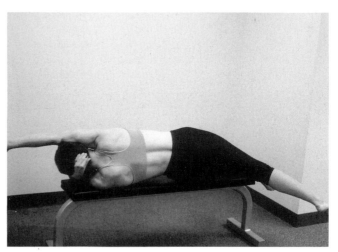

stretched uppermost. The ipsilateral (top) arm is fully abducted overhead and the hip is extended and adducted off the side of the table or bed (Fig. 14.23). A sustained stretch for 20–30 seconds repeated two to three times is recommended.

5. Piriformis. This muscle arises from the anterior surface of sacral segments 2, 3 and 4 and attaches to the greater trochanter of the femur. From extension to 60° of hip flexion the piriformis acts as an external rotator and abductor of the hip. Beyond 60° of hip flexion it still acts as an abductor but is now an internal rotator[6]. Balancing the pull of the piriformis on the sacrum is believed to be important when treating sacroiliac joint dysfunction. Since the muscle has two distinctly different actions, there is no singular exercise which adequately addresses this muscle. Two stretches which are believed to address length restrictions of the piriformis are the 'buttock stretch' and the supine hip rotation stretch. The buttock stretch is described in Chapter 15 for self mobilisation for forward sacral torsion (see Fig. 15.14). The supine hip rotation stretch operates when the muscle is acting as an abductor and external rotator. For the right piriformis the patient is supine and the right hip flexed to less than 60°. The right hip is adducted to place the foot on the lateral side of the left leg. The patient grasps her right knee with her left hand and adducts and medially rotates her right hip. By a series of isometric contract/relax cycles the hip is brought progressively into further adduction and internal rotation (Fig. 14.24).

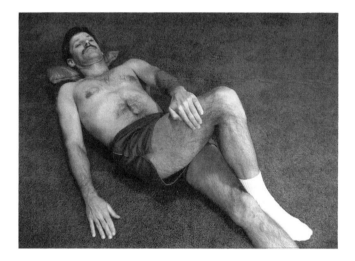

Fig. 14.24 Supine stretch for the right piriformis.

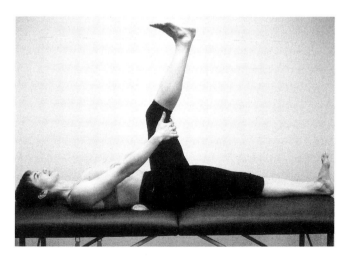

Fig. 14.25 Supine stretch for the right hamstrings.

6. *Hamstrings*. The patient is supine with a small towel roll supporting her lumbar spine. The hip on the side to be stretched is flexed to 90° and held there by the patient clasping her hands behind the thigh. The other leg is held straight actively. The stretch is performed by active quadriceps contraction with the foot dorsiflexed as in the instruction 'reach toward the ceiling with your heel' (Fig. 14.25). The stretch is held for 5–10 seconds and repeated five to six times.

Lower quarter treatment, retraining

Patients with low back pain are commonly found to have weakness of the gluteus maximus, medius and minimus muscles. In addition there is a controversial role for the abdominal musculature in prevention of low back pain. Exercises are described for these muscles specifically in the hope of decreasing the biomechanical stresses placed on the lumbar spine and pelvis.

1. *Gluteus maximus*. Weakness of the gluteus maximus is seen clinically in patients with sacroiliac joint dysfunction; it may be inhibited by reflex mechanisms and/or by a tight or shortened iliopsoas muscle. The iliopsoas should be stretched before attempting to strengthen the gluteus maximus. Strengthening exercises are done in the prone position after careful analysis of the hip extension muscle firing pattern (Fig. 14.26).

Fig. 14.26 Analysis of left hip extension firing pattern.

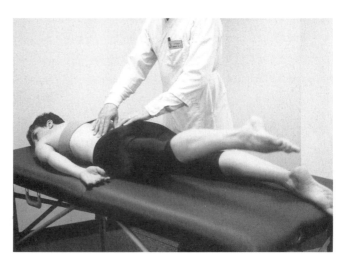

Many patients fail to recruit the gluteus maximus in active hip extension, substituting with the lumbar erector spinae and the hamstring musculature; if this is not recognised the patient may be given an exercise that only reinforces the dysfunctional substitution pattern.

The initial exercise emphasises active recruitment of the gluteus maximus without activation of the lumbar erector spinae (Fig. 14.27a).

Lying prone, with the foot on the ipsilateral side dorsiflexed and resting on the toes, the hip and knee are extended by a strong gluteus maximus contraction. As muscle tone improves, the exercise can be made more challenging by plantar flexing the foot while holding the extended leg off the resting surface for a count of 5–10 seconds (Fig. 14.27b). The leg is then slowly lowered to the floor and the exercise is repeated with the opposite leg.

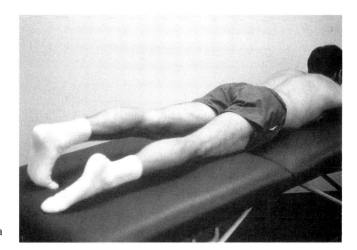

a

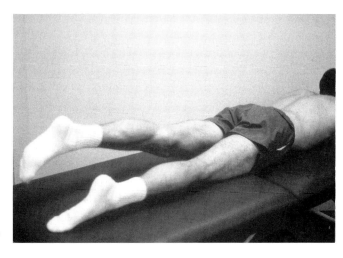

b

Fig. 14.27 (a) Initial exercise for activation of the left gluteus maximus. (b) Progression of left gluteus maximus strengthening.

Once the patient knows how to recruit the gluteus maximus properly, a bridging exercise may be added. The patient is supine with her knees flexed and feet flat on the table (or floor). She performs a posterior pelvic tilt and lifts her buttocks off the table by a strong gluteus maximus contraction, being careful to avoid lumbar spine extension (Fig. 14.28). Initially with this exercise cramping of the hamstrings may occur due to

Fig. 14.28 Supine bridging.

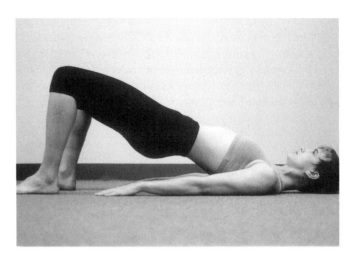

over facilitation (substitution) for lack of active hip extension by the gluteus maximus. Once the gluteus maximus is properly activated cramping of the hamstrings with the bridging exercise ceases.

2. Gluteus medius and minimus. The patient is in side lying with the dysfunctional side uppermost, with emphasis on maintaining a neutral lumbar spine. The leg is abducted, attempting to avoid substitution by the tensor fasciae latae; it may be an advantage to stretch the tensor fasciae latae first.

3. Abdominals. Strengthening exercises for the abdominal muscles include curl-ups which focus on the rectus abdominis and supine leg slides with a posterior pelvic tilt which, according to Kendall[7], can be used to focus more on specific strengthening of the external oblique musculature. The exercises are described as follows.

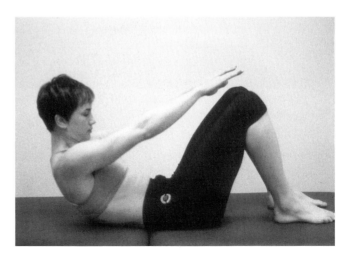

Fig. 14.29 Abdominal curl-ups.

(a) Curl-ups. The patient is supine with the pelvis tilted posteriorly to flatten the low back on the table. With the arms extended forward, the head and shoulders are raised from the table to clear the scapulae (Fig. 14.29). The position is held for 5–10 seconds and repeated five to six times.

(b) Supine leg slides with posterior pelvic tilt. The patient is supine with knees bent and feet flat on the table and the hands are beside her head. She performs a posterior pelvic tilt, to flatten her low back, by pulling up and in with the muscles in the lower abdomen. The low back is held flat against the table and she then slides one leg down to extend the knee and hip as far as possible without losing the posterior pelvic tilt. The leg is brought back up to the starting position, again maintaining a flat back (see Fig. 14.18). The procedure is then repeated with the opposite leg.

Emphasis has been placed on evaluation for restrictions in muscle length, assessment of muscle strength, and observation for faulty movement patterns. Although the role of muscle in the production of pain remains controversial, and the question remains as to whether the joint or the soft tissues need to be addressed first, the truly well-rounded practioner should have the tools to treat all of these parts to the puzzle.

REFERENCES

1. Janda V. (1980). Muscles as a pathogenic factor in back pain. In *The Treatment of Patients,* Proceedings IFOMT 4th Conference, pp.1–23.; Christchurch, N.Z.
2. Janda V. (1977). Muscles, central nervous motor regulation and back problems. In *The Neurobiologic Mechanisms in Manipulative Therapy.* pp. 27–41. Korr I. (ed.), New York: Plenum Press.
3. Lewit K. (1975). *Manipulative Therapy in Rehabilitation of the Motor System.* London: Butterworth.
4. Janda V. (1983). *Muscle Function Testing.* London: Butterworth.
5. Janda V. (1983). In an address to the North American Academy of Manipulative Medicine, Alexandria, Virginia.
6. Kapandji I.A. (1970). *The Physiology of the Joints,* vol II, p.68.; Edinburgh: Churchill Livingstone.
7. Kendall F.P., McCreary E.K. (1983). *Muscle Testing and Function* (3rd edn), Baltimore: Williams and Wilkins.

Chapter 15

Exercises as a complement to manual therapy

This, like Chapter 14, is an entirely new addition to the previously published editions of *Spinal Manipulation*. The authors have learned over the years that exercise not only helps to improve aerobic capacity and cardiovascular function and assists in stress reduction, but can and should be used as an adjunct to manual therapy intervention. Generalised exercise programmes have their place in overall conditioning, but more specific exercises are thought to promote patient self management for some of the chronic and recurring dysfunctions previously discussed in this book.

An understanding of the functional anatomy and biomechanics of the spine is essential to the development of an individualised specific home exercise programme. Positional diagnosis of spinal dysfunction forms the basis for the selection of the specific self mobilising exercises described in this chapter and delineates which movements need to be restored (Table 15.1). Failure to assess and treat adequately the biomechanical dysfunctions of the vertebral column and pelvis prior to the initiation of an exercise programme may be one of the main reasons why some patients find an exercise programme pain provoking.

Controversy still exists as to what tissue(s) serve as the restrictors of segmental mobility. Theories have been advanced describing meniscal entrapment[1], joint capsule adhesions[2], and hypertonicity in the deep spinal musculature due to abnormal afferent activity[3]. In theory any of these restrictors could limit single segment mobility. Lewit believes the most frequent cause of the restriction, which he calls joint blockage, is faulty movement patterns due to muscle imbalances and postural overstrain[4]. Theoretically then, correction of muscle imbalances through a specific home exercise programme may prevent faulty movement patterns and therefore prevent further segmental joint dysfunction (see Chapter 14). This concept served as the basis for the exercises selected in the previous chapter.

Table 15.1 Positional diagnosis versus motion restriction

Positional diagnosis	Motion restriction
Flexed	Extension
Extended	Flexion
Right sidebent	Left sidebending
Right rotated	Left rotation

The exercises described in this chapter are designed as self-mobilising exercises to complement manual therapy treatment for specific joint dysfunctions found in the spinal column and pelvis. The exercises are presented by region even though many will have multiregional implications.

LUMBAR SPINE

The design of the lumbar spine primarily allows motion in the sagittal plane, i.e. flexion and extension. Most exercise programmes for patients with low back pain have advocated restoration of either flexion (Williams[5]) or extension (McKenzie[6]) movements as their major emphasis. McKenzie also advocates the use of side gliding (translation) manoeuvres in select patients as a component in lumbar spine self treatment and should be credited with recognising the importance of self-mobilising exercises in the treatment of low back pain. The reader is referred to McKenzie's book, *The Lumbar Spine – Mechanical diagnosis and therapy*, for further information regarding his specific home exercise approach. Several years ago one of the authors (MRB) noted the biomechanical similarities between McKenzie's approach to a patient with a lumbar scoliosis and lateral shift and the osteopathic muscle energy approach to a patient with an FRS lumbar dysfunction, i.e. McKenzie would treat the patient presenting with an acute right lateral shift and lumbar kyphosis with shift correcting movements (left side gliding in standing) and prone press-ups (for extension) (Figs 15.1 and 15.2). From the osteopathic standpoint, this same patient would most likely be manually treated for an FRS right by

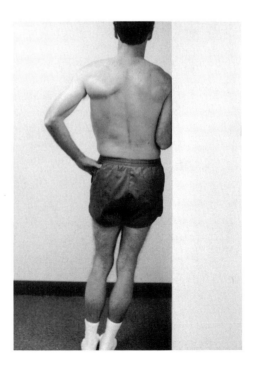

Fig. 15.1 Left side gliding in standing.

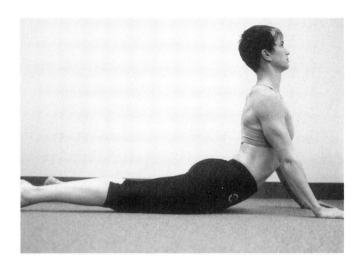

Fig. 15.2 Prone press-ups for lumbar spine extension.

utilising a muscle energy technique that incorporates left side bending and left rotation coupled with lumbar spine extension. The McKenzie approach (standing side gliding coupled with prone press-ups) thus could be used as part of the home exercise programme for patients treated manually for lumbar spine FRS dysfunctions. The challenge is to develop other specific exercises to complement manual therapy for the various spinal and pelvic dysfunctions.

EXERCISES FOR LUMBAR SPINE DYSFUNCTION

For FRS dysfunctions

Extension and side bending
In a lumbar *FRS* right dysfunction the positional diagnosis is *flexed*, right *rotated* and right *sidebent*. Therefore the motion loss is of extension, left rotation and left side bending at that spinal segment. Exercises for this dysfunction include standing side gliding performed against a wall (Fig. 15.1), and performed facing a wall which allows the patient to introduce as much extension as is tolerated before performing the side glide (Fig. 15.3). The extension component can be addressed separately by standing backward bending (Fig. 15.4), by the prone press-ups or when sitting (Fig. 15.5), allowing the exercise to be carried out easily at work or at home.

Rotation
The muscle energy and McKenzie type of exercises address the flexion/extension and side bending components assuming that the rotation will follow as a coupled movement. To address the rotation specifically, one of the authors (MRB) uses other exercises both for self mobilisation by the patient and for neuromuscular re-education, particularly of the deep spinal rotators and the abdominal oblique muscles. Both are performed with the patient supine.

Fig. 15.3 Left side glide in standing facing the wall.

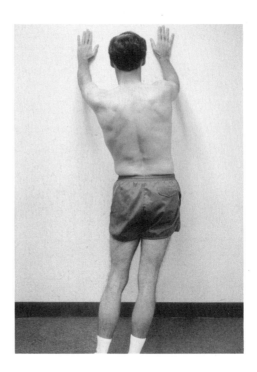

Fig. 15.4 Backward bending in standing.

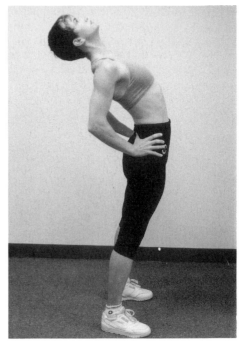

1. For restoration of rotation through the hips, pelvis and lumbar spine. The supine patient crosses one flexed leg over the other and then rotates the legs and pelvis towards the side of the upper (anterior) leg (Fig. 15.6).

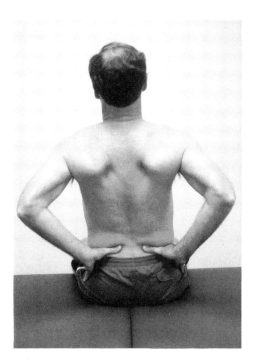

Fig. 15.5 Self mobilising for lumbar spine extension in sitting.

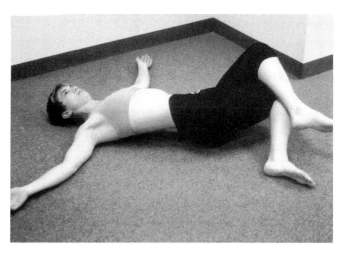

Fig. 15.6 Self mobilisation exercise to restore right rotation through the lumbar spine.

The position is maintained as a static stretch for 20–30 seconds and repeated two to three times to each side.

2. For restoration of rotational control by the spinal and abdominal muscles. The patient is supine with her knees flexed and feet flat on the floor. The legs are dropped first to one side and then the other but when bringing them back to the starting position, the patient tries to bring each spinal segment in turn back to the floor, from craniad to caudad. The purpose is to re-educate the deep rotators of the spine and the

Fig. 15.7 Strengthening exercise for lumbar spine rotation.

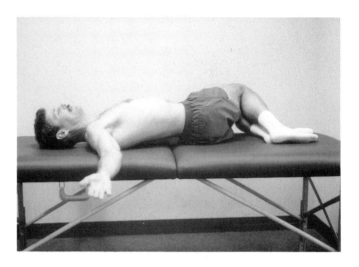

oblique abdominal muscles so that control of rotational movement occurs through the trunk rather than through the hips and lower extremities (Fig. 15.7).

For ERS dysfunctions
With a lumbar *ERS* right dysfunction the positional diagnosis is *e*xtended, right *r*otated and right *s*idebent so that the motion loss is of flexion, left rotation and left side bending.

To restore flexion:

1. Single knee to chest, supine.
2. Bilateral knee to chest, supine.
3. 'Prayer stretch' from hands and knees position (Fig. 15.8).

To restore flexion, rotation and side bending together:

1. Diagonal 'hip sink' movements from the hands and knees position with the right hip directed towards the outside of the right ankle to elongate the right side of the spine and open the facet joints (Fig. 15.9).

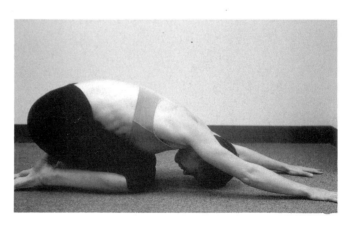

Fig. 15.8 Prayer stretch.

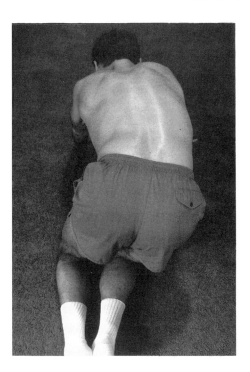

Fig. 15.9 Diagonal hip sink to the right.

2. Forward bending in left step standing as advocated by McKenzie. The patient stands with the left foot up on a chair or stool and places both hands around her left knee. She then slides her hands down her leg to the ankle and rests the middle of her chest on her knee. The stretch is maintained for 5–10 seconds and she then brings her trunk back to the upright position. The stretch is repeated five to six times (Fig. 15.10).

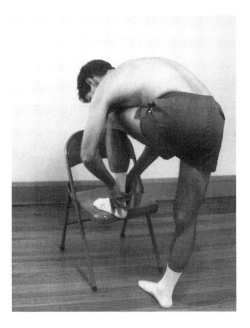

Fig. 15.10 Forward bending in left step standing.

For the long restrictors

Multisegment muscles may also be tight and need to be treated. This is particularly true in the presence of group (type I) dysfunctions where the primary restriction is of side bending. The most important long restrictor muscles in the lumbar region are the erector spinae, the quadratus lumborum and the iliopsoas. These can be screened for tightness by observing for a loss of the smooth symmetrical curve during active sidebending of the spine in standing or by the muscle length tests described in Chapter 14.

Exercises to stretch these three muscles were described in Chapter 14.

A non specific exercise to improve lumbar side bending is the Feldenkrais 'elongation in sitting'. To stretch the whole right side the seated patient lifts her left buttock, shifting her weight to the right ischial tuberosity, at the same time raising her right arm. This is repeated several times in a rhythmical rocking motion (Fig. 15.11).

Fig. 15.11 Elongation in sitting to the right.

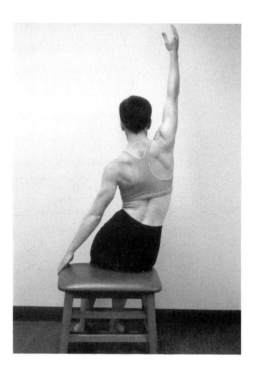

The 'pelvic clock'

This exercise, originally learned from a Feldenkrais practitioner, is useful both for self mobilisation and for neuromuscular re-education for the pelvis as well as the lumbar spine and also has value in diagnosis.

The patient is supine with her knees flexed and is instructed to visualise movements of the pelvis as though taking place on an imaginary clock (Fig. 15.12). Movement towards 6:00 creates lumbar spine extension whereas movement towards 12:00 creates lumbar flexion. Movements across the clock from 3:00 to 9:00 and from 9:00 to 3:00 promote

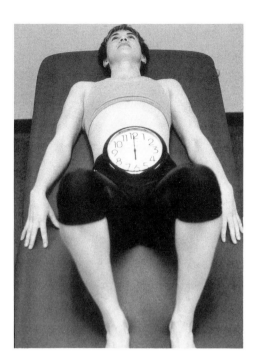

Fig. 15.12 Pelvic clock.

rotation. When the patient is asked to move through each point selectively around the face of the clock, three-dimensional motion takes place, i.e. from 3:00 to 6:00 promoting extension, right side bending and right rotation of the lumbar spine. This particular movement is characteristically restricted if there is a residual FRS left lumbar spine dysfunction present. When a patient can perform a symmetrical full circle pelvic clock both in a clockwise and counter-clockwise direction, then the lumbar spine is fairly clear of any non-neutral (type II) dysfunctions.

Pelvis

Pubic symphysis dysfunctions
The superior and inferior pubis dysfunctions were described and the specific treatment detailed in Chapters 4 and 7.

The symphysis is stabilised by strong ligaments and balanced by muscular attachments from above and below. The superior muscle attachments to the crest and symphysis are the abdominal wall muscles, rectus and transversus abdominis and the internal and external obliques. The inferior attachments to the pubic ramus include the adductors magnus, longus and brevis and the gracilis. Imbalance between these two groups can influence and perpetuate symphysis dysfunction. Treatment for these groups has been described in Chapter 14.

A self-mobilising exercise is similar to the 'blunderbuss' treatment described in Chapter 7. The patient is supine with her knees bent and her feet flat on the floor with the knees separated by at least 15 cm (6 inches) apart by an incompressible object. The patient makes a firm effort

Fig. 15.13 Self correction for pubic dysfunction.

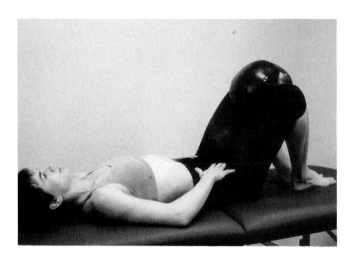

to bring her knees together (Fig. 15.13). The bilateral symmetrical action of the hip adductor muscles disengages the symphysis slightly, allowing correction to occur. This exercise should be followed by appropriate exercises to balance the abdominal and hip adductor musculature (see Chapter 14).

Sacroiliac dysfunctions

The stability of the sacroiliac joint is largely provided by the posterior sacroiliac, sacrospinous and sacrotuberous ligaments. The muscular control is still poorly understood but appears to be important in the overall function and stability of the pelvis. The muscle groups that appear clinically to have the most influence, directly or indirectly, on sacroiliac joint function are the piriformis, the iliacus, the glutei (maximus, medius and minimus) and the lumbar erector spinae all of which have been addressed in Chapter 14.

Four primary dysfunctions of sacral mechanics were described in Chapter 4. These are, on the one hand, anterior sacral torsion and anterior nutation (unilateral sacral flexion) in both of which the major restriction is of posterior nutation of the sacral base, and on the other hand, posterior sacral torsion and posterior nutation (unilateral sacral extension) in which the major restriction is of anterior nutation of the sacral base. In all four the restriction is of anterior or posterior translation of the sacral base on the ilium and these are the movements that the self mobilising exercises will concentrate on attempting to restore.

For correction of a forward translated sacral base

1. Buttock stretch. The patient is in the hands and knees position with the leg on the dysfunctional side externally rotated, flexed, adducted and tucked underneath. The opposite leg slides directly backward while maintaining a level pelvis and a straight spine. The stretch should be felt in the buttocks or posterior thigh. This position stretches the piriformis on that side, as well as opening the posterior aspect of the sacroiliac joint

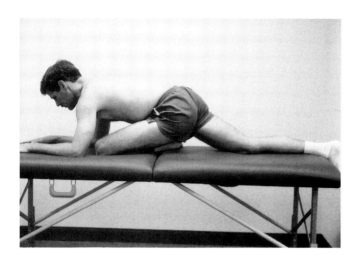

Fig. 15.14 Buttocks stretch for left piriformis.

and induces slight flexion of L5 which encourages the sacrum to nutate posteriorly (Fig. 15.14).

2. Flexion exercises for the lumbar spine for ERS dysfunction as described above.

For correction of a backward translation of the sacral base
1. The patient is prone. For restriction of anterior nutational movement of the right sacral base, the right leg is abducted slightly and externally rotated to loose pack the right sacroiliac joint and open its anterior aspect. The left leg is dropped off the table and flexed at the hip and knee with the foot on the floor so that the left side of the pelvis is stabilised by posterior rotation of the left ilium (Fig. 15.15). The instruction is then to perform a prone press-up while maintaining a relaxed lumbar spine and pelvis. By the selective positioning of the pelvis, the press-up should encourage anterior nutation movement of the right sacral base.

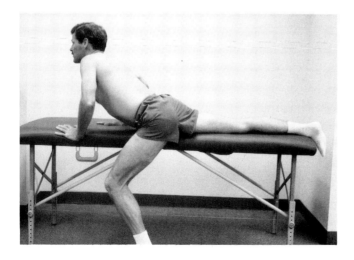

Fig. 15.15 Self mobilisation to correct a posteriorly nutated right sacral base.

2. Extension exercises (prone press-ups) for lumbar spine FRS dysfunctions in the presence of a backward translated sacral base are often painful and clinically do not seem to be effective unless manual therapy has previously been directed to the sacroiliac joint for correction.

Iliosacral dysfunctions
In this text the innominate bone is considered as part of the lower extremity and it is felt that imbalances of muscle length and strength in the lower limbs need to be addressed as they will have a significant influence on iliosacral dysfunctions.

1. Anterior innominate correction. The patient is supine and rotates the innominate posteriorly by bringing the hip on the dysfunctional side into flexion, slight abduction and external rotation using both hands across her knee. She is instructed to contract her gluteus maximus by trying to extend the hip against the resistance of her hands for 5–7 seconds. After each contraction the leg is brought into further flexion, slight abduction and external rotation. This isometric exercise is repeated three to four times (Fig. 15.16).

Fig. 15.16 Correction of a right anteriorly rotated innominate.

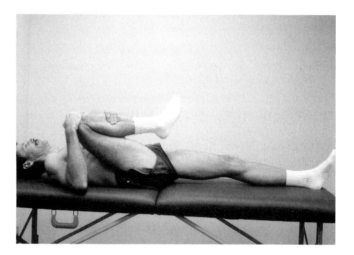

2. Posterior innominate correction. The patient is supine and drops the leg on the dysfunctional side off the table while the opposite lower extremity is held in flexion and posterior rotation with both hands. A series of isotonic contractions of the gluteus maximus on the involved side are made and held for 5–7 seconds to promote correction (Fig. 15.17).

Thoracic spine

Just as lumbar spinal mechanics are influenced by the lower extremities, the thoracic spine is influenced by the upper extremities. For example, in the presence of bilateral shortening of the latissimus dorsi the thoracic

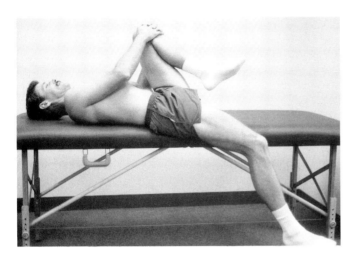

Fig. 15.17 Correction of a right posteriorly rotated innominate.

spine will be in a posture of exaggerated kyphosis which predisposes to FRS dysfunctions. The home exercise programme will need to include both self mobilising spinal exercises and those that address muscular imbalances in the upper quarter as described in Chapter 14.

For thoracic spinal dysfunction
Because multiple 'stacked' ERS and FRS dysfunctions are common in the thoracic spine an exercise to attempt to 'elongate' the spine may be helpful even before specific mobilisation. The standing wall stretch is a suitable exercise (Fig. 15.18).

The patient stands facing the wall with hands placed against the wall, starting at about shoulder height. The feet are positioned 3–4 feet away so that in the stretch position the arms are fully extended. The patient attempts to lengthen the spine by pressing the hips up and back and performing an anterior pelvic tilt. The stretch should be held for 30 seconds or longer and is repeated several times.

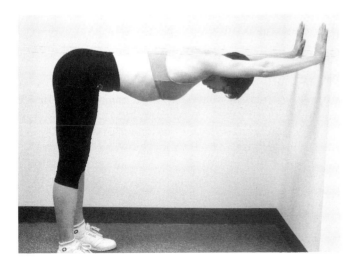

Fig. 15.18 Wall stretch for elongation of the spine and stretch of the posterior legs.

Extension

1. This can be localised to different areas of the spine in the hands and knees position by allowing the spine to sag and then rocking forwards or backwards. When maintaining the sag, rocking forward promotes extension lower in the spine; rocking backward promotes extension higher in the spine (Figs 15.19a and b).

Fig. 15.19 Extension of the spine in the hands and knees position. (a) Rocking forward to increase extension in the lower lumbar area; (b) rocking backward to increase extension in the lower thoracic spine.

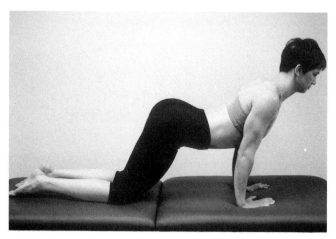

a

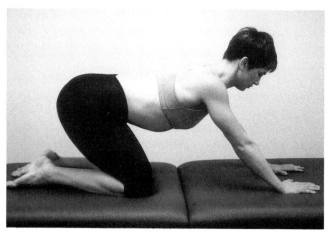

b

2. The patient is supine with knees and hips bent and the feet resting on a chair (Fig. 15.20). She holds on to the front legs of the chair and, during exhalation, presses down with her feet on the chair to extend through the hips and lumbar region up into the thoracic spine. At the same time she should retract her shoulders to increase the stretch in the anterior rib cage and sternum. A blanket folded under the shoulders may be needed to prevent loss of the normal cervical lordosis during the effort. The position is held for a few seconds and repeated four to five times[7]. This exercise serves not only to mobilise the thoracic spine for extension, but also helps to strengthen the erector spinae musculature to prevent recurrence of chronic FRS dysfunctions.

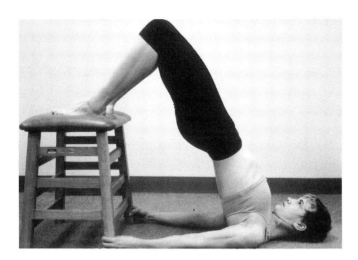

Fig. 15.20 Exercise to promote thoracic spine extension. This patient could benefit from a blanket folded under the shoulders to prevent loss of the normal cervical lordosis.

Flexion

1. ERS dysfunctions in the thoracic spine can be mobilised with a 'cat back' exercise in the hands and knees position and some specificity can be obtained by varying the hand position. The closer the hands are to the knees the higher the apex of the flexion motion induced in the spine (Fig. 15.21).

2. The wall press exercise described by Ward[8] is an excellent exercise to promote flexion in the upper thoracic spine for correction of ERS dysfunctions. It is also useful for neuromuscular re-education of scapular control, particularly in the presence of weakness of the serratus anterior and lower trapezius.

The patient stands facing the wall about 3 feet away with the hands placed on the wall at shoulder level. The scapulae are stabilised against the rib cage as the patient bends the elbows and leans forward to touch her nose to the wall without raising her heels from the floor. She then presses back, extending the elbows, and maximally flexes the cervical and

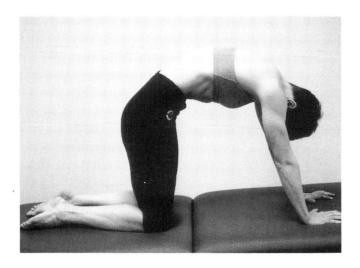

Fig. 15.21 Cat back exercise to increase thoracic spinal flexion. The closer the hands are to the knees, the higher the apex of the flexion induced in the thoracic spine.

Fig. 15.22 (a) The wall press exercise, starting position. (b) Maximal flexion is produced in the upper thoracic spine.

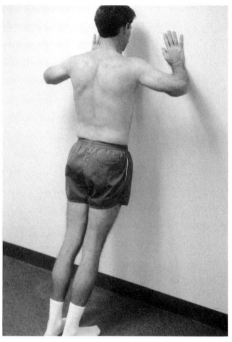

a

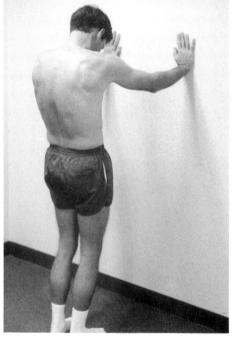

b

upper thoracic spine with the pelvis tucked under (posteriorly tilted) (Fig. 15.22a and b). The entire exercise is repeated four to five times, varying the hand position by placing them higher or lower before repeating the sequence.

Rotation

1. Supine. An exercise to promote rotation can be done supine as illustrated for the lumbar spine in Fig. 15.6.

2. Seated. Rotation in sitting can be performed working from below up to avoid strain on the cervical spine. To improve left rotation the patient sits sideways on a chair with her feet on the floor and the chair back to her left side. She grasps the chair back with both hands and initiates rotation from below up, turning to the left. Breathing is used to enhance the movement, inhalation producing lifting (elongation) and exhalation assisting the turn. A series of four to five gentle turns are performed making sure that the shoulders remain down throughout the turn (Fig. 15.23).

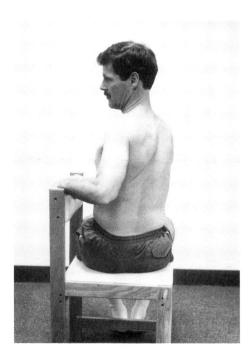

Fig. 15.23 Seated twist.

Cervical spine

Typical joints C2–7 (T1)
Because in these joints rotation and side bending are always coupled to the same side there are only four patterns of dysfunction to be considered. They may be flexed and left or right sidebent/rotated or extended and left or right sidebent/rotated.

For FRS dysfunctions
The patient is sitting and localises to the dysfunctional segment with the index finger contacting the articular pillar of the lower vertebra at the level to be mobilised. She uses a combined movement of extension, sidebending and rotation with her hand on the side to which the sidebending and rotation effort is to be made (Fig. 15.24).

Fig. 15.24 Self mobilisation for cervical spine FRS left dysfunction.

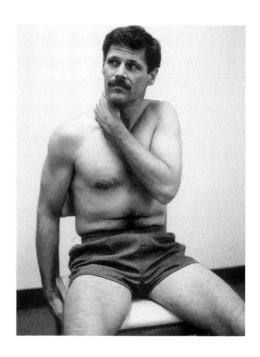

For ERS dysfunctions

The patient is sitting with an index finger on the articular pillar of the superior vertebra of the dysfunctional segment directing and guiding the combined movement of flexion, side bending and rotation with a passive stretch to open the dysfunctional facet joint (Fig. 15.25).

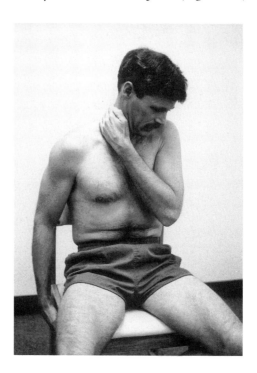

Fig. 15.25 Self mobilisation for cervical spine ERS right dysfunction.

For the long restrictors

When multiple ERS dysfunctions are found in the cervical spine one must be suspicious of long restrictor muscle tightness, particularly if the dysfunctions involve the upper three or four cervical spinal segments. The levator scapulae and the splenius cervicis both produce extension and ipsilateral rotation and side bending of the upper cervical spine and may be implicated when multiple cervical ERS dysfunctions exist. Stretching of the levator scapulae previously described in Chapter 14 and the self-mobilising exercise described above for ERS dysfunctions is also effective in lengthening the splenius cervicis.

Multiple FRS dysfunctions of the cervical spine may also implicate long restrictor involvement particularly of the longus colli muscle. This muscle is best stretched by placing the cervical spine in extension combined with rotation and side bending away from the tight side as was previously shown in Fig. 15.24.

Cervical 1–2

The primary motion is rotation and the exercise is easily performed with the patient sitting. The neck is fully flexed to bring the chin to the chest (to limit the available rotation in the lower joints) and the patient is then asked to rotate her head to whichever is the restricted side (Fig. 15.26). The rotation effort is repeated four to five times.

Occipitoatlantal joint

The primary motion is flexion and extension and a self-mobilising exercise can be done by flexing and extending the head on the neck (nodding), rather than moving the neck itself. This is the active

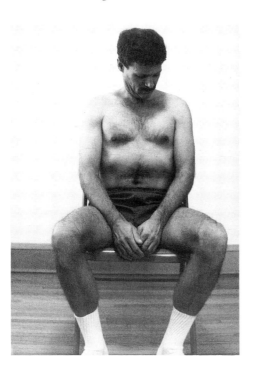

Fig. 15.26 Self mobilisation for rotation of the atlantoaxial joint to the left.

Fig. 15.27 Self mobilisation for the occipitoatlantal joints.

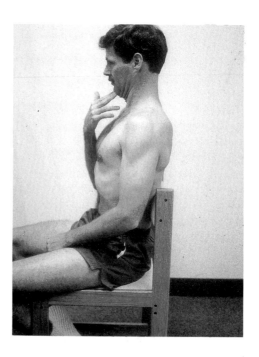

counterpart of the passive movement used in examination of this joint and involves rotation about an axis through the external auditory meatus (Fig. 15.27).

This exercise can be made more specific to one occipitoatlantal joint by rotating the head 30° towards the joint that is to be mobilised before performing the nodding (Fig. 15.28). The facets are set at about a 30° angle to the sagittal plane.

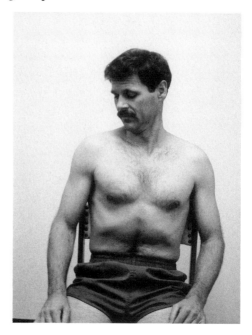

Fig. 15.28 Self mobilisation for the right occipitoatlantal joint.

The list of exercises included in this chapter is by no means exhaustive, but gives suggestions for more specific directions to patients who will take part in a home exercise programme. If the goal is for patients eventually to be capable of managing their own condition, it is essential for them to understand where their dysfunctions are, and how they can be addressed and controlled by exercises. This gives the patient responsibility for his or her own well being. Patient compliance seems to improve when the exercises are designed in a specific fashion.

It is hoped that this chapter will stimulate further interest in specificity of exercises for musculoskeletal problems.

REFERENCES

1. Bogduk N., Jull G. (1985). The theoretical pathology of acute locked back: A basis for manipulative therapy. *Manual Medicine;* **1**:78–82.
2. Stoddard A. (1961). *A Manual of Osteopathic Practice,* p.43. London: Hutchinson.
3. Korr I. (1977). Muscle spindle and the lesioned segment. *Proceedings: IFOMT.* Vail, Colo. **45**:53.
4. Lewit K. (1985). *Manipulative Therapy in Rehabilitation of the Motor System,* p.22; London: Butterworth.
5. Williams P.C. (1953). Conservative management of lesions of the lumbosacral spine. *Instruct. Lect. Amer. Acad. Orth. Surg.;* **10**:90–121.
6. McKenzie R.A. (1981). *The Lumbar Spine: Mechanical Diagnosis and Therapy.* Waikanae, N.Z.: Spinal Publications Ltd.
7. Tobias M., Stewart M. (1985). *Stretch and Relax,* p.45; Tucson: The Body Press.
8. Ward R. (1988). Myofascial Release Course Notes. East Lansing, Mi.

Chapter 16

Clinical observations

It is not easy to practice manual medicine well. The ability to sense blockage in joint movement comes very gradually. At first one despairs of ever being able to localise; as the ability to sense the reduced movement grows, there is another challenge to overcome, that is your lack of confidence that the diagnosis is correct. Once in practice, the instructor is no longer at your side to review your findings and for you to fall back on. The person before you is a patient who is unlikely to be forgiving if your venture into treatment simply results in more pain. The wisest approach is to use muscle energy techniques; indeed it is often the preferable way to manipulate at any time. Unfortunately it also demands the most skill, and other than certain joints such as the sacroiliacs, the novice is unlikely to obtain satisfactory results to start with. Direct thrust is more forgiving of minor errors in localisation and can be very effective, but it is not wise to use thrust if there is uncertainty in the diagnosis, or if there is difficulty in localizing the barrier, or if the patient is apprehensive or nervous.

I remember how grateful I was to the senior author of this book for the inclusion in his first edition[1], that if one was uncertain of which side to manipulate, try one side, and then the other if the first did not give satisfactory results. As far as I was concerned, it meant the difference in getting started in manipulation or not ever taking it up. This advice is no longer included in this book because it is bad practice, but one must remember that most physicians who take up manipulation will find themselves with no one to fall back on when they first start to implement manipulative medicine into their practices. In my circumstances it was good advice; one must take the plunge at some point. The greatest fear is that one will do harm, but it soon becomes apparent that this manoeuvre is remarkably safe despite its physical nature. Far better, of course, to feel secure that one has identified the blocked joint movement correctly. It was not like that for me; I thought that I had mastered palpation when I finally decided to start manipulating, but my confidence eroded rapidly when it quickly became clear that my patient had obtained no benefit when by my careful assessment he should have.

Direct thrust is an efficient technique and, if the barrier has been engaged accurately, minimal force is required to release the joint. It has its own psychological challenges; learning to carry through with an effective thrust requires considerable confidence. It is the common technique, used universally, and in some quarters believed to be manipulation *per se*. Other techniques of manual management are either not known or are placed under some other category not necessarily believed to be manipulation.

I have found pain after treatment to be unpredictable. The immediate result of well carried out treatment is usually a shedding of pain and tension, a remarkable disappearance of complaints that is startling in its rapidity, except in very acute cases. Often this relief is replaced by gradual relapse, and it is clear that one treatment is often not enough. The pain that returns can be of quite a different character and intensity, and at times it seems to be due to a tissue reaction rather than because more treatment is required. If so it usually disappears within a day or so. Some people have chronic problems; relief will be short lived, a matter of weeks before they are in trouble once more. I believed at first that such people had not been treated well in the first place, that something had been missed, and this can happen, but I am more confident now that there are indeed people whose tendency to relapse periodically without obvious triggering factors remains unexplained.

I have been struck by how few of the large numbers of practitioners drawn to the superlative teaching of manual medicine at Michigan State University continuing medical education courses actually do take up the practice of manipulation. These students are without doubt very interested, very motivated, anxious to acquire a skill which will be of immense use in their practices. It is evident that the practice of manipulation is a manual skill which is not easily acquired; some individuals are enormously gifted, but for the majority it comes after long persistent practice, and for some this manual tool will never be gained. Many medical practitioners are accustomed to taking part in an intellectual exercise, and the idea that they will not be equipped after a week's study is not very attractive; after all, they have already invested years in gaining knowledge in the ever expanding field of medicine. Manipulation, in any case, is looked upon by the medical teaching establishment as something almost unclean; it took courage to go to Michigan at all.

I doubt that the conventional medical teaching institutions in North America will ever open their vision to include manipulation in their curricula; one is aware very quickly that the idea never crosses the minds of those who shape the teaching of tomorrow's doctors. The cliché of the ivory tower is really true; informal discussion with the deans of two Canadian medical schools[2] revealed the vast array of musculoskeletal problems which are not attended to by conventional medicine. This in spite of all the implications of industrial costs, lost time from work, the wellbeing of people, and the expensive pursuit of diagnoses which do not include the obvious[3]. This which appears to us as neglect is not viewed as medical deficiencies at all. One of them believes that musculoskeletal problems are adequately managed by the major surgical and medical specialties, orthopaedic surgery and rheumatology.

Osteopathic medicine seems to me to have the best that there is to offer: it adds the magnificent tool of manipulation to all the advances and expanding horizons of the medical world. There are not enough osteopaths to meet the demand, nor will they come to a country like Canada where they face practice as drugless practitioners. Those of us who came by manipulation through the teaching of osteopathic physicians will not forget the generous sharing of knowledge, the opening of doors which seemed to have no handles, from people who have not been treated with equal generosity by orthodox medicine.

Orthodox medicine is leery of opening the door to groups it knows very little about and even less of practices such as manipulation. There are already many extraordinary practices and outright fraud being inflicted on the public, both inside and outside of the medical establishment. It is sobering to see ideas which were taught as sacrosanct in my day as a medical student fall with few defenders in the light of new knowledge, but much more sobering is an examination of the grounds on which these ideas became established in the first place. There is a tendency for medicine to take up fads which seem to have scientific blessings, but this does not extend to practices which are considered fads without scientific justification. Manipulation does not have an imprimatur from those who matter in medicine, and further, it is too difficult to take up simply because it is the 'in-thing' to do. Today's public is much better informed about medical matters than it has been in the past; it is much better equipped to recognise the nonsensical and to weigh the pros and cons of proffered treatment.

Is medicine doing a good job in what it lets in through the door and what is to be officially spurned? There is a huge public demand for manual services, which does not of course mean that it justifies entry, but it does justify close examination without the bias and prejudgment that manual medicine is usually subjected to.

The chiropractic profession is probably one of the most rapidly growing in the health field, and indeed, if a layman thinks that manipulation is required, it is a chiropractor that he is more likely to consult. There are too few osteopaths to meet the demand. One would not ordinarily even seek the service from a medical practitioner, if one was aware that what was needed was manipulation. The chiropractors, however, labour under a burden: if one trains in chiropractic, and a satisfactory level of skill is simply not attainable by that particular individual, he has no alternative in the profession but to manipulate, however poorly, unless he is going to abandon the time and effort he has invested in qualifying. Chiropractors offer an important service and more medical physicians are sending their patients to chiropractors; there is less undignified antagonism, and more recognition of a field in which medicine today has little to offer.

There are considerable differences between the various groups that practice manipulation, in philosophy, in what they consider to be the nature of the manipulable lesion, in the expected results, and in the outlook for the patient, but in the final analysis manipulation is manipulation whoever practices it, and what counts is how good one is at it. Skill does not confine itself to any one profession; indeed, manipulation has survived from ancient times in bone setters and in folk medicine. Manual medicine should be judged on results, not on credentials and qualifications. Results are usually rapid; few medical procedures can be as dramatic. The ability to detect joint dysfunction by rapid manual sensing seems mysterious to those who do not know how it is done, but to the experienced manipulator it is a very simple procedure; and yet, the mystery of what this lesion really is remains. There are strange effects from manipulation whose aetiology can only be speculated on. None stranger is the effect of craniosacral treatment[4,5], difficult in itself to explain to practitioners who would view with scepticism the idea that the cranial bones are movable.

My first grasp of manual medicine still holds: there is blocked movement which is detected by careful digital sensing, and treatment is effective if that blockage is overcome. There is no pathology as far as I know; no inflammatory process; no cause to feel that the disorder will progress with time. There is no reason to feel that arthritis will develop, or that there will be sinister results if the trouble is not attended to immediately. There are also no grounds on which to feel that there is a permanent problem, no 'hard findings' on which to base a poor prognosis. And yet, one knows, in the clinical setting, that the mechanical explanation is too simple. Some people do have chronic problems; manipulation is required frequently. At one time I believed that I had not treated them well in the first place, and perhaps that is so, but it is more than that. There is much about this business which is simply not known. It seems obvious that once joint dysfunction has been acquired, it will make itself manifest again in time, time that is widely variable in different people. Sometimes there is an obvious cause for the recurrence, and often it comes out of the blue. There is no explanation of why this is so. The manifestations of joint dysfunction are of extraordinary variety and pattern; the mimicking of organic disorders demands investigation of the more serious condition first, and it is the more astute clinicians who will cast their thoughts on the possibility of spinal joint aetiology. There seems little doubt that the spinal joints have a close connection with the autonomic nervous system and with the development of the causalgic state. Indeed, the interlinking of mechanical spinal joint disorders, chronic pain and causalgic states seems a fascinating area to research.

The complaints that have their origin in a mechanical disorder of the spine are of remarkable variety. It is not always 'pain'. Fred Mitchell's dictum that 'pain is a liar' is one of the most useful to keep in mind as one examines a patient. Transient numb sensations in a lower limb may suggest a demyelinating disorder, but turn out to have their origin in the lumbosacral area. Inguinal pain, pain into the scrotum, and perianal pain often come from the lumbosacral area as well. Severe agonizing pain radiating down the leg to the foot, accompanied by restricted range of straight leg elevation and paraesthesiae is more likely to be a joint disorder than radicular in source. Coccydynia is more often referred from elsewhere than the coccyx. Trochanteric bursitis is unlikely to be bursitis at all; look at the corresponding sacroiliac joint. It is worth examining the symphysis pubis if one should become aware, in a musculoskeletal practice, that the patient suffers from urinary frequency. Painful intercourse may have the same origin.

Back pain depends on how well the patient has managed to compensate for a mechanical problem; typically it is manifest on physical effort, and only when hard labour is engaged in does there seem to be a problem. A person may complain that he cannot stand for very long before the onset of symptoms; cocktail parties are not looked forward to (that is if you like cocktail parties). Sometimes the individual cannot sit for very long before suffering from something he considers to be 'restless legs'. The burden that is carried is not something that one is always aware of until treatment reveals a novel level of wellbeing. One long distance runner complained that he had no difficulty whatever until he was on his third mile or so.

Abdominal pain can sometimes originate in the spine, often in the lower thoracic section. Constipation is not something that one deliberately treats in a musculoskeletal practice, but the patient will inform you of the effects of treatment, and the benefit is claimed too often not to believe that there is some relationship with the lower thoracic spine.

Chest wall pain is frequently thoracic in origin; costochondritis points directly at a thoracic problem, likely in the corresponding vertebral level. Pain which appears to be cardiogenic can have its origin in the interscapular area. One of my patients went to an Emergency Department with central chest pain, pain in the left shoulder, and paraesthesiae down the left arm. Because his cardiogram was suspicious, he was whisked into intensive care, intensely investigated and monitored over several days, and then discharged as 'pain of non-cardiac origin'. The experience was jolting for a soccer player in his early thirties. The symptoms recur periodically; sometimes costochondritis is present but invariably this man has one or more upper thoracic 'facet syndromes'.

Pain in the shoulder does not always originate there; the upper thoracic spine has enormous influence on shoulder girdle function. T2 and T3 particularly control shoulder function and symptomatology. The presence of adhesive capsulitis should not stop the examiner from looking further and examining the upper thoracic facets. Thoracic outlet syndromes are often not that at all: the cervicothoracic area is probably responsible and as such the symptoms are generated by a mechanical condition rather than an entrapment neuropathy. Truly radicular causes of pain and paraesthesiae in the upper limb are rare; much more common are facet syndromes involving the C7 and T1 vertebral levels. The symptoms can mimic a neurological condition closely; motor loss is not expected in joint dysfunction and finding it immediately points to nerve root compression. In my estimation, the clinical examination carefully done will tell you the likely cause. Relying on nerve conduction studies can be dangerous in the absence of supporting clinical findings; there are too many false positives. The decision to proceed with a Cloward fusion is not taken lightly; it is dangerous surgery, all too often carried out in good faith but in ignorance of the presence of the ubiquitous facet syndrome, which is a much more common cause of what seems to be radicular pain.

Headaches have a wide differential, and include mechanical causes in the neck. One only has to think of the whiplash victim complaining of occipital pain radiating anteriorly over the parietal bone to the retrorbital area; such complaints can be because of a head injury, but more likely is a neck problem which is treatable by manipulative techniques. Of course, finding a blocked joint at, say C1, does not mean that the headaches originate there, but it is highly likely. Sometimes there are complaints of visual interference, such as difficulty in focusing or blurred vision as part of the syndrome, with nothing found abnormal in ophthalmological examination; the blocked facet joint in the upper cervical spine is probably responsible.

It must not be forgotten that joint dysfunction is common, often silent, and finding it does not necessarily mean that the symptoms come from the blocked facets. One tries to correlate the pattern or level of symptoms with the likelihood that the particular vertebral level found to be blocked is the cause. Facet syndromes and pathology can coexist, and rapid relief from treatment of mechanical blockage does not mean that a more sinister process does not hover in the vicinity; it is likely in such cases that it is the pathological process that is silent. One of my patients who had always responded rapidly and well to manual treatment returned one day with back pain incurred in sports. Mobilising a sacroiliac joint for apparent blockage, isometrically, caused a great deal of pain, and repeat mobilisation was just as painful. Other joints may need more than one manipulation, but the sacroiliac joint is almost always released on one treatment; moreover there was simply too much pain to accept a mechanical cause. A bone scan revealed sacroiliitis not evident on plain films. The condition is now under excellent control; he returns at times, not for the low back, but for thoracic problems, because he is an avid sportsman.

Manipulation works well, but there is always the chance that inflammatory joint disease will involve more joints besides the sacroiliacs, and manipulation and inflammatory synovitis do not mix well. Another individual was referred with acute torticollis; the muscle spasm subsided in response to isometric intervention, and facet blockage was then detectable at the cervicothoracic junction. His musculoskeletal condition was much improved but he had nausea, headaches and vertigo. These can arise from joint dysfunction because there is some link with the autonomic system, but one's first thought is of pathology and examination of the eyes showed papilloedema. There was no neurological deficit but the eye signs had him on his way to a neurosurgeon and an intracranial space occupying lesion was found. The joint dysfunction was in this case of little significance except to mislead initial diagnosis into the musculoskeletal system.

Similarly, remember to look at the corresponding sacroiliac joint when osteoarthritis of the hip becomes suddenly painful; it is not always the obvious pathology that is causing the pain, although one does not really know until the immediately remediable mechanical problem has been cleared.

One learns to look closely at certain areas when the patient complains of particular symptoms, and the transitional areas of the spine are always suspect. If there are complaints of neck pain, the cervicothoracic junction is examined carefully; very often the problem is thoracic and not in the cervical spine at all. The thoraco lumbar junction is notorious[6], and should not be neglected because the more obvious and symptomatic problem is lumbosacral. It seems that one is more likely to find dysfunction in transitional areas than elsewhere, but probably more important is to ensure that these areas are examined carefully even when the apparent cause of the complaint has been found in the more distal or proximal areas. For example, identifying T3 as blocked requires a close look at C7 and T1.

The initial screening examination suggests where to look more closely, but one learns to expect certain associations. For example, symptomatic blockage in the lumbosacral area often is accompanied by thoraco-lumbar lesions; assuming that the problem involves one side of the low back only without checking the opposite side before the patient leaves the office will sometimes result in the patient's return the following week with the complaint that the problem has been shifted to the other side. Ensuring that the symphysis pubis is examined in sacroiliac dysfunctions is wise; it is misleading to decide that the sacroiliac is at fault without knowing what the position of the symphysis pubis is; indeed, some practitioners routinely treat that joint by isometric means on the basis that the pelvis is a ring with three joints, and that disruption of one joint makes it highly likely that one of the other two will be involved as well.

The likely link between causalgia and joint dysfunction is a fascinating consideration. If the patient's condition is not so far advanced that palpation is out of the question, joint dysfunction is usually present in causalgic states. Usually manipulative treatment is intolerable in such situations, but at times, perhaps because the problem is less severe, or because the patient has confidence that the treatment will help and will steel himself to bear a most unpleasant intervention, very gratifying results can be achieved. It is this link which is probably responsible for the extra-ordinary mimicking of organic disorders which is so often a part of spinal joint dysfunction. The involvement of the autonomic nervous system in spinal joint disorders is a fertile field for research. Chronic pain is a devastating situation, and here we have one likely and remediable cause. Unfortunately, by the time this state has developed, manual intervention, even by gentle isometric techniques, is not likely to be tolerable. In some cases epidural injections have abated the symptoms enough to permit physical intervention, but in most cases, by the time causalgia has developed, it is too late in my experience.

In the past, practitioners of manipulation treated many conditions which we know now have no bearing on mechanical disorders of the spine. Dr Carl Cook[7], a prominent American osteopathic physician who practised in England makes many such references in his autobiography *You Must Become A Doctor*. But the more experience one has with manual medicine, the more one is aware of effects which are difficult to explain on a mechanical basis. One hesitates to dismiss manipulative intervention in cases in which antibiotics, for example, are more appropriate; there must be an adjunct effect. Recruiting the autonomic nervous system, if that is what it is, must not be dismissed; it seems to me to be a powerful ally. Certainly in the days before antibiotics, manual treatment could have been of great significance. All this is speculation, of course, but manipulative medicine seems to be far more powerful than merely restoring a joint to physiological function.

I have difficulty with the idea of 'preventive manipulation'. Preventive manipulation[8] is advocated by some groups to ensure optimum spinal function, particularly in individuals where minor spinal malfunction can have devastating effects on performance, such as in athletes. Athletes moreover use their bodies fully, and are a group at risk for frequent spinal dysfunction. Such groups should indeed be examined frequently to ensure satisfactory joint movement; dysfunction can be silent, becoming symptomatic when the individual can no longer compensate. Treating small problems before performance is interfered with makes sense. The objection is to the term: the preventive aspect is the routine examination, not the manipulation, because there is no point in manipulating if there is no lesion. It will certainly not prevent a problem from developing later, and manipulating normal joints is almost anathema, at least without some definitive purpose other than the idea that the joint may block at some point.

If an individual has been subjected to enough force to produce a fracture, there is a good chance that there is concurrent joint dysfunction as well. Even if there is not, the immobilisation to allow healing of the fracture is likely to result in dysfunction of the immobilised joints. It is well to search for this possibility once the more serious injury has healed. The problem may be in the peripheral joints, close to the fracture site, particularly where immobilisation has been carried out, but often the spinal joints, remote from the fracture, are the source of grief, perhaps blamed on a fracture which gives every evidence of satisfactory healing. A particular example of this seen on several occasions by one of the authors (JFB) in the course of a busy trauma practice was the association of a wrist fracture, often produced by a fall on the outstretched hand, with spinal joint dysfunction. Many of those with this combination had had a history of previous neck or back symptoms and it does not seem unreasonable to assume that the spinal condition had been aggravated by the force of the fall. The symptoms were often confined to the periphery and, surprisingly, often manifested as a 'trophic' hand. The results of treating the spinal joints in such patients was very gratifying; if they were seen early the condition could be aborted in one or two treatments.

Manual medicine is a very satisfying type of practice. There are few fields in medicine where the patient improves as rapidly and as dramatically, and where one knows almost immediately that things have succeeded, or perhaps that the objective has not been attained. The miraculous restoration that takes place after decompression of a subdural haematoma is more dramatic and means more, because here the patient has been rescued from death or severe brain damage, but it does not occur almost every day like the common musculoskeletal conditions dealt with in manual medicine.

REFERENCES

1. Bourdillon J.F. (1970). *Spinal Manipulation*. London: Heinemann.
2. E.A.D. personal communication.
3. Nachemson A.L. (1979). A critical look at the treatment of low back pain. *Scand J. Rehab. Med.*; **11**:143–147.

4. Magoun H.I. (1976). *Osteopathy in the Cranial Field.* 3rd edn. Kirksville: The Journal Printing Co.
5. Gehin A. (1985). *Atlas of Manipulative Techniques for the Cranium and Face.* Seattle: Eastland Press.
6. Maigne R. (1980). Low back pain of lumbar origin. *Arch. Phys. Med. Rehab.;* **60**:389–395.
7. Cook C.M. (1982). *You Must Become a Doctor.* Oxford: Oxford University Press.
8. Lewit K. (1985). *Manipulative Therapy in Rehabilitation of the Motor System.* London: Butterworth.

Chapter 17

The validation of manipulation

The problem of designing a controlled randomised trial of manipulation that will be acceptable to the sceptics who point out, correctly, that manipulation is not proven is a taxing one[1]. The factors influencing outcome are variable and numerous, and it is well to examine some of these. People cleverer than I may see perhaps a simple answer where I only encounter difficulty. Any such trial will perforce be a measure of skill; manipulators have greatly differing levels of deftness, and in some cases likely perceive themselves as having greater proficiency than an observer would award. The number of practitioners who are truly skilled in manipulation appears to be small, at least those who possess a level of skill that would generate confidence in any trial. There are many practitioners of manipulation who carry out excellent work, but once one is aware of the pitfalls and vagaries of this treatment, it would be foolish to attempt to demonstrate its efficacy with less than top talent. Top talent is not necessarily possessed by those who write knowledgeably about the subject. The outcome of manipulative treatment is directly dependent on the skill of the treating practitioner.

The patient's ability to cooperate with a physical treatment is crucial; not everyone can allow themselves to be twisted and turned without some tendency to guard and tense. Manipulation is not everyone's cup of tea no matter how much it may help them. Muscle guarding will result in failure of treatment. Hypermobile people are at one end of the spectrum, and at the other are the fibrous rigid people; both are hard to manipulate. In the one, reaching end point never seems to occur, just more stretching. In the other, there seems to be no movement at all, so that one wonders if there is a barrier, or whether the physiological barrier and the pathological barrier are almost coincident, and ever so close to the anatomic barrier. Anxiety can rear its head any time, particularly in physical intervention, likely resulting in great difficulty in treating such an individual.

Ideally all symptoms disappear rapidly, but that is not always the case; how does one measure relief in variable pain thresholds and variable perceptions of residual pain? It is the subjectiveness of measurement that presents the greatest difficulty. One could perhaps design a task that is to be performed as a measurement, but it would have to be something that could not be done before treatment, and from experience the ability to perform physically will vary from day to day in the same individual, depending on how well he or she has managed to compensate.

Injured workers would seem to present a wonderful opportunity to measure the results of manipulative treatment, by noting the percentages that return to work after a long absence, a period of enough length to be statistically suggestive that the chance of resuming remunerative employment is minimal. Workers' Compensation Board statistics indicate that after 2 years of being off the job for a work injury, the number of workers who manage to get back to work is in the order of 1 to 2%[2]. Even a small improvement in these figures would be significant. Unfortunately, even passing acquaintance with third party involvement and the possibility of secondary gain will dispel any notion that a trial involving injured workers is likely to succeed. Any investigator shies away from a group in which there are multiple other factors operative besides the claimed reason that work cannot be resumed. Secondary gain is not necessarily monetary, and the intrusion of an organisation that appears to direct, perhaps in an indirect way, where and how individuals are to be treated is less than helpful. But perhaps I am being too cynical; nobody does trials in workers' compensation cases because of the influence of secondary gain, not because it is known for certain, but because it seems obvious. The influence of secondary gain could be factored in, but then one has to deal with the intervention of a third party. Even so, people carrying out heavy physical labour are particularly susceptible to joint dysfunction, and more so, to relapse after successful treatment. Some individuals manage to remain at work, but do so only by means of repeated treatment. Surely this need for repeated treatment will not look very good in a statistical analysis. One very difficult aspect is the apparent tendency for recurrence, within very variable time periods and circumstances. In some cases it appears that the problem was not satisfactorily resolved in the first place, and perhaps that is correct; it certainly spoils a trial. The different perceptions of patients in any measurement which takes into account of how they feel is a significant obstacle; some individuals are utterly grateful for a month's respite of pain that has been borne for years, whereas others will stoutly maintain that treatment made no difference because the pain was back in the same pattern as before in a month.

Whiplash injuries seem to be another area that could be explored as a subject for a study. It is much more complex than injured workers, and the influence of secondary gain much more malignant. The time taken to return to work under different management programmes is a good measurement, however. This is a subject on which senior surgeons of distinction do not hesitate to express firm opinions with nothing to back them up except anecdotal episodes and personal perceptions. There is considerable literature on whiplash, but a dearth of controlled studies. Opinions of far reaching consequence are expressed daily in courts of law; the medical evidence is crucial to the outcome. One can be forgiven for believing that the question is decided on the chemistry of greed and anxiety in the victims, the machinations of lawyers, and the ignorance and naivete of doctors. One is dealing in such cases with widely distributed symptoms, including headaches, neck pain, shoulder pain, paraesthesiae in the extremities, claims of weakness, sometimes perceptions which seem bizarre. The approach using computer-aided diagnosis certainly suggests that at least in the low back surgical procedures are only rarely justified[3]. The practitioner of manual medicine has a far better understanding of how these symptoms could arise, or at least what they relate to, than other practitioners, and I believe that the intervention of manual medicine is likely to have more significance for the victim than the usual approach, but of course that is what has been set out to demonstrate. Work-related injuries and whiplash are attractive areas for study precisely because they have not been studied adequately and because a satisfactory demonstration of the efficacy of manipulation would stand out, provided that happens. The cards are stacked against such a result.

The key factor is determining a measurement which is less subjective than pain. Pain charts are not of much value; how much credence can one put on a pain chart that will vary from day to day as the patient manages to compensate, or decompensate, for a mechanical problem which remains unresolved throughout? Physical performance will also vary from day to day; some people manage to carry out rather heavy physical performances with unresolved joint dysfunction, to a degree because they have compensated, to another because they are stoics, to another because not to has devastating effects on their economic status. The answer is not simple. Measuring loss of tension, a newfound feeling of wellbeing, absence of paraesthesiae, and elimination of pain of variable character requires tests for subjective sensations which are not very convincing. I appreciate well the respected practitioner of manual medicine who told me that it would be a waste of time to map out a trial; he had much more experience and was well aware of the vagaries and of the unknowns in this business of manipulation, and I have come to fully appreciate why he said what I then thought was a rather cavalier way of disposing of a gnawing problem. On the other hand was the remark of a friend and fellow practitioner's that such a trial would be 'easy'; just compare any group treated with manual medicine to a group that is treated in the usual way, which begs the question of why it has not been done already.

The diagnosis of joint dysfunction rests on the perception of blocked joint movement, sensed by palpation and careful digital examination for obstruction[4]. Standard radiographs do not assist in such a diagnosis, nor is there any laboratory or blood test that helps. Localized tenderness helps but it is not essential; pain is not part of the diagnosis. The decision regarding the success or failure of treatment also rests on the same criteria, and the patient must be re-examined to determine what if anything has been gained. Removing an obstruction successfully does not tell us whether the patient will feel or do anything different, although the clinician knows that such treatment will likely have far reaching effects. To demonstrate the effectiveness of this treatment to someone who knows little of manipulation one must measure one or more of these effects in such a manner that it satisfies critical appraisal.

The evaluator should have some understanding and experience of manipulation; I would think that he should be able to examine a patient for joint dysfunction, coupling his findings with some measure of physical performance and of spinal kinetics. The control group poses great difficulty: does one carry out a false manipulation, or does one keep the control group well separated from the treated group so that notes are not compared? It is hard to disguise manipulation, and it is not ethical to manipulate a joint that is normal.

Injured workers still present an opportunity, despite the difficulties and the pervasive influence of a third party. Statistics from that same third party suggest that not more than 2% of injured workers return to work after being off work for 2 years. Surely it would not take many successes to show a difference in these statistics? A shift towards the better should take place even in the presence of secondary gain, which after all would be just as prevalent in the control group, and of those who will not return to work regardless of intervention, who also would be found in the control group. Perhaps it would not turn out so, but this group of patients seems to be the most promising.

Physicians who manipulate are by and large solo practitioners. They may have won some respect from the local medical community, but there is certain to be a body of antagonism which would make it difficult to gain access to academic facilities, essential if any clinical trial is to be planned with the care and the deliberations of critical intelligent minds. Without an academic base, it is unlikely that such a study would have an audience. The journals shy away from controversial studies coming out of the wilderness. Clinicians in academic settings are unlikely to want to take part in studies in something they would think of as alien, have no acquaintance with, regard with suspicion, and perhaps risk tainting themselves with unorthodox and condemned practices. The barrier is formidable, and there is no point in railing at it. Medicine may remain aloof, but the patients abound, and after a while one simply gets on with one's work, knowing that the majority obtain relief, and that one is practising something as old as medicine itself.

Careful analysis should come up with a means of measuring outcome. Focusing on failure, because of the large part played by motivation, is destructive. As an example, it has been traditional to state that the complaints resulting from a whiplash injury will disappear once the process of litigation is over. This claim is simply not true. One does not ignore it altogether nevertheless; I have seen many injured people whose motivation in a litigation suit appears to be vindictiveness rather than anything else. But the influence of secondary gain has perhaps been overstated; surely some of the victims of accidents are honest and sincere. Most of the injured people I see in my practice are sincere, and even a degree of resentment should not stop recovery. It is natural to feel anger for an injury caused by someone else, but to feign persistent distress where there is none is too cynical a view of society. Influence of this nature will certainly be present, but it should also be present in the control group.

The question remains: what is a satisfactory measurement for the outcome of manipulative treatment? It becomes easier if one does not think in terms of a 'cure', but rather that the result is likely to be better than the outcome of the usual way of managing back or neck injuries. Ability to return to work seems to be one valid approach. A less indicative means, but one that should be included in the observations, is the amount of time that one remains pain free, or remains with much abated pain. Ability to resume exercise is another, although the standard of what can be resumed will vary widely; perhaps it should be individual standards, i.e. weight lifting for one, jogging for another, aerobics for someone else. A measurement of spinal kinetics before and after may be helpful. A hard look at any of these is not encouraging; the only one that is likely to impress anyone is a documented resumption of remunerative employment. Everything else is too subjective, too variable, and of little significance in things that matter.

A study should include certain basic laboratory studies, not because the diagnosis of joint dysfunction rests on any of these, but because of certain associations which have been traditionally claimed to be significant. Degenerative changes in spinal X-rays are believed by many physicians to be associated with the symptoms, either by joint involvement or nerve root impingement, despite the absence of any study which has managed to make a correlation[5]. But perhaps there is a bearing on outcome in the degree of degeneration present, and it is well to either confirm it or refute it. Bone scans seem a sensible thing to include: occult inflammatory activity will certainly have a bearing on how manipulative treatment is received. I have been aware of one radiologist who became excited when he believed that he was demonstrating through serial bone scans undisplaced vertebral fractures after whiplash, with disappearance of 'hot spots' correlating with the abatement of pain and presumably healing. Persistent increased uptake after months of pain supposedly indicated failure to heal. Such considerations would certainly not encourage a manipulative approach to the victims of whiplash accidents, and yet it is in precisely this group that the benefit of manual medicine is very apparent. The presence of certain disorders would be prejudicial to the success of manual treatment, and some broad laboratory screening is necessary to ensure a level playing field. Thermography has been discredited as a means of measuring pain, which it clearly is not by any clear headed thinking, but it has been admitted to some courts of law as evidence, and it occurs to me that showing its irrelevancy, if that is what turns out, is not just a foolish inclusion in a study.

A history of depression, or of manic manifestations, or of paranoia or hostility, or of frail personalities of whatever appellation, should be excluded. Previous manipulative treatment should probably be a reason for exclusion as well; any such person would be unlikely to settle for inclusion in the control group if it does not involve manipulative treatment, and would be positively influenced if included in the treatment group; or perhaps it would be the reverse. One does not experience manipulation without developing rather definite views on the subject. Inability to tolerate manual intervention is without question a reason for exclusion, but some individuals cannot assess this without experiencing the process; conversely, experience of the treatment can show people that their fears were groundless. Restriction of treatment to certain techniques is unwise: muscle energy is so gentle and so widely applicable to wide age groups that it is the preferred route; but it demands greater skill, and in some joints results are unobtainable if another technique is not allowed.

Previous spinal surgery should likely be excluded, certainly anything involving a fusion; laminectomies sometimes result in the loss of anatomical structures used to make a diagnosis, and there is a good chance that spinal joint dysfunction is only a minor reason for persistent pain.

The first difficulty in mapping out a study is establishing a workable hypothesis. If chronic back pain is to be the subject to be investigated then a definition is needed as to what the aetiology is[1]. 'Non specific back pain' is simply an acknowledgement that one does not know what is being treated. The idea of mechanical interference in joint movement is attractive; at least the determination of such a lesion is the object of this book. The obstruction can be palpated, and its presence before and absence after successful treatment is something that the investigator can determine. Describing the problem in such limited terms is far too simplistic, nevertheless, and the complex factors involved in disordered spinal movement have been well described by other authors. The simplification is workable however; one can make a diagnosis. The problem of low back pain in the absence of pathology can be brought down to obstruction in one or more of the sacroiliac, lumbar, and thoraco-lumbar joints. Whether the obstruction is in the joint, or in the surrounding muscle, or in the ligaments, or whether there is a reflex neurological mechanism at work does not prevent the establishment of a diagnosis which can be confirmed by another individual with adequate palpatory skills.

The method depends on which population is to be evaluated. If injured workers are to be used, then the subjects to be included must have been unable to return to work for at least 2 years because of their injuries, because then one hopes for significant results by success in only a fraction of the sample. One could even say that a control group is not necessary, because success could be measured against prevailing statistics, although that is probably an unwise way to formulate the study. The subjects must not be suffering from systemic disorders or pathology, or musculoskeletal complaints in areas other than the low back, but pain known to commonly originate in the back, such as sciatica, must not be a cause of exclusion. Those with neurological deficit must not be included, but one must be cautious here: pseudo sensory deficit can occur from joint dysfunction, and distinguishing a disc herniation from a mechanical lesion can be confusing. Worse, joint dysfunction and pathology can co-exist. The pool from which patients would be selected will include 'disc herniation' because that diagnosis is frequently made on the strength of pain in sciatic distribution alone. Motor deficit is a clear signal that the problem is unlikely to be joint dysfunction. Systemic disease, advanced demineralization, spinal instability, possible metastatic disease, pregnancy, osteoarthritis of the hip, inflammatory joint disease should all be excluded; some because manipulation is contraindicated and others because they would confuse the issue.

Besides disc herniation, the diagnoses with which patients with back pain are likely to be labelled include lumbosacral sprain, ligamentous tear, degenerative disc disease, muscular sprain, soft tissue injury, facet syndrome, even osteoarthritis. None of these should be excluded, but the presence of a manipulable lesion likely to be responsible for the symptoms must be established before inclusion. Buerger and Greenman's excellent summary of what has been done in *Empirical Approaches to the Validation of Spinal Manipulation*[1] includes a number of papers in which one is uncertain whether the investigators had a firm idea of what a manipulable lesion consisted of. The book clearly establishes how difficult it is to study the subject.

It seems a good idea to include a carefully crafted questionnaire, or a series of questionnaires, to be answered pretreatment and at set periods thereafter. Psychological screening is important, because success and failure are dependent on mental stability.

The control group poses difficulty. Sham manipulation is not convincing to anyone with a little knowledge of what to expect in manipulative treatment, and deliberately manipulating a normal joint is unethical. Using a treatment quite different to manual medicine is probably best; back education classes have a credible status and are a respectable choice. Physiotherapy must be defined very specifically, otherwise a good therapist will be using his or her hands to great effect in a procedure which may not be considered to be manipulation, but in effect is. Massage is not a good choice; it is a valuable adjunct to manipulation and can be considered to have profound effects on connective tissue; its relationship to manipulation is too close to risk using it in a control group. Most physiotherapy consists of a variety of heat modalities and an exercise programme, and if limited to this, would do very well.

The problem of non compliance is more significant in the control group than in the manipulated group: manipulation works fast and benefit is likely to be perceived much more rapidly than in routine exercise regimens, or education in what to do and what not to do. Patients are after all looking for relief, and if there are no gains after what is deemed a fair trial period, will go elsewhere. The loss in patients will be greater in the control group than in the treated group, but here again I am making predictions based on my own bias.

There is bound to be failure in the manipulation group; sometimes a given joint will not release, however many times one tries, perhaps because the operator is repeatedly committing the same error. The effect on the study can be far reaching; ideally there is no trouble in releasing the blocked joints. The occasional and unpredictable reaction to manipulation, experienced in the first couple of days after treatment, is likely to discourage the affected patient from pursuing further treatment of that nature if not advised of the possibility, or if the reaction is deemed to be unacceptable.

The study could incorporate an examination of commonly held beliefs, none of which have any scientific basis. For example, is there a correlation between degenerative disc disease and pain or not? What relationship does obesity have? Structural anomalies and anatomic variants are often blamed for back pain, some on hearsay and some because it appears to make sense; scoliosis, leg length discrepancy, spondylolisthesis and transitional vertebrae all come under that category. The relationship of age to back symptoms has been examined many times, but assessing the outcome of manipulation to age could be interesting. Strengthening exercises are traditional in the management of back problems, but the necessity for them remains unclear. Is exercise of equal or better value than manipulation, or is it a valuable adjunct?

The questions that arise may make the study cumbersome, but if the sample is large enough, the questionnaires designed well, and the treatment group managed by a practitioner with 'good hands', the results could be very useful, not only to document the effects of expert manipulation, but to examine the largely anecdotal world of soft tissue musculoskeletal injury.

REFERENCES

1. Buerger A., Greenman P.E. (1985). *Empirical Approaches to the Validation of Spinal Manipulation*. Springfield, Ill.: Charles C. Thomas.
2. Anderson G.B. (1981). Epidemiologic aspects of low back pain in industry. *Spine;* **6**:53–60.
3. Hudgins W. (1983). Computer aided diagnosis in lumbar disc herniation. *Spine;* **8**:604–615.
4. Greenman P.E. (1989). *Principles of Manual Medicine*. Baltimore: Williams and Wilkins.
5. Nachemson A.L. (1979). A critical look at the treatment of low back pain. *Scand. J. Rehab. Med.;* **11**:143–147.

Index

Also Available–a Companion Videotape!

Spinal Manipulation

Featuring John Bourdillon
describing and demonstrating his techniques

In this new video, renowned orthopedic surgeon and osteopath, Dr. John F. Bourdillon, explains and demonstrates his manipulative techniques for examining and manipulating the pelvis; lumbar, thoracic, and cervical spine; and the thoracic cage to alleviate loss of mobility and musculoskeletal pain.

Dr. Bourdillon's focus is on diagnosis, believing that spinal problems often show up in places other than the spine. This system deals with assessment, treatment, and evaluation. The tape details instructions for a variety of techniques, covering almost if not all the dysfunctions of the axial skeleton and rib cage.

This video will provide valuable insight into manipulative medicine for all professionals dealing with the relief of musculoskeletal pain.

Available Summer 1992   Approx. 4 hour running time: VHS cassette   7506-9425-4

NTSC version available from Butterworth-Heinemann's US office:

    80 Montvale Avenue
    Stoneham, MA 02180
    USA
Toll Free 1-800-366-2665
Telephone 617-438-8464
Fax 617-279-4851

PAL version available from Butterworth-Heinemann's UK office:

    Reed Book Services Ltd.
    PO Box 5
    Rushden Northants
    NN109YX UK
Telephone (0933) 58521
Fax (0933) 50284

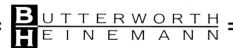

BUTTERWORTH
HEINEMANN

WITHDRAWN FROM
Genesee
Library